NEPHROLOGY MCQs

for Postgraduate and Superspecialty Medical Entrance Examinations

Celebrating 50 years
Passion, Quality and Innovation in Healthcare Publishing

NEPHROLOGY MCQs

for Postgraduate and Superspecialty Medical Entrance Examinations

Based on 20th Edition of Harrison's Prinicples of Internal Medicine

Dr Ajay Mathur
Senior Professor
Department of Medicine
SMS Medical College and Hospital
Jaipur, Rajasthan, India

Foreword
Ramesh Roop Rai

JAYPEE

JAYPEE BROTHERS MEDICAL PUBLISHERS
The Health Sciences Publisher
New Delhi | London

Jaypee Brothers Medical Publishers (P) Ltd

Headquarters
Jaypee Brothers Medical Publishers (P) Ltd
4838/24, Ansari Road, Daryaganj
New Delhi 110 002, India
Phone: +91-11-43574357
Fax: +91-11-43574314
Email: jaypee@jaypeebrothers.com

Overseas Office
J.P. Medical Ltd
83 Victoria Street, London
SW1H 0HW (UK)
Phone: +44 20 3170 8910
Fax: +44 (0)20 3008 6180
Email: info@jpmedpub.com

Website: www.jaypeebrothers.com

Website: www.jaypeedigital.com

Nephrology MCQs for Postgraduate and Superspecialty Medical Entrance Examinations

First Edition: **2019**

ISBN: 978-93-89188-80-6

Printed at Sanat Printers

Foreword

As a professional who has been practicing medicine for over four decades now, I appreciate the value this book brings to the table in times like today. As we move from a largely descriptive era to the bullet-point generation, this academic initiative appears profoundly relevant.

Dr Mathur is bringing to the students and others, Nephrology MCQs in an individual book format. This would be more handy and subject specific. The book has been a reference point for many medical entrance examinations and has left an impact on medical professionals who look for high quality of academic material.

Knowledge is a more processed form of information. Dr Mathur stays true to his pledge by presenting well-digested bytes of knowledge across different fields of medicine. His relying on good old word-of-mouth to make this book a success rather than enthusiastic marketing adds further credibility to his initiative. I recommend this book, without a shadow of doubt, to every medical professional who is looking to continue learning.

Dr Ramesh Roop Rai
Former, Professor and Head
Department of Gastroenterology
SMS Medical College and Hospital, Jaipur
Past President, Indian Society of Gastroenterology (2008)

Preface

Medicine, in all its vastness, needs to be understood in a way that makes most sense to how it is applied today. Memorizing each word is elusive and therefore, testing knowledge of a discipline remains an evergreen challenge.

It is a widely accepted fact that taking a quiz soon after studying helps one retain knowledge better and apply the lessons in practice. Multiple Choice Questions (MCQs) are an effective way of remembering the gist of the matter. This is precisely the reason why most examinations today follow this format. This book is committed to honing your skills to retain knowledge, help diagnose medical conditions, and maximize your impact, as a doctor.

A tremendous volume of questions has been generated over the past ten years. As it stands today, the approach needs to be adjusted according to the knowledge available at hand. This time around, my team has decided that each specialism merits its own edition. This will help you to study existing literature with recent advances in medicine and glean deeper insights into the subject matter. Based on the epic 20th edition of Harrison's Principles of Internal Medicine, published by The McGraw-Hill Companies, Inc., this book is dedicated to the field of Nephrology in all its endless scope. This book caters to medical professionals at all levels. Not only can this be used by aspiring doctors to prepare for medical entrance examinations, but also by seasoned physicians to update knowledge long after it has been acquired. The book is sign-posted with references should the reader require elaboration on any given topic.

The book contains 2101 questions and still counting, I continue to keep my promise to continually refine the content of my book and chronicle the advances of medical science.

Dr Ajay Mathur

Contents

Azotemia and Urinary Abnormalities

1. Broad casts in urinary sediment is a diagnostic clue for which of the major nephrology syndromes?

Harrison's 20th Ed. Chapter 48 Page 289 Table 48-1

A. Acute nephritis
B. Nephrotic syndrome
C. Chronic renal failure
D. All of the above

2. Nocturia is a diagnostic clue for which of the major nephrology syndromes?

Harrison's 20th Ed. Chapter 48 Page 289 Table 48-1

A. Urinary tract obstruction
B. Renal tubule defects
C. Chronic renal failure
D. All of the above

3. Lipiduria is a diagnostic clue for which of the major nephrology syndromes?

Harrison's 20th Ed. Chapter 48 Page 289 Table 48-1

A. Acute nephritis
B. Nephrotic syndrome
C. Chronic renal failure
D. Renal tubular defects

4. Which of the following is a common finding in chronic renal failure?

Harrison's 20th Ed. Chapter 48 Page 289 Table 48-1

A. Hypocalcemia
B. Hyperphosphatemia
C. Hyperparathyroidism
D. All of the above

5. Azotemia for more than how many months is labeled as chronic renal failure?

Harrison's 20th Ed. Chapter 48 Page 289 Table 48-1

A. > 1 month
B. > 3 months
C. > 6 months
D. > 12 months

Azotemia for > 3 months is labeled as chronic renal failure.

6. Which of the following is a typical finding in chronic renal failure?

Harrison's 20th Ed. Chapter 48 Page 289 Table 48-1

A. Kidneys reduced in size bilaterally
B. Broad casts in urinary sediment
C. Azotemia for >3 months
D. All of the above

7. Renal osteodystrophy is a finding in?

Harrison's 20th Ed. Chapter 48 Page 289 Table 48-1

A. Acute nephritis
B. Nephrotic syndrome
C. Chronic renal failure
D. Renal tubular defects

8. Hypercoagulable state is a finding in?

Harrison's 20th Ed. Chapter 48 Page 289 Table 48-1

A. Acute nephritis
B. Nephrotic syndrome
C. Chronic renal failure
D. Renal tubular defects

9. Flank tenderness is a finding in?

Harrison's 20th Ed. Chapter 48 Page 289 Table 48-1

A. Acute nephritis
B. Nephrolithiasis
C. Urinary tract obstruction
D. All of the above

10. Large kidneys are a finding in?

Harrison's 20th Ed. Chapter 48 Page 289 Table 48-1

A. Acute nephritis
B. Nephrolithiasis
C. Urinary tract obstruction
D. Renal tubular defects

11. Renal calcification is a finding in?

Harrison's 20th Ed. Chapter 48 Page 289 Table 48-1

A. Acute nephritis
B. Chronic renal failure
C. Urinary tract obstruction
D. Renal tubular defects

12. "Tubular" proteinuria (<1 gram/24 hours) is a finding in?

Harrison's 20th Ed. Chapter 48 Page 289 Table 48-1

A. Urinary tract obstruction
B. Renal tubule defects
C. Chronic renal failure
D. All of the above

13. Which of the following is not a finding in renal tubule defects?

Harrison's 20th Ed. Chapter 48 Page 289 Table 48-1

A. Renal calcification
B. Electrolyte disorders
C. Hypoalbuminemia
D. Large kidneys

14. Circulatory congestion is a typical finding in?
Harrison's 20th Ed. Chapter 48 Page 289 Table 48-1

A. Acute nephritis
B. Chronic renal failure
C. Nephrotic syndrome
D. All of the above

15. Normal combined kidney volume is about?
Can J Kidney Health Dis. 2017;4:1-6

A. 100 to 150 cm^3
B. 150 to 200 cm^3
C. 200 to 300 cm^3
D. 250 to 400 cm^3

Normal combined kidney volume is about 250 to 400 cm^3.

16. Formula for calculation of total kidney volume (TKV) is?
Can J Kidney Health Dis. 2017;4:1-6

A. Length × width × thickness × (π/2)
B. Length × width × thickness × (π/4)
C. Length × width × thickness × (π/6)
D. Length × width × thickness × (π/8)

Ellipsoid formula to calculate TKV is length × width × thickness × (π/6).

17. Which of the following is the primary metric for kidney "function"?
Harrison's 20th Ed. Chapter 48 Page 288

A. Creatinine clearance
B. Glomerular filtration rate
C. Fractional excretion of sodium
D. Albumin-to-creatinine ratio

GFR is the primary metric for kidney "function".

18. Which of the following is used as a surrogate to estimate GFR?
Harrison's 20th Ed. Chapter 48 Page 289

A. Blood urea
B. Plasma creatinine
C. Urine creatinine
D. Creatinine clearance

As direct GFR measurement is not feasible, plasma creatinine is used as a surrogate to estimate GFR.

19. Value of GFR is expressed in?
Harrison's 20th Ed. Chapter 48 Page 289

A. mL/minute
B. mL/hour
C. mL/day
D. mL/kg/minute

20. Value of creatinine clearance is expressed in?
Harrison's 20th Ed. Chapter 48 Page 289

A. mL/minute
B. mL/hour
C. mL/day
D. mL/kg/minute

Creatinine clearance & GFR is calculated for a defined time period (24 hours) & is expressed in mL/minute.

21. In general, patients do not develop symptomatic uremia until GFR is?
Harrison's 20th Ed. Chapter 48 Page 289

A. < 15 mL/minute
B. < 45 mL/minute
C. < 60 mL/minute
D. < 90 mL/minute

In general, patients do not develop symptomatic uremia until renal insufficiency is usually quite severe (GFR < 15 mL/minute).

22. Azotemia best relates to?
Harrison's 20th Ed. Chapter 48 Page 289

A. Retention of nitrogenous waste products
B. Decreased urine output
C. Circulatory overload
D. All of the above

Azotemia is defined as retention of nitrogenous waste products.

23. Azotemia may result from?
Harrison's 20th Ed. Chapter 48 Page 289

A. Reduced renal perfusion
B. Intrinsic renal disease
C. Postrenal processes
D. All of the above

Azotemia may result from reduced renal perfusion (40-80% of cases of acute renal failure), intrinsic renal disease or postrenal processes (ureteral obstruction).

24. In a patient of azotemia due to chronic renal failure, which of the following is false?
Harrison's 20th Ed. Chapter 48 Page 290 Figure 48-1

A. Small kidneys, thin cortex
B. Bland sediment
C. Isosthenuria
D. None of the above

25. In patient of prerenal azotemia, which of the following is false?
Harrison's 20th Ed. Chapter 48 Page 290 Figure 48-1

A. Normal urinalysis with oliguria
B. FeNa < 1%
C. Urine osmolality > 500 mOsmol
D. None of the above

26. In a patient of acute tubular necrosis, which of the following is false?
Harrison's 20th Ed. Chapter 48 Page 290 Figure 48-1

A. Normal urinalysis with oliguria
B. FeNa > 1%
C. Urine osmolality < 350 mOsmol
D. None of the above

27. Which of the following is the first observation in investigations that helps in arriving at the cause of azotemia?
Harrison's 20th Ed. Chapter 48 Page 290 Figure 48-1

A. Renal size
B. Hydronephrosis
C. Cortical thickness
D. Urinary sediment

28. In azotemia, RBC cast with proteinuria point towards the diagnosis of?

Harrison's 20th Ed. Chapter 48 Page 290 Figure 48-1

A. Glomerulonephritis
B. Renal artery occlusion
C. Interstitial nephritis
D. All of the above

29. In azotemia, muddy brown cast with proteinuria point towards the diagnosis of?

Harrison's 20th Ed. Chapter 48 Page 290 Figure 48-1

A. Glomerulonephritis
B. Prerenal azotemia
C. Interstitial nephritis
D. Acute tubular necrosis

30. In azotemia, WBC cast with eosinophilia point towards the diagnosis of?

Harrison's 20th Ed. Chapter 48 Page 290 Figure 48-1

A. Glomerulonephritis
B. Prerenal azotemia
C. Interstitial nephritis
D. Acute tubular necrosis

31. Which of the following is false about creatinine?

Harrison's 20th Ed. Chapter 48 Page 290

A. Small, freely filtered solute, not reabsorbed by tubules
B. Produced from muscle
C. Excreted at a relatively constant rate
D. None of the above

32. For a 20- to 50-year-old man, creatinine excretion should be?

Harrison's 20th Ed. Chapter 48 Page 290

A. 6.5–15.0 mg/kg body weight
B. 18.5–25.0 mg/kg body weight
C. 28.5–35.0 mg/kg body weight
D. 36.5–44.0 mg/kg body weight

For a 20 to 50 year old man, creatinine excretion should be 18.5–25.0 mg/kg body weight. For a woman of the same age, it should be 16.5–22.4 mg/kg body weight.

33. Creatinine clearance (CrCl) is calculated by?

Harrison's 20th Ed. Chapter 48 Page 290

A. $(P_{cr} X T_{min})/(U_{vol} X U_{cr})$
B. $(U_{vol} X U_{cr})/(P_{cr} X T_{min})$
C. $(U_{vol} X P_{cr})/(U_{cr} X T_{min})$
D. $(P_{cr} X U_{cr})/(U_{vol} X T_{min})$

Creatinine clearance (CrCl) is calculated by $(U_{vol} X U_{cr})/(P_{cr} X T_{min})$

34. Which of the following variable is not included in the Cockcroft-Gault formula?

Harrison's 20th Ed. Chapter 48 Page 290

A. Age
B. Weight
C. Plasma creatinine
D. Blood urea

Cockcroft-Gault formula is as follows : CrCl (mL/min) = (140 – age (years) × weight (kg) × [0.85 if female])/(72 × PCr (mg/dL).

35. For calculating GFR by Cockcroft-Gault formula, the value is multiplied by what factor for women?

Harrison's 20th Ed. Chapter 48 Page 290

A. 0.55
B. 0.65
C. 0.75
D. 0.85

For calculating GFR by Cockcroft-Gault formula, the value is multiplied by 0.85 for women a lower fraction of the body weight is composed of muscle.

36. Which of the following variable is not included in the Modification of Diet in Renal Disease (MDRD) formula?

Harrison's 20th Ed. Chapter 48 Page 290

A. Age
B. Gender
C. Ethnicity
D. Height

MDRD formula is as follows : eGFR (mL/min per 1.73 m^2) = 186.3 × PCr ($e^{-1.154}$) × age ($e^{-0.203}$) × (0.742 if female) × (1.21 if black).

37. Which of the following is not used to estimate GFR?

Harrison's 20th Ed. Chapter 48 Page 290

A. Insulin clearance
B. MDRD (modification of diet in renal disease)
C. Cockcroft-Gault formula
D. CKD-EPI

38. MDRD equation better correlates with true GFR when GFR is?

Harrison's 20th Ed. Chapter 48 Page 290

A. < 90 mL/min per 1.73 m^2
B. < 60 mL/min per 1.73 m^2
C. < 30 mL/min per 1.73 m^2
D. < 15 mL/min per 1.73 m^2

The MDRD equation is better correlated with true GFR when the GFR is < 60 mL/min per 1.73 m^2.

39. Cystatin C estimation is a renal function equivalent of?

N Engl J Med. 2006;354:2473-83

A. Urea
B. Creatinine
C. Ammonium
D. Inulin

40. Which of the following is false about Cystatin C?

Harrison's 20th Ed. Chapter 48 Page 290

A. Member of cysteine protease inhibitors
B. Produced from all nucleated cells
C. Production not affected by diet or nutritional status
D. None of the above

Cystatin C is a member of cystatin superfamily of cysteine protease inhibitors, produced at a relatively constant rate from all nucleated cells. Cystatin C production is not affected by diet or nutritional status. It provides a more sensitive indicator of GFR than the plasma creatinine concentration.

41. Laboratory abnormalities characteristic of chronic renal failure include?

Harrison's 20th Ed. Chapter 48 Page 291

A. Anemia
B. Hypocalcemia
C. Hyperphosphatemia
D. All of the above

42. Abnormalities characteristic of chronic renal failure include?

Harrison's 20th Ed. Chapter 48 Page 291

A. Isosthenuria
B. Small kidneys on ultrasound
C. Cortical thinning
D. All of the above

Laboratory abnormalities characteristic of chronic renal failure include anemia, hypocalcemia and hyperphosphatemia. Radiographic evidence of renal osteodystrophy is also characteristic of chronic renal failure but is a very late finding. Other typical findings include proteinuria, nonconcentrated urine (isosthenuria; isosmotic with plasma) and small kidneys on ultrasound with increased echogenicity and cortical thinning.

43. Decreased circulating blood volume due to volume sequestration occurs in?

Harrison's 20th Ed. Chapter 48 Page 291

A. Pancreatitis
B. Peritonitis
C. Rhabdomyolysis
D. All of the above

44. Profound renal vasoconstriction occurs in?

Harrison's 20th Ed. Chapter 48 Page 291

A. Severe heart failure
B. Hepatorenal syndrome
C. Nonsteroidal antiinflammatory drugs (NSAIDs) use
D. All of the above

45. There occurs a steep decline in GFR when mean arterial pressure falls below?

Harrison's 20th Ed. Chapter 48 Page 291

A. 80 mm Hg
B. 90 mm Hg
C. 100 mm Hg
D. 110 mm Hg

Once the mean arterial pressure falls below 80 mm Hg, there is a steep decline in GFR.

46. Which of the following statements is false?

Harrison's 20th Ed. Chapter 48 Page 291

A. Prostaglandin dilate afferent arterioles of glomerulus
B. Angiotensin II constricts efferent arterioles of glomerulus
C. Arterial hypovolemia leads to release of vasopressin (AVP)
D. None of the above

47. Patients are most susceptible to hemodynamically mediated acute renal failure from which drug combinations?

Harrison's 20th Ed. Chapter 48 Page 291

A. NSAIDs + aminoglycosides
B. NSAIDs + ACE inhibitors/ARBs
C. NSAIDs + Azithromycin
D. NSAIDs + Alcohol

Patients taking NSAIDs and/or ACE inhibitors/ARBs are most susceptible to hemodynamically mediated acute renal failure when blood volume is reduced for any reason.

48. The BUN/P_{Cr} ratio in prerenal azotemia is?

Harrison's 20th Ed. Chapter 48 Page 291 Table 48-2

A. > 5:1
B. > 10:1
C. > 15:1
D. > 20:1

BUN/P_{Cr} ratio in prerenal azotemia is > 20:1. It is 10–15:1 in oliguric acute renal failure.

49. Which of the following is false in prerenal azotemia?

Harrison's 20th Ed. Chapter 48 Page 291 Table 48-2

A. Urine sodium (U_{Na}) <20 mEq/L
B. Urine osmolality >500 mOsmol/L H_2O
C. Fractional excretion of sodium (FE_{Na}) >2%
D. Urine/plasma creatinine (U_{Cr}/P_{Cr}) >40

In prerenal azotemia, Fractional excretion of sodium (FE_{Na}) is <1%. In prerenal conditions, renal tubules are intact capable of concentrating urine (>500 mOsmol), avid Na retention (urine Na concentration <20 mmolfL, fractional excretion of Na < 1%) and U_{cr}/P_{cr} >40. The prerenal urine sediment is usually normal or has hyaline and granular casts whereas the sediment of ATN usually is filled with cellular debris, tubular epithelial casts and dark (muddy brown) granular casts.

50. Which of the following formula is correct to calculate fractional excretion of sodium (FE_{Na})?

Harrison's 20th Ed. Chapter 48 Page 291 Table 48-2

A. $U_{Na} + U_{cr} \times 100 \div (P_{Na} + P_{cr})$
B. $U_{Na} \times P_{cr} \times 100 \div (P_{Na} \times U_{cr})$
C. $U_{Na} \times P_{cr} \times 100 - (P_{Na} \times U_{cr})$
D. $U_{Na} \times P_{cr} \times 100 + (P_{Na} \times U_{cr})$

51. Which of the following is a radiopharmaceutical used for evaluation of the kidneys?

J Nucl Med 1996; 37:1883-1890

A. Technetium-99m mercaptoacetyl triglycine (MAG3)
B. Technetium-99m diethylene triamine penta-acetic acid (DTPA)
C. Technetium-99m dimercaptosuccinic acid (DMSA)
D. All of the above

52. Intrinsic renal disease can arise from processes involving which of the following?

Harrison's 20th Ed. Chapter 48 Page 291

A. Large renal vessels
B. Intrarenal microvasculature
C. Glomeruli or the tubulo-interstitium
D. All of the above

Intrinsic renal disease can arise from processes involving large renal vessels, intrarenal microvasculature and glomeruli or the tubulointerstitium.

53. Enhanced reabsorption of Na^+ by collecting duct occurs due to?
Harrison's 20th Ed. Chapter 48 Page 291

A. Increased aldosterone
B. Increased AVP secretion
C. Suppressed atrial natriuretic peptide secretion
D. All of the above

Enhanced reabsorption of Na^+ by collecting duct is in response to increased aldosterone, increased AVP secretion & suppressed atrial natriuretic peptide secretion.

54. Ischemic and toxic ATN account for what percentage of cases of acute intrinsic renal failure?
Harrison's 20th Ed. Chapter 48 Page 291

A. ~ 10%
B. ~ 40%
C. ~ 60%
D. ~ 90%

Ischemic and toxic ATN account for -90% of cases of acute intrinsic renal failure.

55. Evidence of which of the following is present in ATN?
Harrison's 20th Ed. Chapter 48 Page 291

A. Structural collecting duct injury
B. Structural glomerular injury
C. Structural tubule injury
D. All of the above

Prerenal azotemia and ATN are part of a spectrum of renal hypoperfusion. Prolonged renal hypoperfusion can lead to acute tubular necrosis (ATN) and evidence of structural tubule injury is present in ATN.

56. Renal blood flow constitutes what percentage of cardiac output?
Harrison's 20th Ed. Chapter 48 Page 291

A. 5%
B. 10%
C. 15%
D. 25%

Renal blood flow is approximately 25% of cardiac output, or 1000 mL/minute.

57. Medications cause nephrotoxic ATN by?
Harrison's 20th Ed. Chapter 48 Page 292

A. Intrarenal vasoconstriction
B. Direct tubule toxicity
C. Tubular obstruction
D. All of the above

Medications cause nephrotoxic ATN by inducing a combination of intrarenal vasoconstriction, direct tubule toxicity, and/or tubular obstruction.

58. Process that can cause acute kidney injury (AKI) is?
Harrison's 20th Ed. Chapter 48 Page 292

A. Drug-induced interstitial nephritis
B. Infections
C. Systemic diseases
D. All of the above

Acute kidney injury (AKI) is a subtype of acute renal failure due to involvement of tubules & interstitium. These processes include drug-induced interstitial nephritis (antibiotics, NSAIDs, diuretics), severe infections (bacterial and viral), systemic diseases (systemic lupus erythematosus) and infiltrative disorders (sarcoidosis, lymphoma or leukemia).

59. To demonstrate urinary eosinophils, which of the following stains is used?
Harrison's 20th Ed. Chapter 48 Page 292

A. Periodic acid–Schiff (PAS) stain
B. Hansel's stain
C. Warthin-Starry stain
D. Gram stain

To demonstrate urinary eosinophils, Wright's or Hansel's stain is used. The classic sediment finding in allergic interstitial nephritis is a predominance (>10%) of urinary eosinophils.

60. Renal arteries can be occluded due to?
Harrison's 20th Ed. Chapter 48 Page 292

A. Atheroemboli
B. Thromboemboli
C. In situ thrombosis
D. All of the above

Renal arteries can be occluded with atheroemboli, thromboemboli, in situ thrombosis, aortic dissection or vasculitis.

61. Atheroembolic renal failure most often is associated with?
Harrison's 20th Ed. Chapter 48 Page 292

A. Blunt abdominal trauma
B. Recent aortic instrumentation
C. Acute pancreatitis
D. All of the above

Atheroembolic renal failure can occur spontaneously but most often is associated with recent aortic instrumentation.

62. Stigmata of atheroemboli is?
Harrison's 20th Ed. Chapter 48 Page 292

A. Livedo reticularis
B. Distal peripheral infarcts
C. Eosinophilia
D. All of the above

Stigmata of atheroemboli are livedo reticularis, distal peripheral infarcts, eosinophilia.

63. Which of the following statements is false?
Harrison's 20th Ed. Chapter 48 Page 292

A. Renal artery thrombosis leads to mild proteinuria & hematuria
B. Renal vein thrombosis leads to heavy proteinuria & hematuria
C. Eosinophils in urine suggest atheroembolic renal disease
D. None of the above

Eosinophils in urine suggest allergic interstitial nephritis or atheroembolic renal disease.

64. Diseases of the renal microvasculature include?
Harrison's 20th Ed. Chapter 48 Page 292

A. Hemolytic-uremic syndromes
B. Thrombotic thrombocytopenic purpura
C. Malignant hypertension
D. All of the above

Diseases of the renal microvasculature include hemolytic-uremic syndromes, thrombotic thrombocytopenic purpura and malignant hypertension.

65. Oliguria refers to a 24-hour urine output of?

Harrison's 20th Ed. Chapter 48 Page 292

A. < 200 mL
B. < 300 mL
C. < 400 mL
D. < 500 mL

Oliguria refers to a 24-hour urine output of < 400 mL.

66. Anuria refers to a 24-hour urine output of?

Harrison's 20th Ed. Chapter 48 Page 292

A. < 300 mL
B. < 200 mL
C. < 100 mL
D. < 50 mL

Anuria is the complete absence of urine formation (< 100 mL).

67. Urine output of > 400 mL/day in acute or chronic azotemia is called?

Harrison's 20th Ed. Chapter 48 Page 292

A. False anuria
B. Nonanuria
C. Nonoliguria
D. False azotemia

Nonoliguria refers to urine output >400 mL/day in patients with acute or chronic azotemia.

68. Which of the following statements is false?

Harrison's 20th Ed. Chapter 48 Page 292

A. Oliguria is never normal
B. RBC casts are highly specific for glomerulonephritis
C. Hematuria without RBC casts can be an indication of glomerular disease
D. None of the above

69. Which of the following is false about dipstick measurement of proteinuria?

Harrison's 20th Ed. Chapter 48 Page 293

A. False-positive when urine pH is > 7.0
B. False-positive when urine is very concentrated
C. False-positive when urine is contaminated with blood
D. None of the above

Dipstick measurement detects albumin and gives false-positive results when urine pH > 7.0, urine is very concentrated or contaminated with blood.

70. Unit of expression of albumin-to-creatinine ratio (ACR) is?

Harrison's 20th Ed. Chapter 48 Page 293

A. mg/mg
B. mg/dL
C. mg/gram
D. mg%

Albumin-to-creatinine ratio (ACR) is expressed in mg/gram. 24-hour albumin excretion rate (AER) is expressed as mg/24 hour.

71. Proteins of what size are freely filtered by the kidneys?

Harrison's 20th Ed. Chapter 48 Page 293

A. < 20 kDa
B. < 30 kDa
C. < 40 kDa
D. < 50 kDa

Smaller proteins (<20 kDa) are freely filtered but are readily reabsorbed by the proximal tubule.

72. Normal individuals excrete what amount of total protein in urine?

Harrison's 20th Ed. Chapter 48 Page 293

A. < 150 mg/day
B. < 200 mg/day
C. < 250 mg/day
D. < 300 mg/day

73. Normal individuals excrete what amount of albumin in urine?

Harrison's 20th Ed. Chapter 48 Page 293

A. < 30 mg/day
B. < 100 mg/day
C. < 200 mg/day
D. < 300 mg/day

Normal individuals excrete <150 mg/day of total protein and <30 mg/day of albumin.

74. Which of the following is secreted by renal tubules?

Harrison's 20th Ed. Chapter 48 Page 293

A. Tamm-Horsfall protein
B. IgA
C. Urokinase
D. All of the above

75. Which of the following is not secreted by renal tubules?

Harrison's 20th Ed. Chapter 48 Page 293

A. Tamm-Horsfall protein
B. IgA
C. Urokinase
D. β_2-microglobulin

Tamm-Horsfall, IgA, and urokinase in urine is secreted by the tubules. Small amounts of β_2-microglobulin, apoproteins, enzymes, and peptide hormones are filtered.

76. Size of pores of normal glomerular endothelial cell is?

Harrison's 20th Ed. Chapter 48 Page 293

A. ~50 nm
B. ~100 nm
C. ~150 nm
D. ~200 nm

Normal glomerular endothelial cell forms a barrier composed of pores of ~100 nm that hold back blood cells but allow passage of most proteins.

77. Disease that allows "selective" loss of albumin is?

Harrison's 20th Ed. Chapter 48 Page 293

A. Diabetes
B. Focal segmental glomerulosclerosis (FSGS)
C. Minimal change disease
D. Hypertension

"Selective" loss of albumin is seen in minimal change disease. Diabetes & FSGS lead to "nonselective" loss of all plasma proteins. Hypertension, CRF cause increased tubular protein loss.

78. Urinary protein excretion of >3.5 grams/day can occur without the features of nephrotic syndrome in?

Harrison's 20th Ed. Chapter 48 Page 293

A. Diabetes
B. Amyloidosis
C. Minimal change disease
D. All of the above

79. Urinary protein excretion of >3.5 grams/day can occur without the features of nephrotic syndrome in?

Harrison's 20th Ed. Chapter 48 Page 293

A. Focal segmental glomerulosclerosis (FSGS)
B. Membranous glomerulopathy
C. Membranoproliferative glomerulonephritis (MPGN)
D. All of the above

80. Mechanism of renal failure due to plasma cell dyscrasias is?

Harrison's 20th Ed. Chapter 48 Page 293

A. Fusion of glomerular epithelial cell foot processes
B. Disruption of basement membrane & slit diaphragms
C. Tubule obstruction (cast nephropathy)
D. All of the above

Renal failure from plasma cell dyscrasias (multiple myeloma) occurs due to tubule obstruction (cast nephropathy) and light chain deposition.

81. Mechanisms of edema formation in hypoalbuminemia is the activation of?

Harrison's 20th Ed. Chapter 48 Page 293

A. Renin-angiotensin system
B. Antidiuretic hormone
C. Sympathetic nervous system
D. All of the above

Hypoalbuminemia in nephrotic syndrome is due to excessive urinary losses & increased proximal tubule catabolism of filtered albumin. Edema forms from renal sodium retention & reduced plasma oncotic pressure. Mechanisms include activation of renin-angiotensin system, antidiuretic hormone, & sympathetic nervous system, all of which promote excessive renal salt & water reabsorption.

82. In nephrotic syndrome, which of the following protein is lost?

Harrison's 20th Ed. Chapter 48 Page 293

A. Thyroxine-binding globulin
B. Cholecalciferol-binding protein
C. Transferrin
D. All of the above

In nephrotic syndrome, thyroxine-binding globulin, cholecalciferol-binding protein, transferrin, metal-binding proteins, antithrombin III, proteins S & C, fibrinogen and IgG are lost.

83. Hypercoagulable state in nephrotic syndrome is due?

Harrison's 20th Ed. Chapter 48 Page 293

A. Urinary loss of Antithrombin III
B. Urinary loss of Proteins S & C
C. Hyperfibrinogenemia
D. All of the above

Hypercoagulable state in severe nephrotic syndrome is due to urinary losses of antithrombin III, proteins S & C, hyperfibrinogenemia and enhanced platelet aggregation.

84. Normal red blood cell excretion in urine is?

Harrison's 20th Ed. Chapter 48 Page 294

A. ~ 2 million RBCs per day
B. ~ 3 million RBCs per day
C. ~ 4 million RBCs per day
D. ~ 5 million RBCs per day

Normal red blood cell excretion is up to 2 million RBCs per day.

85. Hematuria is defined as how many RBCs per high-power field?

Harrison's 20th Ed. Chapter 48 Page 294

A. 2–5
B. 5–8
C. 8–12
D. 12–15

Hematuria is defined as 2 to 5 RBCs per high-power field (HPF) & can be detected by dipstick.

86. Persistent or significant hematuria means?

Harrison's 20th Ed. Chapter 48 Page 294

A. > 3 RBCs/HPF on three urinalyses
B. Single urinalysis with > 100 RBCs
C. Gross hematuria
D. All of the above

Persistent or significant hematuria means >3 RBCs/HPF on three urinalyses, or a single urinalysis with >100 RBCs, or gross hematuria.

87. Isolated hematuria may be a feature of all except?

Harrison's 20th Ed. Chapter 48 Page 294

A. Urogenital neoplasms
B. Hypercalciuria
C. Hyperoxaluria
D. Hyperuricosuria

Urogenital neoplasms present as isolated painless hematuria with nondysmorphic RBCs. Hypercalciuria & hyperuricosuria are risk factors for unexplained isolated hematuria in children & adults.

88. Isolated glomerular hematuria can occur in?

Harrison's 20th Ed. Chapter 48 Page 294

A. IgA nephropathy
B. Hereditary nephritis
C. Thin basement membrane disease
D. All of the above

Common etiologies of isolated glomerular hematuria are IgA nephropathy, hereditary nephritis, and thin basement membrane disease.

89. Which of the following urinary feature is diagnostic of glomerulonephritis?

Harrison's 20th Ed. Chapter 48 Page 294

A. Hematuria with dysmorphic RBCs
B. RBC casts
C. Protein excretion >500 mg/day
D. All of the above

Hematuria with dysmorphic RBCs, RBC casts, and protein excretion >500 mg/day is virtually diagnostic of glomerulonephritis. RBC casts form as RBCs that enter tubule fluid become trapped in a cylindrical mold of gelled Tamm-Horsfall protein.

90. In urine, WBCs and/or WBC casts are seen in?

Harrison's 20th Ed. Chapter 48 Page 294

A. Interstitial nephritis
B. Systemic lupus erythematosus
C. Transplant rejection
D. All of the above

WBCs and/or WBC casts in urine are seen in tubulointerstitial diseases like interstitial nephritis, SLE and transplant rejection.

91. Urinary sediment of ATN has which of the following?

Harrison's 20th Ed. Chapter 48 Page 294

A. Cellular debris
B. RBC cast
C. Waxy cast
D. Broad cast

Urinary sediment of ATN is filled with cellular debris & dark (muddy brown) granular casts.

92. Waxy casts refer to?

Harrison's 20th Ed. Chapter 48 Page 294

A. Lipid bodies
B. Oval fat bodies
C. Degenerated cellular casts
D. All of the above

In chronic renal diseases, degenerated cellular casts called waxy casts can be seen in the urine.

93. Broad casts are diagnostic of?

Harrison's 20th Ed. Chapter 48 Page 294

A. Pyelonephritis
B. Chronic renal failure
C. Membranoproliferative glomerulonephritis (MPGN)
D. All of the above

Broad casts arise in dilated tubules of enlarged nephrons that have undergone compensatory hypertrophy in response to reduced renal mass as in chronic renal failure.

94. Which of the following statements is false?

Harrison's 20th Ed. Chapter 48 Page 294

A. Normal individuals excrete < 150 mg/day of total protein
B. Normal individuals excrete ~ 30 mg/day of albumin
C. Polyuria is defined as urine output of > 3 L/day
D. None of the above

95. Polyuria is defined as a 24-hour urine output of?

Harrison's 20th Ed. Chapter 48 Page 294

A. > 2 L/day
B. > 3 L/day
C. > 4 L/day
D. > 5 L/day

Polyuria is defined as a 24-hour urine output of >3 L/day.

96. Polyuria results from which of the following mechanisms?

Harrison's 20th Ed. Chapter 48 Page 294

A. Excretion of nonabsorbable solutes
B. Defect in AVP production
C. Defect in AVP renal responsiveness
D. All of the above

Polyuria results from excretion of nonabsorbable solutes (glucose) or excretion of water due to a defect in AVP production or defect in AVP renal responsiveness. Estimation of urine osmolality distinguishes them.

97. An average person excretes how much of solutes per day?

Harrison's 20th Ed. Chapter 48 Page 294

A. 200–600 mOsmol/day
B. 600–800 mOsmol/day
C. 800–1400 mOsmol/day
D. 1400–1800 mOsmol/day

Average person excretes 600 - 800 mOsmol of solutes per day, primarily as urea & electrolytes.

98. In polyuria (>3 L/day) with dilute urine (<250 mOsmol/L), the cause is?

Harrison's 20th Ed. Chapter 48 Page 294

A. Polydipsia
B. Central diabetes insipidus
C. Nephrogenic diabetes insipidus
D. All of the above

99. In polyuria (>3 L/day) with urine osmolality >300 mOsmol/L, the cause is?

Harrison's 20th Ed. Chapter 48 Page 294

A. Polydipsia
B. Central diabetes insipidus
C. Nephrogenic diabetes insipidus
D. Solute diuresis

In polyuria (>3 L/day) with dilute urine (<250 mOsmol/L), the cause can be polydipsia, central diabetes insipidus, or nephrogenic diabetes insipidus. If the urine volume is >3 L/day and urine osmolality is >300 mOsmol/L, a solute diuresis is present.

100. Which of the following is a poorly reabsorbed solute?

Harrison's 20th Ed. Chapter 48 Page 294

A. Glucose
B. Mannitol
C. Urea
D. All of the above

Poorly reabsorbed solutes are glucose, mannitol or urea.

101. Which of the following is a "salt-wasting disorder"?

Harrison's 20th Ed. Chapter 48 Page 294

A. Cystic renal diseases
B. Bartter's syndrome
C. Resolving ATN
D. All of the above

Cystic renal diseases, Bartter's syndrome, or a resolving ATN are salt-wasting disorders.

102. Which of the following drugs can cause primary polydipsia?

Harrison's 20th Ed. Chapter 48 Page 294 Figure 48-4

A. Thioridazine
B. Chlorpromazine
C. Anticholinergic agents
D. All of the above

103. Which of the following can cause solute diuresis?

Harrison's 20th Ed. Chapter 48 Page 294 Figure 48-4

A. Lithium
B. Demeclocycline
C. Diuretics
D. Ethanol

104. Which of the following can cause central diabetes insipidus (vasopressin-sensitive)?

Harrison's 20th Ed. Chapter 48 Page 294 Figure 48-4

A. Sheehan's syndrome
B. Guillain-Barre syndrome
C. Empty sella syndrome
D. All of the above

105. In psychogenic polydipsia, which of the following is false?

Harrison's 20th Ed. Chapter 48 Page 294 Figure 48-4

A. Polyuria
B. Urine osmolality < 250 mOsmol
C. Low serum sodium
D. None of the above

Urine osmolality is maximally dilute at 50 mOsmol/L.

106. Which of the following is the best method to distinguish between central & nephrogenic diabetes insipidus?

Harrison's 20th Ed. Chapter 48 Page 294

A. Urine osmolality
B. Plasma AVP level
C. Water deprivation test
D. All of the above

Estimation of plasma AVP level is the best method for distinguishing between central & nephrogenic diabetes insipidus. Water deprivation test along with exogenous vasopressin may distinguish primary polydipsia from central & nephrogenic diabetes insipidus.

Fluid and Electrolyte Disturbances

107. Water comprises what percentage of body weight in women?
Harrison's 20th Ed. Chapter 49 Page 295

A. ~ 50%
B. ~ 60%
C. ~ 70%
D. ~ 80%

108. Water comprises what percentage of body weight in men?
Harrison's 20th Ed. Chapter 49 Page 295

A. ~ 50%
B. ~ 60%
C. ~ 70%
D. ~ 80%

Water comprises ~50% of body weight in women and ~60% in men.

109. What percentage of total body water is found as intracellular fluid (ICF)?
Harrison's 20th Ed. Chapter 49 Page 295

A. 15–35%
B. 35–55%
C. 55–75%
D. 75–95%

110. What percentage of total body water is found as extracellular fluid (ECF)?
Harrison's 20th Ed. Chapter 49 Page 295

A. 15–25%
B. 25–45%
C. 45–55%
D. 55–75%

55–75% of body water is present as intracellular fluid (ICF) & 25–45% as extracellular fluid (ECF).

111. Ratio of water in intravascular and extravascular spaces is?
Harrison's 20th Ed. Chapter 49 Page 295

A. 1:2
B. 2:1
C. 1:3
D. 3:1

Ratio of intravascular (plasma water) & extravascular (interstitial) ECF water is 1:3.

112. Which of the following is true for Osmolality?
Harrison's 20th Ed. Chapter 49 Page 295

A. Osmoles of solute per milligram of water (Osm/mg)
B. Osmoles of solute per milliliter of water (Osm/mL)
C. Osmoles of solute per kilogram of water (Osm/kg)
D. Osmoles of solute per liter of water (Osm/L)

Osmolality is defined as the concentration of all solutes in a given weight of water and is expressed as milliosmoles or osmoles of solute per kilogram of water (mOsm/kg H_2O). Osmolarity is the measure of osmoles of solute per liter of water (mOsm/L H_2O). Osmolarity = Osmolality × 0.995

113. Plasma osmolality (mOsm/kg H_2O) is calculated by?
Harrison's 20th Ed. Chapter 49 Page 295

A. 2 × plasma [Na^+ + K^+] + glucose/18 + BUN/1.8
B. 2 × plasma [Na^+ + K^+] + glucose/18 + BUN/2.8
C. 2 × plasma [Na^+ + K^+] + glucose/18 + BUN/3.8
D. 2 × plasma [Na^+ + K^+] + glucose/18 + BUN/4.8

Plasma osmolality (mOsm/kg H_2O) is calculated as 2 × plasma [Na^++K^+](mEq/L) + glucose(mg/dL)/18 + BUN(mg/dL)/2.8.

114. Which of the following is correct?
Harrison's 20th Ed. Chapter 49 Page 295

A. ECF osmolality = ICF osmolality
B. ECF osmolality < ICF osmolality
C. ECF osmolality > ICF osmolality
D. All of the above

Osmotic equilibrium refers to ECF osmolality = ICF osmolality.

115. Which of the following is a reflection of ECF volume?
Harrison's 20th Ed. Chapter 49 Page 296

A. Total body Na^+
B. Total body K^+
C. Total body Cl^-
D. Total body HCO_3^-

Total body Na^+ content reflects ECF volume as it is restricted to extracellular compartment.

116. Difference between ICF and ECF composition is due to?
Harrison's 20th Ed. Chapter 49 Page 295

A. Transporters
B. Channels
C. ATP-driven membrane pumps
D. All of the above

117. Which of the following is an organic phosphate ester?
Harrison's 20th Ed. Chapter 49 Page 295

A. ATP
B. Creatine phosphate
C. Phospholipids
D. All of the above

Apart from potassium, the predominant ICF osmoles are organic phosphate esters like ATP, creatine phosphate, and phospholipids.

118. A change in ICF osmolality is due to a change in?
Harrison's 20th Ed. Chapter 49 Page 295

A. ICF water content
B. ICF Na^+ content
C. ICF K^+ content
D. ICF Cl^- content

A change in ICF osmolality is usually due to a change in ICF water content.

119. Which of the following is known as "ineffective osmole"?
Harrison's 20th Ed. Chapter 49 Page 295

A. Inositol
B. Phospholipids
C. Urea
D. All of the above

An osmole is the number of moles that a solute contributes to the osmotic pressure of a solution. Water travels from a low solute concentration to a high solute concentration in order to establish equilibrium. Osmotic pressure is what drives osmosis. It's the force that pulls water from areas of low solute concentration to high solute concentration. Solutes like urea do not contribute to water shift across cell membranes and are known as ineffective osmoles. Ineffective osmoles like urea & glucose do not play a role in stimulating thirst.

120. Regulation of water balance is governed by a high-gain feedback mechanism involving?
N Engl J Med. 2015;372:1349-58

A. Hypothalamus
B. Neurohypophysis
C. Kidneys
D. All of the above

121. AVP gene codes for?
N Engl J Med. 2015;372:1349-58

A. 9–amino acid peptide arginine vasopressin
B. Carrier protein neurophysin-2
C. Glycoprotein copeptin
D. All of the above

AVP gene codes for three peptides — the 9–amino acid peptide arginine vasopressin, a carrier protein called neurophysin-2, and a small glycoprotein called copeptin.

122. Which of the following is considered as a second "antidiuretic hormone"?
N Engl J Med. 2015;372:1349-58

A. Copeptin
B. Oxytocin
C. Neurophysin-2
D. All of the above

Oxytocin gene has a structure that is very similar to that of the arginine vasopressin gene expressed in oxytocinergic cells in the supraoptic & paraventricular nuclei of hypothalamus. Vasopressin secretion is increased by osmotic stimuli. It binds to vasopressin receptors in kidney and produces similar, although weaker, responses than AVP. Consequently, oxytocin is considered to be a second "antidiuretic hormone".

123. Transient vasopressin-resistant diabetes insipidus of pregnancy is due to?
N Engl J Med. 2015;372:1349-58

A. Aquanase
B. Nephrinase
C. Vasopressinase
D. Vasopressinine

Rarely, in III trimester of pregnancy, a syndrome called transient vasopressin-resistant diabetes insipidus of pregnancy occurs as a result of placental secretion of vasopressinase (also called oxytocinase), which hydrolyzes circulating vasopressin and oxytocin. Affected patients have a response to desmopressin acetate, which is resistant to this enzyme.

124. Which of the following collaborate to maintain human body fluid osmolality?
Harrison's 20th Ed. Chapter 49 Page 295

A. Water ingestion
B. Vasopressin secretion
C. Renal water transport
D. All of the above

Vasopressin secretion, water ingestion & renal water transport collaborate to maintain human body fluid osmolality between 280 & 295 mOsm/kg.

125. Osmotic threshold for AVP release is?
Harrison's 20th Ed. Chapter 49 Page 295 Figure 49-1

A. 275 mOsmol/kg
B. 285 mOsmol/kg
C. 295 mOsmol/kg
D. 305 mOsmol/kg

AVP secretion is stimulated as systemic osmolality increases above a threshold level of ~285 mOsm/kg. It maintains plasma osmolality within a 1–2% range. Plasma AVP becomes detectable in euvolemic, healthy individuals at a threshold of ~285 mOsm/kg, above which there is a linear relationship between osmolality and circulating AVP.

126. In hypothalamus, vasopressin (AVP) is synthesized in?
Harrison's 20th Ed. Chapter 49 Page 295

A. Neuroendocrine cells of the periventricular nucleus
B. Neuroendocrine cells of the preoptic area
C. Magnocellular neurons
D. Parvocellular neurosecretory cells of paraventricular nucleus

Vasopressin (AVP) is synthesized in magnocellular neurons within the hypothalamus.

127. Thirst is mediated by?
Harrison's 20th Ed. Chapter 49 Page 295

A. Increase in effective osmolality
B. Decrease in ECF volume
C. Decrease in blood pressure
D. All of the above

Primary stimulus for water ingestion is thirst mediated either by an increase in effective osmolality or a decrease in ECF volume or blood pressure.

128. 'Osmoreceptors' are located in?
Harrison's 20th Ed. Chapter 49 Page 295

A. Posterior pituitary
B. Anterolateral hypothalamus
C. Posteromedial hypothalamus
D. All of the above

Osmoreceptors, located in the anterolateral hypothalamus, are stimulated by a rise in tonicity.

129. Arginine vasopressin is synthesized in?
Harrison's 20th Ed. Chapter 49 Page 295

A. Hypothalamus
B. Anterior pituitary gland
C. Posterior pituitary gland
D. All of the above

130. Arginine vasopressin (AVP) is secreted by?
Harrison's 20th Ed. Chapter 49 Page 295

A. Hypothalamus
B. Anterior pituitary gland
C. Posterior pituitary gland
D. All of the above

Arginine vasopressin (AVP) or antidiuretic hormone (ADH) is a polypeptide synthesized in supraoptic & paraventricular nuclei of hypothalamus & secreted by posterior pituitary gland.

131. Thirst is mediated by?

Harrison's 20th Ed. Chapter 49 Page 295

A. Increase in effective osmolality
B. Decrease in ECF volume
C. Decrease in blood pressure
D. All of the above

Primary stimulus for water ingestion is thirst mediated either by an increase in effective osmolality or a decrease in ECF volume or blood pressure.

132. Half-life of AVP in the circulation is?

Harrison's 20th Ed. Chapter 49 Page 295

A. 1–2 minutes
B. 2–4 minutes
C. 4–8 minutes
D. 10–20 minutes

AVP has a half-life in the circulation of only 10–20 minutes.

133. Nonosmotic factors that regulate AVP secretion include?

Harrison's 20th Ed. Chapter 49 Page 295

A. Nausea
B. Serotonin
C. Intracerebral angiotensin II
D. All of the above

Nonosmotic factors that regulate AVP secretion include effective circulating (arterial) volume, nausea, pain, stress, hypoglycemia, pregnancy, intracerebral angiotensin II, serotonin and multiple drugs.

134. Receptor to which AVP binds in renal collecting ducts is?

Harrison's 20th Ed. Chapter 49 Page 295

A. U_2 receptor
B. V_2 receptor
C. W_2 receptor
D. X_2 receptor

AVP acts on renal V2 type receptors in the thick ascending limb of Henle and principal cells of the collecting duct (CD), increasing intracellular levels of cyclic AMP and activating protein kinase A (PKA) - dependent phosphorylation of multiple transport proteins.

135. Which of the following about V2 vasopressin receptor is false?

N Engl J Med. 2015;372:1349-58

A. G protein–coupled receptor
B. Functions mediated by the heterotrimeric G-protein G_s
C. Located chiefly in renal epithelia
D. None of the above

136. V2 receptor acts chiefly in?

N Engl J Med. 2015;372:1349-58

A. Principal cells of renal collecting duct
B. Distal convoluted tubule cells
C. Cells of the thick ascending limb of Henle
D. All of the above

V2 receptor acts chiefly in the principal cells of the renal collecting duct, the connecting tubule cells, the distal convoluted tubule cells, and the cells of the thick ascending limb of Henle.

137. Which of the following aquaporin is present in renal proximal tubule & thin descending limb of the loop of Henle?

N Engl J Med. 2015;372:1349-58

A. Aquaporin-1 gene
B. Aquaporin-2 gene
C. Aquaporin-3 gene
D. Aquaporin-4 gene

138. Which of the following aquaporin is present in renal connecting tubule & collecting duct?

N Engl J Med. 2015;372:1349-58

A. Aquaporin-2 gene
B. Aquaporin-3 gene
C. Aquaporin-4 gene
D. All of the above

139. Water channels in collecting ducts activated by AVP are encoded by?

Harrison's 20th Ed. Chapter 49 Page 295

A. Aquaporin-1 gene
B. Aquaporin-2 gene
C. Aquaporin-3 gene
D. Aquaporin-4 gene

AVP binds to V_2 receptors on basolateral membrane of principal cells in the collecting duct activating the water channels which are encoded by aquaporin-2 gene.

140. Loss or gain of approximately how much water will change plasma Na^+ concentration by ~1 mmol per liter?

N Engl J Med. 2015;372:55-65

A. 1 mL per kilogram of body weight
B. 2 mL per kilogram of body weight
C. 3 mL per kilogram of body weight
D. 4 mL per kilogram of body weight

Loss or gain of approximately 3 mL of water per kilogram of body weight will change the plasma sodium concentration by approximately 1 mmol per liter.

141. Site where AVP exerts its principal effect is?

Lancet 2005;365:417-430

A. Proximal convoluted tubule
B. Loop of Henle
C. Distal convoluted tubule
D. Cortical & papillary portions of collecting duct

142. Site of action of loop diuretics is?

Lancet 2005;365:417-430

A. Proximal convoluted tubule
B. Thin ascending limb of Henle's loop
C. Medullary thick ascending limb of Henle
D. All of the above

Na:K:2Cl cotransporter is the site of action of the powerful loop diuretics in the medullary thick ascending limb of Henle, and its mutations give rise to Bartter's syndrome.

143. Normally, major quantity of phosphate is reabsorbed in?
Lancet 2005;365:417-430

A. Proximal convoluted tubule
B. Loop of Henle
C. Distal convoluted tubule
D. Collecting duct

144. The principle site of action of parathyroid hormone (PTH) is?
Lancet 2005;365:417-430

A. Proximal convoluted tubule
B. Loop of Henle
C. Distal convoluted tubule
D. Collecting duct

145. Fluid that enters the distal convoluted tubule is always?
N Engl J Med. 2015;372:55-65

A. Isoosmotic
B. Hypoosmotic
C. Hyperosmotic
D. None of the above

146. The terminal segment of the distal nephron is?
N Engl J Med. 2015;372:55-65

A. Cortical collecting tubule
B. Papillary collecting duct
C. Terminal duct
D. None of the above

147. Calcium reabsorption in cortical thick ascending limb of Henle's loop (cTAL) requires which of the following?
N Engl J Med. 2015;372:55-65

A. PTH
B. $1{,}25(OH)_2D$
C. Paracellin-1
D. Calbindin-D28k

Mutations in CLDN16 encoding paracellin-1, a transmembrane protein located within the tight junction complex, leads to familial hypomagnesemia with hypercalciuria & nephrocalcinosis, suggesting that the ion conductance of the paracellular pathway in thick limb is regulated.

148. In cells & in ECF, phosphorus exists in which form?
N Engl J Med. 2015;372:55-65

A. $H_2PO_4^-$
B. $NaHPO_4^-$
C. HPO_4^{2-}
D. All of the above

149. In adults, above what level of fasting serum phosphate concentration is called hyperphosphatemia?
N Engl J Med. 2015;372:55-65

A. 2.5 mg/dL
B. 3.5 mg/dL
C. 4.5 mg/dL
D. 5.5 mg/dL

Hyperphosphatemia is defined in adults as a fasting serum phosphate concentration > 1.8 mmol/L or 5.5 mg/dL. It results from impaired glomerular filtration, hypoparathyroidism, excessive delivery of phosphate into the ECF from bone, gut, or parenteral phosphate therapy. Upper limit of normal serum phosphate concentrations is higher in children & neonates (2.4 mmol/L or 7 mg/dL).

150. Normally, the concentration of magnesium in serum is?
N Engl J Med. 2015;372:55-65

A. 0.7 to 1.2 mg/dL
B. 1.2 to 1.6 mg/dL
C. 1.5 to 2.0 mg/dL
D. 2.4 to 2.9 mg/dL

The concentration of magnesium in serum is closely regulated within the range of 0.7 - 1 mmol!L or 1.5 - 2 mEq/L. One-half of the 25 gram (1000 mmol) of total body magnesium is located in bone and only 1% of body magnesium resides in the ECF. Almost all extraskeletal magnesium is present within cells, where the total concentration is 5 mM.

151. Which of the following should be supplemented in patients with hypomagnesemia?
N Engl J Med. 2015;372:55-65

A. Calcium
B. Potassium
C. Phosphate
D. All of the above

152. Maximal urine osmolality can be?
Harrison's 20th Ed. Chapter 49 Page 296, N Engl J Med. 2015;372:55-65

A. 500 mOsmol/kg
B. 800 mOsmol/kg
C. 1000 mOsmol/kg
D. 1200 mOsmol/kg

Under "antidiuretic" conditions, with increased circulating AVP, kidneys reabsorbs water filtered at glomerulus, equilibrating the osmolality across CD epithelium to excrete a hypertonic or concentrated urine (osmolality of up to 1200).

153. Minimum urine osmolality in humans can be?
Harrison's 20th Ed. Chapter 49 Page 296, N Engl J Med. 2015;372:55-65

A. 50 mOsmol/kg
B. 100 mOsmol/kg
C. 150 mOsmol/kg
D. 200 mOsmol/kg

In the absence of circulating AVP, insertion of aquaporin-2 channels & water absorption across CD is essentially abolished, resulting in secretion of a hypotonic, dilute urine (osmolality as low as 30-50 mOsm/kg).

154. Maximally dilute urine occurs in which of the following?
N Engl J Med. 2015;372:55-65

A. Untreated diabetes insipidus
B. Spontaneous recovery from hyponatremia
C. Administration of a vasopressin antagonist
D. All of the above

155. Individuals eating a typical western diet consume what amount of NaCl daily?
N Engl J Med. 2015;372:55-65

A. ~ 50 mmol
B. ~ 150 mmol
C. ~ 250 mmol
D. ~ 500 mmol

Individuals eating a typical western diet consume ~150 mmol of NaCl daily.

156. Major regulatory mechanism controlling sodium excretion is?
Harrison's 20th Ed. Chapter 49 Page 296

A. GFR
B. Tubule Na^+ reabsorption
C. Tubule water reabsorption
D. All of the above

Tubule Na^+ reabsorption, and not GFR, is the major regulatory mechanism controlling Na^+ excretion.

157. Kidneys filter how many millimoles of Na^+ per day?
Harrison's 20th Ed. Chapter 49 Page 296

A. 20,200
B. 25,200
C. 30,200
D. 35,200

Kidneys filter ~25,200 mmol of Na^+ per day. This is equivalent to ~1.5 kg of salt.

158. How many millimoles of Na^+ is excreted per day?
Harrison's 20th Ed. Chapter 49 Page 296

A. 100 mM
B. 400 mM
C. 800 mM
D. 1000 mM

99.6% of filtered Na^+-Cl^- is reabsorbed to excrete 100 mM per day.

159. Which of the following play a role in the renal absorption of sodium?
Harrison's 20th Ed. Chapter 49 Page 296

A. Na^+-K^+-2Cl^- cotransporter (NKCC2)
B. Na^+-Cl^- cotransporter (NCC)
C. Epithelial Na^+ channels (ENaC)
D. All of the above

160. Majority of filtered sodium is reabsorbed in?
Harrison's 20th Ed. Chapter 49 Page 296

A. Proximal convoluted tubule
B. Thick ascending limb of loop of Henle
C. Distal convoluted tubule
D. Cortical and medullary collecting ducts

161. Reabsorption of filtered sodium mediated by 'Na^+ - K^+ - 2Cl^- cotransporter' occurs in?
Harrison's 20th Ed. Chapter 49 Page 296

A. Proximal convoluted tubule
B. Thick ascending limb of the loop of Henle (TALH)
C. Distal convoluted tubule
D. Cortical and medullary collecting ducts

162. Reabsorption of filtered sodium mediated by 'thiazide - sensitive Na^+ - Cl^- cotransporter' occurs in?
Harrison's 20th Ed. Chapter 49 Page 296

A. Proximal convoluted tubule
B. Thick ascending limb of loop of Henle (TALH)
C. Distal convoluted tubule
D. Cortical & medullary collecting ducts

Almost two-thirds of filtered Na^+ is reabsorbed in the proximal convoluted tubule. 25-30% occurs in TALH via apical furosemide-sensitive Na^+-K^+-2Cl^- co-transporter. 5% occurs in DCT mediated by thiazide-sensitive Na^+-Cl^- co-transporter. Na^+ reabsorption also occurs in cortical and medullary collecting ducts.

163. Distal nephron comprises of?
Harrison's 20th Ed. Chapter 49 Page 296

A. Distal convoluted tubule (DCT)
B. Connecting tubule (CNT)
C. Collecting ducts (CD)
D. All of the above

164. Amiloride-sensitive epithelial Na^+ channels (ENaC) are located in?
Harrison's 20th Ed. Chapter 49 Page 296

A. Proximal convoluted tubule
B. Thin descending limb of loop of Henle
C. Thick ascending limb of loop of Henle (TALH)
D. Collecting ducts (CD)

165. Chloride ions are primarily reabsorbed by?
Harrison's 20th Ed. Chapter 49 Page 296

A. Principal cells
B. β–intercalated cells
C. Macula densa
D. All of the above

Cl^- ions are primarily reabsorbed by intercalated cells, via apical Cl^- exchange (Cl^--OH^- and Cl^--HCO_3^- exchange, mediated by the SLC26A4 anion exchanger.

166. Angiotensin II acts at which of the following?
Harrison's 20th Ed. Chapter 49 Page 296

A. Proximal convoluted tubule
B. Thick ascending limb of loop of Henle (TALH)
C. Distal convoluted tubule
D. Cortical & medullary collecting ducts

Angiotensin II activates proximal Na^+ - Cl^- reabsorption like adrenergic receptors under the influence of renal sympathetic innervation. Locally generated dopamine has a natriuretic effect.

167. Aldosterone-sensitive distal nephron comprises of?
Harrison's 20th Ed. Chapter 49 Page 296

A. Distal convoluted tubule (DCT)
B. Connecting tubule (CNT)
C. Collecting duct (CD)
D. All of the above

Aldosterone-sensitive distal nephron comprises of distal convoluted tubule (DCT), Connecting tubule (CNT) and collecting duct (CD). Aldosterone primarily activates Na-Cl reabsorption within the aldosterone-sensitive distal nephron.

168. Na^+ absorption and promoting K^+ excretion is a function of?
Harrison's 20th Ed. Chapter 49 Page 296

A. Na^+–K^+–2Cl^- cotransporter
B. Thiazide–sensitive Na^+–Cl^- cotransporter
C. Epithelial Na^+ channels (ENaC)
D. All of the above

Aldosterone activates ENaC channel in principal cells inducing Na^+ absorption & promoting K^+ excretion.

169. AVP maintains circulatory integrity by?

Harrison's 20th Ed. Chapter 49 Page 297

A. Inducing vasoconstriction
B. Increasing sympathetic nervous system tone
C. Increasing renal retention of water and Na^+–Cl^-
D. All of the above

AVP maintains circulatory integrity by inducing vasoconstriction, increasing sympathetic nervous system tone, increasing renal retention of both water and Na - Cl and modulating the arterial baroreceptor reflex. Most of these responses involve activation of systemic V_{1A} AVP receptors but concomitant activation of V2 receptors in the kidney can result in renal water retention and hyponatremia.

170. Aquaporin-2 dysregulation occurs in?

N Engl J Med. 2015;372:1349-58

A. Congestive heart failure
B. Hepatic cirrhosis
C. Syndrome of inappropriate antidiuretic hormone secretion
D. All of the above

Aquaporin-2 dysregulation occurs in syndromes associated with renal water retention & dilutional hyponatremia, mainly severe congestive heart failure, hepatic cirrhosis, and the syndrome of inappropriate antidiuretic hormone secretion (SIADH).

171. Type I Bartter's syndrome is associated with?

N Engl J Med. 2015;372:1349-58

A. Bumetanide-sensitive sodium-potassium-chloride cotransporter
B. Thiazide-sensitive sodium-chloride cotransporter
C. Vasopressin receptor V2
D. Vasopressin-regulated urea channel

In the thick ascending limbs of Henle, transport of sodium & chloride from lumen is mediated by the bumetanide-sensitive sodium–potassium–chloride cotransporter. Vasopressin upregulates this cotransporter by increasing the expression of SLC12A1, which codes for the cotransporter protein. Up-regulation of sodium–potassium–chloride cotransporter does not affect salt excretion, primarily because thick ascending limb is upstream from macula densa, which compensates for changes in salt delivery by adjusting glomerular filtration rate. This compensatory process is called glomerulotubular feedback. Bumetanide and other loop diuretics increase salt excretion because they inhibit sodium–potassium–chloride cotransporter in macula densa, thereby blocking the feedback to the glomerulus. Type I Bartter's syndrome is due to loss-of-function mutations in SLC12A1 and is manifested by a salt-losing syndrome rather than by a simple defect in water balance.

172. Gitelman's syndrome is associated with?

N Engl J Med. 2015;372:1349-58

A. Bumetanide-sensitive sodium-potassium-chloride cotransporter
B. Thiazide-sensitive sodium-chloride cotransporter
C. Vasopressin receptor V2
D. Vasopressin-regulated urea channel

Vasopressin also regulates salt transport in distal convoluted tubule by upregulating apical thiazide-sensitive sodium–chloride cotransporter,. It transports salt at a high rate but is impermeable to water and thereby contributes to dilution of the tubular fluid. This cotransporter is also regulated by aldosterone. Inactivating mutations in thiazide-sensitive sodium–chloride cotransporter cause Gitelman's syndrome, which is manifested by hypotension, hypokalemia, hypomagnesemia, hypocalciuria, and metabolic alkalosis.

173. Deafness is invariably associated with which type of Bartter's syndrome?

N Engl J Med. 2015;372:1349-58

A. Type 1
B. Type 2
C. Type 3
D. Type 4

Bartter type 4 is due to mutations in barttin which is also expressed in inner ear. Deafness is invariably associated with Bartter type 4.

174. Which of the following is false for Bartter's syndrome?

N Engl J Med. 2015;372:1349-58

A. Inherited as autosomal recessive trait
B. Due to abnormality in renal tubule transport proteins
C. Prostaglandin E production is low
D. Metabolic abnormalities similar to diuretic abuse

In Bartter's syndrome, RAS activation causes increased levels of cyclooxygenase 2 (COX-2) & marked overproduction of renal prostaglandins (PGE2).

175. Hyperprostaglandin E syndrome is related to?

N Engl J Med. 2015;372:1349-58

A. Bartter's syndrome
B. Gitelman's syndrome
C. Liddle's syndrome
D. All of the above

Hyperprostaglandin E syndrome is a severe form of Bartter's syndrome. Neonates present with pronounced volume depletion, fever, vomiting and diarrhea from PGE_2 overproduction.

176. Protein affected in Bartter's syndrome is?

N Engl J Med. 2015;372:1349-58

A. NKCC2
B. ROMK
C. Barttin
D. All of the above

Bartter's syndrome is the result of mutations in ion transport proteins in TAL. Type 1 is due to apical loop-diuretic sensitive sodium-potassium-chloride co-transporter protein NKCC2, type 2 is due to apical potassium channel ROMK, type 3 is due to basolateral chloride channel ClC-Kb and Bartter type 4 results from mutations in barttin, an essential subunit of ClC-Ka and ClC-Kb that enables transport of the chloride channels to the cell surface.

177. Which of the following electrical situations occur in Bartter's syndrome?

N Engl J Med. 2015;372:1349-58

A. Loss of lumen-positive electrical transport potential
B. Loss of lumen-negative electrical transport potential
C. Loss of cell-positive electrical transport potential
D. Loss of cell-negative electrical transport potential

In Bartter's syndrome, loss of lumen-positive electrical transport potential that normally drives paracellular reabsorption of sodium, calcium & magnesium causes NaCl wasting, hypercalciuria & mild hypomagnesemia.

178. Gitelman's syndrome is due to mutations in?

N Engl J Med. 2015;372:1349-58

A. Apical loop-diuretic sensitive Na-K-Cl co-transporter
B. Apical potassium channel
C. Thiazide-sensitive Na-Cl co-transporter (NCCT)
D. Basolateral chloride channel ClC-Kb

Gitelman's syndrome is due to mutations in thiazide-sensitive Na-Cl co-transporter (NCCT) in DCT.

179. Gitelman's syndrome is distinguished from Bartter's syndrome by?

N Engl J Med. 2015;372:1349-58

A. Hypokalemia
B. Metabolic alkalosis
C. Elevated renin and aldosterone levels
D. Hypomagnesemia

Severe magnesium wasting occurs in Gitelman's syndrome.

180. Gitelman's syndrome is distinguished from Bartter's syndrome by?

N Engl J Med. 2015;372:1349-58

A. Hypokalemia
B. Metabolic alkalosis
C. Elevated renin and aldosterone levels
D. Hypocalciuria

Gitelman's syndrome is distinguished from Bartter's syndrome by presence of severe hypomagnesemia & hypocalciuria. Hypercalciuria marked overproduction of renal prostaglandins (PGE2) occurs in Bartter's syndrome.

181. Carpopedal spasm, cramps & tetany are clinical features of?

N Engl J Med. 2015;372:1349-58

A. Bartter's syndrome
B. Gitelman's syndrome
C. Liddle's syndrome
D. Von Hippel-Lindau disease

Gitelman's syndrome is characterized by hypocalciuria, severe hypomagnesemia resulting in carpopedal spasm, cramps and tetany. Autosomal recessive familial hypomagnesemia with hypercalciuria and nephrocalcinosis (FHHNC), autosomal recessive hypomagnesemia with secondary hypocalcemia (HSH), autosomal dominant hypomagnesemia, and autosomal dominant hypoparathyroidism can also produce such presentation.

182. Which of the following best relate to Liddle's syndrome?

N Engl J Med. 2015;372:1349-58

A. Unregulated sodium reabsorption
B. Overactive ENaC in cortical collecting duct
C. Chloride-independent sodium reabsorption
D. All of the above

183. Which of the following is false for Liddle's syndrome?

N Engl J Med. 2015;372:1349-58

A. Hypertension
B. Hypokalemia
C. High aldosterone levels
D, Metabolic alkalosis

Liddle's syndrome mimics a state of aldosterone excess. Features include early and severe hypertension, hypokalemia & metabolic alkalosis. Plasma aldosterone & renin levels are low.

184. Which of the following drug is ineffective in treatment of Liddle's syndrome?

N Engl J Med. 2015;372:1349-58

A. Spironolactone
B. Amiloride
C. Triamterene
D. All of the above

Amiloride or triamterene block ENaC and, combined with salt restriction, provide effective therapy for hypertension and hypokalemia.

185. Polyuria is a prominent feature of all except?

N Engl J Med. 2015;372:1349-58

A. ADPKD
B. Medullary cystic kidney disease (MCKD)
C. Bartter's syndrome
D. Gitelman's syndrome

186. During antenatal period, fetal polyuria causes maternal polyhydramnios and premature labor in?

N Engl J Med. 2015;372:1349-58

A. ADPKD
B. Medullary cystic kidney disease (MCKD)
C. Bartter's syndrome
D. Gitelman's syndrome

In antenatal period, fetal polyuria may cause maternal polyhydramnios & premature labor in Bartter's syndrome.

187. ENaC best relates to?

N Engl J Med. 2015;372:1349-58

A. Amiloride-sensitive epithelial sodium channel
B. Thiazide-sensitive Na-Cl co-transporter
C. Na-K-2Cl co-transporter
D. Sodium-bicarbonate co-transporter

ENaC is an amiloride-sensitive epithelial sodium channel.

188. Which of the following about aquaporin-1 is false?

N Engl J Med. 2015;372:1349-58

A. Expressed in proximal tubule
B. Expressed in thin descending limb of the loop of Henle
C. Not regulated by vasopressin
D. None of the above

189. Which of the following about aquaporin-2 is false?

N Engl J Med. 2015;372:1349-58

A. Expressed throughout the collecting-duct system
B. Regulated by vasopressin
C. Half-life of aquaporin-2 protein is increased by vasopressin
D. None of the above

Aquaporin-2 is expressed throughout collecting-duct system i.e., in the region of renal tubule where vasopressin regulates osmotic transport of water. Aquaporin-2 mediates "apical" component of transepithelial water transport, and its regulation by vasopressin controls the overall rate of water permeation across the collecting-duct epithelium.

190. Which of the following about aquaporin-3 is false?

N Engl J Med. 2015;372:1349-58

A. Localized to the basolateral plasma membrane
B. Present in collecting-duct principal cells, connecting-tubule cells, and inner medullary collecting-duct cells
C. Conducts glycerol in addition to water
D. None of the above

Like aquaporin-2, aquaporin-3 is regulated by vasopressin.

191. Which of the following about aquaporin-4 is false?

N Engl J Med. 2015;372:1349-58

A. Localized to the basolateral plasma membrane
B. Present in the collecting-duct system
C. Not regulated by vasopressin
D. None of the above

192. In erythrocytes, aquaporin-3 is responsible for which of the following blood-group antigen?

N Engl J Med. 2015;372:1349-58

A. KEL
B. GIL
C. MNS
D. LU

Aquaporin-3 is widely expressed throughout body. In RBCs, it is responsible for GIL blood-group antigen.

193. Urea-channel proteins (UT-A1 & UT-A3) are produced from which of the following gene?

N Engl J Med. 2015;372:1349-58

A. SLC12A2
B. SLC13A2
C. SLC14A2
D. SLC15A2

Urea-channel proteins (UT-A1 & UT-A3) are produced from the same gene, SLC14A2. In the inner medullary collecting duct, vasopressin rapidly & reversibly increases transepithelial urea permeability, allowing urea to exit and become trapped within countercurrent exchange system. Accumulation of urea in the medullary interstitium by this mechanism contributes to the high osmolality in the inner medulla.

194. Amiloride-sensitive epithelial Na^+ channel (ENaC) best relates to?

N Engl J Med. 2015;372:1349-58

A. Nedd4-1
B. Nedd4-2
C. Nedd4-3
D. Nedd4-4

The activity of ENaC is increased by SGK1-mediated phosphorylation of Nedd4-2, a protein that promotes recycling of the Na+ channel from the plasma membrane.

195. Which of the following channels is regulated by vasopressin?

N Engl J Med. 2015;372:1349-58

A. Epithelial Sodium Channel
B. Urea Channel
C. Aquaporin-2
D. All of the above

196. X-linked nephrogenic diabetes insipidus is associated with?

N Engl J Med. 2015;372:1349-58

A. Bumetanide-sensitive sodium-potassium-chloride cotransporter
B. Thiazide-sensitive sodium-chloride cotransporter
C. Vasopressin receptor V2
D. Vasopressin-regulated urea channel

Most patients with non–X-linked nephrogenic diabetes insipidus have mutations in AQP2.

197. Autosomal nephrogenic diabetes insipidus is associated with?

N Engl J Med. 2015;372:1349-58

A. Epithelial sodium channel Beta subunit
B. Epithelial sodium channel Gamma subunit
C. Vasopressin receptor V2
D. Aquaporin-2

198. Which of the following is false about hereditary nephrogenic diabetes insipidus (NDI)?

N Engl J Med. 2015;372:1349-58

A. High plasma levels of vasopressin
B. Hyponatremia
C. Polyuria
D. Seizures & mental retardation

Hereditary nephrogenic diabetes insipidus (NDI) presents in infancy with severe vasopressin-resistant polyuria, dehydration, failure to thrive, and dilute urine despite the presence of hypernatremia.

Hypovolemia

199. True volume depletion or hypovolemia refers to?

Harrison's 20th Ed. Chapter 49 Page 297

A. Salt loss
B. Water loss
C. Contraction of ECFV
D. All of the above

True volume depletion, or hypovolemia, refers to a state of combined salt & water loss, leading to contraction of the ECFV. The loss of salt & water may be renal or nonrenal in origin.

200. Which of the following can cause osmotic diuresis?

Harrison's 20th Ed. Chapter 49 Page 297

A. Glucose
B. Urea
C. Mannitol
D. All of the above

201. Which of the following causes natriuresis by inhibiting proximal tubular Na^+ - Cl^- absorption?

Harrison's 20th Ed. Chapter 49 Page 297

A. Acetazolamide
B. Trimethoprim
C. Pentamidine
D. All of the above

Acetazolamide induces natriuresis as a side effect by inhibiting proximal tubular Na^+ - Cl^- absorption.

202. Which of the following causes natriuresis by inhibiting distal tubular amiloride-sensitive ENaC channel?

Harrison's 20th Ed. Chapter 49 Page 297

A. Acetazolamide
B. Trimethoprim
C. Doxycycline
D. All of the above

Trimethoprim & pentamidine inhibit distal tubular Na^+ reabsorption through amiloride-sensitive ENaC channel leading to urinary Na^+-Cl^- loss.

203. Which of the following reduce Na^+-Cl^- reabsorption by the aldosterone-sensitive distal nephron?

Harrison's 20th Ed. Chapter 49 Page 297

A. Mineralocorticoid deficiency
B. Mineralocorticoid resistance
C. Inhibition of mineralocorticoid receptor (MLR)
D. All of the above

204. What quantity of fluid enters gastrointestinal tract daily as secretions?

Harrison's 20th Ed. Chapter 49 Page 297

A. ~ 3 liters
B. ~ 5 liters
C. ~ 7 liters
D. ~ 9 liters

~ 9 liters of fluid enters GI tract daily, 2 by ingestion & 7 liters by secretion.

205. Fecal fluid loss is?

Harrison's 20th Ed. Chapter 49 Page 297

A. 100–200 mL/day
B. 200–300 mL/day
C. 300–400 mL/day
D. 400–500 mL/day

Fecal fluid loss is 100 - 200 mL/day.

206. Which of the following secretions is alkaline?

Harrison's 20th Ed. Chapter 49 Page 297

A. Biliary
B. Pancreatic
C. Intestinal
D. All of the above

Biliary, pancreatic and intestinal secretions are alkaline.

207. What is the magnitude of "insensible losses" in healthy adults?

Harrison's 20th Ed. Chapter 49 Page 297

A. 250–500 mL/day
B. 500–650 mL/day
C. 750–1000 mL/day
D. 1000–1500 mL/day

"Insensible losses" refers to the evaporation of water from skin and respiratory tract. They are a major route for loss of solute-free water. It is typically 500-650 mL/day in healthy adults.

208. Reliable sign of hypovolemia is?

Harrison's 20th Ed. Chapter 49 Page 297

A. Decreased jugular venous pressure (JVP)
B. Orthostatic tachycardia
C. Orthostatic hypotension
D. All of the above

Diminished skin turgor & dry oral mucous membranes are less reliable markers of a decreased ECFV in adult patients. More reliable signs of hypovolemia include a decreased jugular venous pressure (JVP), orthostatic tachycardia (increase of >15-20 beats/minute upon standing) and orthostatic hypotension (>10-20 mm Hg drop in blood pressure on standing).

209. In nonrenal hypovolemia, which of the following is true?

Harrison's 20th Ed. Chapter 49 Page 298

A. Urine Na^+ <20 mM, Urine osmolality >450 mOsm/kg
B. Urine Na^+ >20 mM, Urine osmolality <450 mOsm/kg
C. Urine Na^+ <20 mM, Urine osmolality <450 mOsm/kg
D. Urine Na^+ >20 mM, Urine osmolality >450 mOsm/kg

In nonrenal hypovolemiaurine, urine Na^+ concentration is typically <20 mM with a urine osmolality of >450 mOsm/kg. This is because neurohumoral response to hypovolemia stimulates an increase in renal tubular Na^+ and water reabsorption.

210. In hypovolemia and hypochloremic alkalosis, which of the following is true?

Harrison's 20th Ed. Chapter 49 Page 298

A. Urine Na^+ <20 mM, urine pH <7.0
B. Urine Na^+ >20 mM, urine pH >7.0
C. Urine Na^+ >20 mM, urine pH <7.0
D. Urine Na^+ <20 mM, urine pH >7.0

Patients with hypovolemia and hypochloremic alkalosis due to vomiting, diarrhea or diuretics will typically have a urine Na^+ concentration >20 mM and urine pH of >7.0, due to the increase in filtered HCO_3^-. Urine Cl^- concentration in therefore a more accurate indicator of volume status, with a level <25 mM suggestive of hypovolemia.

211. Isotonic, "normal" saline (0.9% NaCl) contains what amount of sodium?

Harrison's 20th Ed. Chapter 49 Page 298

A. 134 mM
B. 144 mM
C. 154 mM
D. 164 mM

212. Red cell transfusion is given to hypovolemic patients due to severe hemorrhage/anemia keeping hematocrit levels below?

Harrison's 20th Ed. Chapter 49 Page 298

A. 25%
B. 35%
C. 45%
D. 55%

Hypovolemic patients due to severe hemorrhage or anemia should receive red cell transfusions, without increasing the hematocrit beyond 35%.

213. Plasma osmolality is calculated by?

Harrison's 20th Ed. Chapter 49 Page 297

A. Na^+ + (Glucose/18) + (BUN/2.8)
B. $2Na^+$ + (Glucose/18) + (BUN/2.8)
C. $3Na^+$ + (Glucose/18) + (BUN/2.8)
D. $4Na^+$ + (Glucose/18) + (BUN/2.8)

BUN are expressed in milligrams per deciliter: Posm = $2Na^+$ + Glucose/18 + BUN/2.8.

214. What level of BUN : creatinine ratio distinguishes pre-renal azotemia (PRA) from acute tubular necrosis (ATN)?

Clin Kidney J. 2012;5(2):187-191

A. 5:1
B. 10:1
C. 15:1
D. 20:1

The blood urea nitrogen (BUN)/creatinine ratio (BCR) is used to distinguish pre-renal azotemia (PRA) and acute tubular necrosis (ATN), with a typical threshold of 20 (0.081 in international units).

215. An increased BUN : creatinine ratio may be due to?

Clin Kidney J. 2012;5(2):187-191

A. Prerenal azotemia
B. GI bleeding
C. Glucocorticoid therapy
D. All of the above

Increased BUN (relative to creatinine) may be due to prerenal azotemia, increased urea production as in hyperalimentation (high-protein), glucocorticoid therapy, and gastrointestinal bleeding.

216. Which of the following statements is false?
Clin Kidney J. 2012;5(2):187-191

A. A 70 gram protein diet produces about 12 gram of urea/day
B. BUN is roughly one-half of the blood urea
C. >99% of urea synthesis occurs in liver
D. None of the above

Hyponatremia

217. Much of the sodium in the body is bound to?
N Engl J Med. 2015;372:55-65

A. Bone
B. Cartilage
C. Connective tissue
D. All of the above

A substantial amount of sodium is bound to large polyanionic macromolecules called proteoglycans, which make up the ground substance of bone, connective tissue, cartilage and skin. These tissues could serve as sodium reservoirs, taking up or releasing sodium in response to the needs of the body.

218. Hyponatremia is defined as a plasma Na^+ concentration of?
Harrison's 20th Ed. Chapter 49 Page 298

A. < 115 mM
B. < 125 mM
C. < 135 mM
D. < 145 mM

Hyponatremia is defined as a plasma Na^+ concentration <135 mM. This is almost always the result of an increase in circulating AVP and/or increased renal sensitivity to AVP, combined with an intake of free water.

219. Hyponatremia can be?
Harrison's 20th Ed. Chapter 49 Page 298

A. Hypovolemic
B. Euvolemic
C. Hypervolemic
D. All of the above

Hyponatremia is subdivided diagnostically into three groups, depending on clinical history and volume status—hypovolemic, euvolemic & hypervolemic.

220. Which of the following is the cause of hypovolemic hyponatremia with U_{Na} > 20?
Harrison's 20th Ed. Chapter 49 Page 298 Figure 49-5

A. Diuretic excess
B. Mineral corticoid deficiency
C. Salt losing deficiency
D. All of the above

221. Which of the following is the cause of hypovolemic hyponatremia with U_{Na} > 20?
Harrison's 20th Ed. Chapter 49 Page 298 Figure 49-5

A. Ketonuria
B. Osmotic diuresis
C. Cerebral salt wasting syndrome
D. All of the above

222. Which of the following is the cause of euvolemic hyponatremia with U_{Na} > 20?
Harrison's 20th Ed. Chapter 49 Page 298 Figure 49-5

A. Glucocorticoid deficiency
B. Hypothyroidism
C. SIADH
D. All of the above

223. Which of the following is the cause of hypervolemic hyponatremia with U_{Na} > 20?
Harrison's 20th Ed. Chapter 49 Page 298 Figure 49-5

A. Hyperthyroidism
B. Cushing's syndrome
C. Acromegaly
D. Acute or chronic renal failure

224. Which of the following is the cause of hypervolemic hyponatremia with U_{Na} < 20?
Harrison's 20th Ed. Chapter 49 Page 298 Figure 49-5

A. Nephrotic syndrome
B. Cirrhosis
C. Cardiac failure
D. All of the above

225. In hypovolemic hyponatremia, AVP helps preserve blood pressure via?
Harrison's 20th Ed. Chapter 49 Page 299

A. V1A receptors
B. V1B receptors
C. V1C receptors
D. V1D receptors

In hypovolemic hyponatremia, increase in circulating AVP helps preserve blood pressure via vascular & baroreceptor V1A receptors and increases water reabsorption via renal V2 receptors.

226. In nonrenal hypovolemic hyponatremia, without adequate oral replacement, urine Na^+ concentration is typically?
Harrison's 20th Ed. Chapter 49 Page 299

A. < 10 mM
B. < 20 mM
C. < 30 mM
D. < 40 mM

227. In renal hypovolemic hyponatremia, urine Na^+ concentration is typically?
Harrison's 20th Ed. Chapter 49 Page 299

A. > 10 mM
B. > 20 mM
C. > 30 mM
D. > 40 mM

228. Hyperkalemia & hyponatremia in a hypotensive and/or hypovolemic patient with high urine Na^+ strongly suggests?
Harrison's 20th Ed. Chapter 49 Page 299

A. Alcoholic ketoacidosis
B. Medullary cystic disease
C. Thiazide diuretics use
D. Primary adrenal insufficiency

229. Which of the following is a salt-losing nephropathy?

Harrison's 20th Ed. Chapter 49 Page 299

A. Interstitial nephropathies
B. Medullary cystic disease
C. Recovery phase of acute tubular necrosis
D. All of the above

Typical causes of salt-losing nephropathies include reflux nephropathy, interstitial nephropathies, postobstructive uropathy, medullary cystic disease and the recovery phase of acute tubular necrosis.

230. 'Diuretic-induced hyponatremia' is almost always due to?

Harrison's 20th Ed. Chapter 49 Page 299

A. Thiazide diuretics
B. Loop diuretics
C. Aldosterone antagonists
D. All of the above

Diuretic-induced hyponatremia is almost always due to thiazide diuretics which lead to Na^+ & K^+ depletion & AVP-mediated water retention. Thiazides do not inhibit the renal concentrating mechanism. Loop diuretics decrease tonicity of medullary interstitium & impair maximal urinary concentrating capacity which limits ability of AVP to promote water retention.

231. Which of the following can cause hypovolemic hyponatremia?

Harrison's 20th Ed. Chapter 49 Page 299

A. Glycosuria
B. Ketonuria
C. Bicarbonaturia
D. All of the above

232. Syndrome of "cerebral salt wasting" is due to?

Harrison's 20th Ed. Chapter 49 Page 299

A. Subarachnoid hemorrhage
B. Traumatic brain injury
C. Meningitis
D. All of the above

Syndrome of "cerebral salt wasting" is due to subarachnoid hemorrhage, traumatic brain injury, craniotomy, encephalitis and meningitis. Unlike SIADH, it typically responds to aggressive Na^+-Cl^- repletion.

233. Which of the following is false in hypervolemic hyponatremia?

Harrison's 20th Ed. Chapter 49 Page 299

A. Reduced plasma Na^+ concentration
B. Increase in total body Na^+-Cl^-
C. Increase in total body water
D. None of the above

Patients with hypervolemic hyponatremia develop an increase in total-body Na^+-Cl^- that is accompanied by a "proportionately greater" increase in total body water, leading to a reduced plasma Na^+ concentration.

234. Which of the following is an 'osmolyte'?

Harrison's 20th Ed. Chapter 49 Page 300, N Engl J Med. 2015;372:55-65

A. Myo-inositol
B. Betaine
C. Creatine
D. All of the above

Organic solutes, also called osmolytes are creatine, betaine, glutamate, myo-inositol & taurine. These are small intracellular molecules regulated through osmolyte-accumulating transporters (taurine transporter TauT and the myo-inositol transporter SMIT).

235. Which of the following is not a secretory diarrhea?

Harrison's 20th Ed. Chapter 49 Page 299

A. Cholera
B. Carcinoid
C. Lactulose induced
D. VIPoma

236. Which of the following conditions can cause hyponatremia?

Harrison's 20th Ed. Chapter 49 Page 299

A. Hypothyroidism
B. Hyperthyroidism
C. Cushing's disease
D. Pheochromocytoma

Adrenal insufficiency & hypothyroidism may cause hyponatremia. Hypothyroidism decreases cardiac output and GFR and thus increased AVP secretion leading to hyponatremia.

237. Which of the following statements is false?

Harrison's 20th Ed. Chapter 49 Page 299

A. Glucocorticoids exert a negative feedback on AVP release
B. Thiazides do not inhibit renal concentrating mechanism
C. SIAD is the most frequent cause of euvolemic hyponatremia
D. None of the above

238. Which of the following is the most common pattern of AVP secretion recognized in patients with SIAD?

Harrison's 20th Ed. Chapter 49 Page 300

A. Unregulated, erratic AVP secretion
B. Failure to suppress AVP secretion at lower serum osmolalities
C. "Reset osmostat," with a lower threshold osmolality
D. No detectable circulating AVP

Four distinct patterns of AVP secretion have been recognized in patients with SIAD, independent of the underlying cause. First, unregulated, erratic AVP secretion seen in about a third of patients, with no obvious correlation between serum osmolality & circulating AVP levels. Second, patients fail to suppress AVP secretion at lower serum osmolalities, with a normal response curve to hyperosmolar conditions. Third, a "reset osmostat" with a lower threshold osmolality and a left-shifted osmotic response curve. Fourth, patients with essentially no detectable circulating AVP, suggesting either a gain in function in renal water reabsorption or a circulating antidiuretic substance that is distinct from AVP.

239. Drugs that stimulate release of AVP or enhance its action include?

Harrison's 20th Ed. Chapter 49 Page 299 Table 49-1

A. SSRIs
B. Tricyclic antidepressants
C. Antipsychotic drugs
D. All of the above

240. Drugs that stimulate release of AVP or enhance its action include?

Harrison's 20th Ed. Chapter 49 Page 299 Table 49-1

A. Nicotine
B. Nonsteroidal antiinflammatory drugs
C. Narcotics
D. All of the above

241. Drugs that stimulate release of AVP or enhance its action include?

Harrison's 20th Ed. Chapter 49 Page 299 Table 49-1

A. Vincristine
B. Cyclophosphamide
C. Ifosfamide
D. All of the above

242. Drugs that either stimulate AVP secretion or enhance its action on the kidney includes all except ?

Harrison's 20th Ed. Chapter 49 Page 299 Table 49-1

A. Chlorpropamide
B. Clofibrate
C. Carbamazepine
D. Phenytoin

Drugs that either stimulate AVP secretion or enhance its action on kidney are chlorpropamide, clofibrate, carbamazepine and NSAIDs.

243. Which of the following can cause syndrome of inappropriate antidiuresis (SIAD)?

Harrison's 20th Ed. Chapter 49 Page 299 Table 49-1

A. Endurance exercise
B. General anesthesia
C. Nausea, pain
D. All of the above

244. Which of the following can cause syndrome of inappropriate antidiuresis (SIAD)?

Harrison's 20th Ed. Chapter 49 Page 299 Table 49-1

A. Guillain-Barré syndrome
B. Acute intermittent porphyria
C. Meningitis
D. All of the above

245. Which of the following can cause syndrome of inappropriate antidiuresis (SIAD)?

Harrison's 20th Ed. Chapter 49 Page 299 Table 49-1

A. Asthma
B. Bacterial pneumonia
C. Respiratory failure associated with positive-pressure breathing
D. All of the above

246. Which of the following can cause syndrome of inappropriate antidiuresis (SIAD)?

Harrison's 20th Ed. Chapter 49 Page 299 Table 49-1

A. Aspergillosis
B. Cystic fibrosis
C. Tuberculosis
D. All of the above

247. Syndrome of inappropriate antidiuresis (SIAD) is most common with which of the following malignancies?

Harrison's 20th Ed. Chapter 49 Page 300

A. Small-cell lung carcinoma
B. Lymphoma
C. Pancreatic cancer
D. Prostate cancer

248. Syndrome of inappropriate antidiuresis (SIAD) is most common with which of the following drugs?

Harrison's 20th Ed. Chapter 49 Page 300

A. SSRIs
B. Narcotics
C. Nonsteroidal antiinflammatory drugs
D. Carbamazepine

249. Which of the following is useful in distinguishing between hypervolemic & euvolemic hyponatremia?

Harrison's 20th Ed. Chapter 49 Page 300

A. Serum triglyceride
B. Serum uric acid
C. Serum lipase
D. Serum amylase

Serum uric acid is low (<4 mg/dL) in patients with SIAD, consistent with suppressed proximal tubular transport in the setting of increased distal tubular Na-Cl and water transport. In contrast, patients with hypovolemic hyponatremia will be hyperuricemic, due to a shared activation of proximal tubular Na-Cl and urate transport.

250. Phenomenon of 'hyponatremia' in beer drinkers is called?

Harrison's 20th Ed. Chapter 49 Page 300

A. Beer syndrome
B. Beer flush
C. Beer potomania
D. Beer psychosis

Beer is very low in protein and salt content, containing only 1-2 mM of Na^+. Beer drinkers who consume large volumes of beer, which may exceed renal excretory capacity and result in hyponatremia. This is referred to as beer potomania. Saline hydration corrects causative plasma Na^+ concentration deficit.

251. Which of the following statements about hyponatremia is false?

Harrison's 20th Ed. Chapter 49 Page 300

A. Hyponatremia induces generalized cellular swelling
B. Symptoms of hyponatremia are primarily neurologic
C. Normocapneic or hypercapneic respiratory failure
D. None of the above

252. Urine osmolality is calculated with which of the following formula?

Am J Nephrol. 1990;10(2):89-102

A. $2 \times (U_{Na}) + U_K$ + (urinary urea nitrogen/2.8) + (urine glucose/18)
B. $3 \times (U_{Na}) + U_K$ + (urinary urea nitrogen/2.8) + (urine glucose/18)
C. $4 \times (U_{Na}) + U_K$ + (urinary urea nitrogen/2.8) + (urine glucose/18)
D. $5 \times (U_{Na}) + U_K$ + (urinary urea nitrogen/2.8) + (urine glucose/18)

Urine Osmolality = 2 x (urine Na) + Urine K + (urinary urea nitrogen/2.8) + (urine glucose/18)

253. Which of the following statements is false?

Am J Nephrol. 1990;10(2):89-102

A. Osmolarity refers to concentration per liter of solution
B. Osmolality refers to concentration per kilogram of solution
C. Osmolarity is affected by temperature & pressure, whereas osmolality is not
D. None of the above

Osmolality measures only the number of particles present in a solution, while specific gravity determines not only the number but also weight of the particles in a solution.

254. Urine tonicity is calculated by?

Am J Nephrol. 1990;10(2):89-102

A. $[Na^+] + [K^+] - [Cl^-]$
B. $[Na^+] \times [K^+]$
C. $[Na^+] \times [K^+] \div [Cl^-]$
D. $[Na^+] + [K^+]$

Urine tonicity is calculated as the sum of concentrations of Na^+ and K^+. The normal 24-hour urine osmolality is 500 - 800 mOsm/kg of water. Random urine osmolality should average 300—900 mOsm/kg of water. After 12–14 hours of fluid intake restriction, the urine osmolality should exceed 850 mOsm/kg of water.

255. 'Syndrome of inappropriate antidiuretic hormone secretion' (SIADH) causes?

Harrison's 20th Ed. Chapter 49 Page 300

A. Normovolemic hyponatremia
B. Hypovolemic hyponatremia
C. Hypervolemic hyponatremia
D. All of the above

Syndrome of inappropriate antidiuretic hormone secretion (SIADH) is the most common cause of normovolemic or euvolemic hyponatremia. The urine sodium value of 50 mEq/L conferred the best accuracy in separating SIADH from hypovolemic hyponatremia.

256. 'Osmotic diuresis' is defined as a solute excretion rate of more than?

Harrison's 20th Ed. Chapter 49 Page 300

A. ~ 250 mOsmol/day
B. ~ 450 mOsmol/day
C. ~ 550 mOsmol/day
D. ~ 750 mOsmol/day

Osmotic diuresis refers to a solute excretion rate of > ~750 mOsmol/day.

257. Organic osmolytes include which of the following?

Harrison's 20th Ed. Chapter 49 Page 300

A. Creatine
B. Betaine
C. Glutamate
D. All of the above

Organic osmolytes include creatine, betaine, glutamate, myoinositol and taurine.

258. Hyponatremia lasting for how many hours is termed as chronic hyponatremia?

Harrison's 20th Ed. Chapter 49 Page 300

A. 24 Hours
B. 48 Hours
C. 60 Hours
D. 72 Hours

259. Stupor, seizures, and coma occur when plasma sodium concentration falls below?

Harrison's 20th Ed. Chapter 49 Page 300

A. 125 mM
B. 127 mM
C. 129 mM
D. 131 mM

Stupor, seizures & coma occur when plasma Na^+ concentration falls below 125 mM.

260. In hyponatremia, plasma Na^+ concentration during the first 24 hours should not be more than?

Harrison's 20th Ed. Chapter 49 Page 300

A. 2–3 mM
B. 4–6 mM
C. 6–8 mM
D. 8–10 mM

Overly rapid correction of hyponatremia (>8–10 mM in 24 hours or 18 mM in 48 hours) is associated with a disruption in integrity of the blood-brain barrier, allowing the entry of immune mediators that may contribute to demyelination.

261. In a 70 kg man, to raise plasma Na^+ concentration from 110 to 120 mmol/L, what is the amount of Na^+ required?

Harrison's 20th Ed. Chapter 49 Page 300

A. 420 mmol
B. 440 mmol
C. 460 mmol
D. 480 mmol

To raise plasma Na^+ concentration from 110 to 120 mmol/L in a 70-kg man requires 420 mmol [(120 – 110)x70x0.6] of Na^+. Total body water is 50 & 60% of lean body weight in women or men respectively.

262. Osmotic demyelination syndrome (ODS) includes?

Harrison's 20th Ed. Chapter 49 Page 300

A. Flaccid paralysis
B. Dysarthria
C. Dysphagia
D. All of the above

If hyponatremia is corrected too rapidly, osmotic demyelination syndrome (ODS) develops which is characterized by paraparesis or quadriparesis, dysphagia, dysarthria, diplopia, a "locked-in syndrome," and/or loss of consciousness (central pontine myelinolysis). Patients with chronic hyponatremia are most susceptible to development of ODS.

263. The lesions of ODS classically affects which of the following?

Harrison's 20th Ed. Chapter 49 Page 301

A. Pons
B. Cerebellum
C. Thalamus
D. Cerebral cortex

The lesions of ODS classically affect the pons. Clinically, patients with central pontine myelinolysis present 1 or more days after overcorrection of hyponatremia with paraparesis or quadriparesis, dysphagia, dysarthria, diplopia, a "locked-in syndrome" and/or loss of consciousness. Other regions of the brain can also be involved in ODS, most commonly in association with lesions of the pons but occasionally in isolation. In order of frequency, the lesions of extrapontine myelinolysis can occur in the cerebellum, lateral geniculate body, thalamus, putamen and cerebral cortex or subcortex.

264. Risk factors for ODS include?

Harrison's 20th Ed. Chapter 49 Page 301

A. Rapid or overcorrection of hyponatremia
B. Prior cerebral anoxic injury
C. Hypokalemia
D. All of the above

Besides, rapid or overcorrection of hyponatremia, risk factors for ODS include prior cerebral anoxic injury, menstruating women, prepubescent children, hypokalemia, and malnutrition.

265. Which of the following is related to central pontine myelinolysis?
Harrison's 20th Ed. Chapter 49 Page 301

A. Cerebral oedema
B. Cerebral dehydration
C. Cerebral atrophy
D. None of the above

Acute brain dehydration produced by rapid correction disrupts the tight junctions of blood-brain barrier. Disruption of BBB results in an influx of activated complement into brain which is toxic to oligodendrocytes that produce and maintain myelin in CNS. Clinical symptoms of central pontine myelinolysis do not occur until a few days after rapid Na^+ correction. The classic presentation is pseudobulbar palsy & spastic quadriparesis.

266. Rapid correction of hyponatremia leads to?
N Engl J Med. 2015;372:55-65

A. Triggering apoptosis
B. Disrupts blood–brain barrier
C. Brain demyelination
D. All of the above

Rapid correction of hyponatremia is a hypertonic stress to astrocytes that are depleted of osmolytes, triggering apoptosis, disruption of the blood–brain barrier, and, eventually, brain demyelination.

267. Pseudohyponatremia is defined as the coexistence of?
Harrison's 20th Ed. Chapter 49 Page 301

A. Hyponatremia with increased plasma tonicity
B. Hyponatremia with decreased plasma tonicity
C. Normonatremia with increased plasma tonicity
D. Normonatremia with decreased plasma tonicity

Pseudohyponatremia is defined as the coexistence of hyponatremia with a normal or increased plasma tonicity.

268. Which of the following about pseudohyponatremia is false?
Harrison's 20th Ed. Chapter 49 Page 301

A. Iso-osmolar & isotonic hyponatremia
B. Severe hypertriglyceridemia or paraproteinemia
C. Increase in solid phase of plasma
D. None of the above

Pseudohyponatremia is a spurious form of iso-osmolar & isotonic hyponatremia when severe hypertriglyceridemia or paraproteinemia increases substantially the solid phase of plasma.

269. Patients with hyponatremia have an effective osmolality of?
Harrison's 20th Ed. Chapter 49 Page 301

A. < 295 mOsm/kg
B. < 285 mOsm/kg
C. < 275 mOsm/kg
D. < 265 mOsm/kg

Patients with hyponatremia have an effective osmolality of < 275 mOsm/kg.

270. Plasma sodium concentration falls by how much for every 100 mg/dL rise in plasma glucose concentration?
Harrison's 20th Ed. Chapter 49 Page 301

A. 1.1–1.6 mM
B. 1.6–2.4 mM
C. 2.4–3.2 mM
D. 3.2–4.4 mM

Plasma Na^+ concentration falls by ~ 1.6 - 2.4 mM for every 100 mg/dL increase in glucose due to glucose-induced water efflux from cells. This "true" hyponatremia resolves after correction of hyperglycemia.

271. Which of the following is a cause of hypovolemic hyponatremia?
Harrison's 20th Ed. Chapter 49 Page 301

A. Hypothyroidism
B. Secondary adrenal failure due to pituitary insufficiency
C. Primary adrenal failure
D. All of the above

272. "Gold standard" for diagnosis of hypovolemic hyponatremia is plasma Na^+ correction after?
Harrison's 20th Ed. Chapter 49 Page 301

A. Hydration with normal saline
B. Intake of oral salt
C. Restriction of water intake
D. All of the above

Ultimate "gold standard" for the diagnosis of hypovolemic hyponatremia is the demonstration that plasma Na^+ concentration corrects after hydration with normal saline.

273. Which of the following statements is false?
Harrison's 20th Ed. Chapter 49 Page 301

A. Urine osmolality <100 mOsm/kg is suggestive of polydipsia
B. Urine osmolality >400 mOsm/kg indicates AVP excess
C. Urine Na^+ is <20 mM in beer potomania
D. None of the above

274. Which of the following is a cause of euvolemic hyponatremia?
Harrison's 20th Ed. Chapter 49 Page 301

A. Hypothyroidism
B. Secondary adrenal failure due to pituitary insufficiency
C. SIAD
D. All of the above

275. Syndrome of inappropriate antidiuretic hormone secretion (SIADH) is also called?
Ther Adv Endocrinol Metab. 2012;3(2):61-73

A. Achard-Thiers syndrome
B. Liebenberg syndrome
C. Schwartz-Bartter syndrome
D. Donnai-Barrow syndrome

Schwartz-Bartter described SIADH as hyponatremia with corresponding hypo-osmolality, continued renal excretion of sodium, urine less than maximally dilute, absence of clinical evidence of volume depletion, absence of other causes of hyponatremia and correction of hyponatremia by fluid restriction.

276. Patients with which of the following conditions have a very high risk of developing ODS?
Harrison's 20th Ed. Chapter 49 Page 301

A. Beer potomania
B. CHF
C. Hypothyroidism
D. Secondary adrenal failure

Patients with beer potomania have a very high risk of developing ODS due to the associated hypokalemia, alcoholism, malnutrition and high risk of overcorrecting plasma Na^+ concentration.

277. Which of the following are modalities to correct plasma Na^+ concentration?

Harrison's 20th Ed. Chapter 49 Page 301

A. Fluid restriction
B. Potassium replacement
C. Increased solute intake
D. All of the above

Modalities to correct plasma Na^+ concentration include fluid restriction, potassium replacement, oral urea and/or increased solute intake.

278. Which of the following are modalities to correct plasma Na^+ concentration in patients with SIAD?

Harrison's 20th Ed. Chapter 49 Page 301

A. Oral furosemide
B. Demeclocycline
C. Oral urea
D. All of the above

279. Which of the following statements about SIADH is false?

Harrison's 20th Ed. Chapter 49 Page 301

A. Hypoosmotic hyponatremia
B. Urine osmolality >100 mOsmol/kg
C. Hypervolemia
D. Normal sodium balance

Patients with SIADH are usually euvolemic.

280. Which of the following statements about SIADH is false?

Harrison's 20th Ed. Chapter 49 Page 301

A. Normal renal, adrenal, and thyroid function
B. Normal potassium and acid-base balance
C. Hypouricemia
D. None of the above

SIADH is characterized by hypoosmotic hyponatremia in the setting of an inappropriately concentrated urine (urine osmolality >100 mOsmol/kg). Patients are typically normovolemic & have normal Na^+ balance. They tend to be mildly volume-expanded secondary to water retention & have a urine Na^+ excretion rate equal to intake (urine Na^+ concentration usually >40 mmol/L). By definition, they have normal renal, adrenal & thyroid function & usually have normal K^+ & acid-base balance. Hypouricemia in SIADH is due to uricosuric state induced by volume expansion. In contrast, hypovolemic patients tend to be hyperuricemic secondary to increased proximal urate reabsorption.

281. What percentage of increase in brain volume can be fatal?

Cleveland clinic J of Medicine 2007;74(5):377-383

A. 2% to 4%
B. 4% to 6%
C. 6% to 8%
D. 8% to 10%

If plasma is dilute, water diffuses into brain by osmosis causing dilution of extracellular fluid in brain & swelling of brain cells. An increase in brain volume of 8% to 10% can be fatal. By cerebral osmoregulatory (adaptive) mechanism brain cells pump out myoinositol, glutamine, glycerophosphoryl-choline, betaine, creatine & taurine to restore osmolality of cerebral ECF & limiting swelling of brain cells. Acute hyponatremia may cause cerebral edema due to underlying osmotic interactions between brain cells and the extracellular fluid compartment.

282. Sodium required to correct hyponatremia can be estimated by multiplying the deficit in plasma sodium concentration by?

Ther Adv Endocrinol Metab. 2012;3(2):61-73

A. Weight
B. Height
C. Total body water
D. Urine output in liters

Quantity of Na^+ required to increase plasma Na^+ concentration by a given amount can be estimated by multiplying the deficit in plasma Na^+ concentration by total body water.

283. Which of the following formula is used to calculate the change in serum sodium expected from a saline infusion?

Ther Adv Endocrinol Metab. 2012;3(2):61-73

A. Holliday-Segar formula
B. Adrogué-Madias formula
C. Schmidt formula
D. Buckley-Leblanc formula

284. Quantity of sodium in 0.9% (normal, isotonic) saline is?

Ther Adv Endocrinol Metab. 2012;3(2):61-73

A. 77 mM
B. 154 mM
C. 256 mM
D. 513 mM

285. Quantity of sodium in 3% (hypertonic) saline is?

Ther Adv Endocrinol Metab. 2012;3(2):61-73

A. 77 mM
B. 154 mM
C. 256 mM
D. 513 mM

286. Physiologic functions of AVP include?

Lancet 2008;371:1624-32

A. Contraction of vascular smooth muscle
B. Stimulation of liver glycogenolysis
C. Regulation of corticotropin release
D. All of the above

Physiologic functions of AVP or antidiuretic hormone include contraction of vascular smooth muscle, stimulation of liver glycogenolysis, regulation of corticotropin release and renal antidiuresis.

287. Inappropriately elevated levels of AVP are found in?

Drugs. 2007;67(6):847-58

A. Congestive heart failure
B. Cirrhosis of liver
C. SIADH
D. All of the above

Inappropriately elevated levels of AVP occur in CHF, cirrhosis liver, treatment with diuretics & SIADH.

288. Which of the following is a arginine-vasopressin-receptor subtype?

Lancet 2008;371:1624-32

A. V1a
B. V1b
C. V2
D. All of the above

Arginine vasopressin (AVP) is a neuropeptide hormone. Three arginine-vasopressin-receptor subtypes V1a, V1b, and V2 belong to the large rhodopsin-like G-protein-coupled receptor family. V1A & V1B receptors are linked to phosphoinositol signaling pathway, with intracellular calcium acting as the second messenger, whereas V2 receptors are linked to adenylate cyclase signaling pathway, with intracellular cyclic adenosine monophosphate (cAMP) acting as second messenger.

289. V(1A) receptors located in?
Lancet 2008;371:1624-32

A. Vascular smooth muscle cells & myocardium
B. Collecting tubules
C. Anterior pituitary
D. All of the above

290. V(2) receptors located in?
Lancet 2008;371:1624-32

A. Vascular smooth muscle cells & myocardium
B. Collecting tubules
C. Anterior pituitary
D. All of the above

291. V(1B) receptors located in?
Lancet 2008;371:1624-32

A. Vascular smooth muscle cells & myocardium
B. Collecting tubules
C. Anterior pituitary
D. All of the above

Activation of V(1A) receptors located in vascular smooth muscle cells & myocardium results in vasoconstriction & increased afterload & hypertrophy. V(2) receptors located in principal cells of renal-collecting-duct system & mediate free water absorption. V(1B) receptors are located in anterior pituitary & mediate adrenocorticotropin hormone release. Cardiovascular & renal effects of AVP are mediated primarily by V(1A) and V(2) receptors.

292. Which of the following is a combined V(1A)/V(2)-receptor antagonist?
Lancet 2008;371:1624-32

A. Mozavaptan
B. Tolvaptan
C. Conivaptan
D. Lixivaptan

Conivaptan is a combined V(1A)/V(2)-receptor antagonist (non-selective) that induces diuresis as well as haemodynamic improvement.

293. Which of the following is a selective V(1A) receptor antagonist?
Lancet 2008;371:1624-32

A. Mozavaptan
B. Tolvaptan
C. Relcovaptan
D. Lixivaptan

Relcovaptan is a selective V1a-receptor antagonist used in the treatment of Raynaud's disease, dysmenorrhoea, and tocolysis.

294. Which of the following is a V2-receptor antagonist?
Lancet 2008;371:1624-32

A. Mozavaptan
B. Satavaptan
C. Tolvaptan
D. All of the above

V2-receptor antagonists—mozavaptan, lixivaptan, satavaptan & tolvaptan, induce a highly hypotonic diuresis without substantially affecting excretion of electrolytes (by contrast with effects of diuretics). These are effective in the treatment of euvolaemic & hypervolaemic hyponatraemia.

295. Which of the following is administered intravenously?
Lancet 2008;371:1624-32

A. Mozavaptan
B. Tolvaptan
C. Conivaptan
D. Lixivaptan

Conivaptan is available for intravenous (IV) administration, whereas the other three agents are for oral administration.

296. Which of the following is a Benzodiazepine derivative?
Lancet 2008;371:1624-32

A. Mozavaptan
B. Tolvaptan
C. Conivaptan
D. Lixivaptan

Tolvaptan, Mozavaptan & Conivaptan are benzazepine derivative, Satavaptan is N-arylsulfonyl oxindole derivative, Lixivaptan is a Benzodiazepine derivative.

297. Vaptans are metabolised by which of the following hepatic cytochrome enzymes?
Lancet 2008;371:1624-32

A. CYP2D6
B. CYP2C9
C. CYP3A4
D. CYP2C19

298. Vaptans are excreted through?
Lancet 2008;371:1624-32

A. Urine
B. Faeces
C. Lungs
D. All of the above

299. V2-receptor antagonists are contraindicated in which of the following conditions?
Lancet 2008;371:1624-32

A. Hypovolaemic hyponatraemia
B. Euvolaemic hyponatraemia
C. Hypervolaemic hyponatraemia
D. None of the above

Conivaptan & other V2-receptor antagonists are contraindicated in patients with hypovolaemic hyponatraemia, since it is an aquaretic.

300. Non-peptide vasopressin receptor antagonists are called?
Lancet 2008;371:1624-32

A. Captans
B. Vaptans
C. Naptans
D. Saptans

Vaptans are orally & intravenously active non-peptide vasopressin receptor antagonists. AVP receptor antagonists induces free water diuresis without natriuresis or kaliuresis, an effect termed aquaresis.

301. Na^+ deficit is calculated by?

Lancet 2008;371:1624-32

A. 0.3 × body weight × (target plasma Na^+–starting plasma Na^+ concentration)
B. 0.4 × body weight × (target plasma Na^+–starting plasma Na^+ concentration)
C. 0.5 × body weight × (target plasma Na^+–starting plasma Na^+ concentration)
D. 0.6 × body weight × (target plasma Na^+–starting plasma Na^+ concentration)

Na^+ deficit = 0.6 x body weight x (target plasma Na^+ concentration - starting plasma Na^+ concentration.

302. AVP antagonists do not have an approved role in the management of?

Lancet 2008;371:1624-32

A. Acute hyponatremia
B. Heart failure
C. Cirrhosis
D. SIAD

AVP antagonists do not have an approved role in the management of acute hyponatremia. AVP antagonists (vaptans) are highly effective in SIAD and in hypervolemic hyponatremia due to heart failure or cirrhosis.

Hypernatremia

303. Hypernatremia is defined as a plasma sodium concentration more than?

Harrison's 20th Ed. Chapter 49 Page 302

A. 135 mmol/L
B. 140 mmol/L
C. 145 mmol/L
D. 150 mmol/L

Hypernatremia is defined as a plasma Na^+ concentration >145 mmol/L.

304. Which of the following about hypernatremia is false?

Harrison's 20th Ed. Chapter 49 Page 302

A. Associated with mortality rates of 40–60%
B. Result due to losses of H_2O in excess of Na^+
C. Diarrhea is the most common gastrointestinal cause
D. None of the above

305. Which of the following about hypernatremia is false?

Harrison's 20th Ed. Chapter 49 Page 302

A. State of iso-osmolality
B. Results in ICF volume contraction
C. Stimulates thirst
D. Excretion of minimum volume of maximally concentrated urine

Hypernatremia is a state of hyperosmolality.

306. Which of the following is a cause of adipsic diabetes insipidus?

Harrison's 20th Ed. Chapter 49 Page 302

A. Primary or metastatic tumor
B. Occlusion or ligation of the anterior communicating artery
C. Hydrocephalus
D. All of the above

Causes of adipsic DI include primary or metastatic tumor, occlusion or ligation of the anterior communicating artery, trauma, hydrocephalus & inflammation.

307. Which of the following causes osmotic diuresis?

Harrison's 20th Ed. Chapter 49 Page 303

A. Hyperglycemia
B. Excess urea
C. Mannitol
D. All of the above

308. Which of the following can cause nephrogenic diabetes insipidus (NDI)?

Harrison's 20th Ed. Chapter 49 Page 303

A. Loss of function mutations in X-linked V2 receptor
B. Mutations in AVP-responsive aquaporin-2 water channel
C. Recessive deficiency of aquaporin-1 water channel
D. All of the above

309. Which of the following can cause polyuria and NDI?

Harrison's 20th Ed. Chapter 49 Page 303

A. Hypercalcemia
B. Hypokalemia
C. Lithium
D. All of the above

In hypercalcemia, calcium signals directly through calcium-sensing receptor to downregulate Na^+, K^+ & Cl^- transport by TALH & water transport in principal cells, thus reducing renal concentrating ability. In hypokalemia, the renal response to AVP are inhibited and aquaporin-2 expression is downregulated.

310. Which of the following best relates to lithium therapy?

Harrison's 20th Ed. Chapter 49 Page 303

A. (Lif)/Stat3
B. Mapk1/3
C. Glycogen synthase kinase-3 (GSK3)
D. All of the above

311. Which of the following when used with lithium can mitigate lithium associated NDI?

Harrison's 20th Ed. Chapter 49 Page 303

A. Triamterene
B. Amiloride
C. Spironolactone
D. All of the above

Lithium causes NDI by direct inhibition of renal glycogen synthase kinase-3 (GSK3). GSK3 is required for the response of principal cells to A VP. Entry of lithium through amiloride-sensitive Na^+ channel ENaC is required for the effect of the drug on principal cells, such that combined therapy of lithium and amiloride can mitigate lithium associated NDI.

312. Which of the following about glycogen synthase kinase-3 (GSK3) is false?

Curr Opin Nephrol Hypertens. 2012;21(5):541-546

A. Serine/threonine protein kinase
B. Inhibits glycogen synthase
C. Exists in two isoforms–GSK3α and GSK3β
D. None of the above

Lithium is a reversible & highly specific inhibitor of GSK3. Glycogen synthase kinase-3 (GSK3) inhibition by LiCl increases cyclooxygenase 2 expression and reduces aquaporin 2 expression.

313. Which of the following about nephrogenic diabetes insipidus is false?

Harrison's 20th Ed. Chapter 49 Page 303

A. Congenital Nephrogenic diabetes insipidus (NDI) is X-linked recessive trait due to mutations in V2 receptor gene
B. Congenital Nephrogenic diabetes insipidus (NDI) may be due to mutation in autosomal aquaporin-2 gene
C. Lithium, hypercalcemia & hyperkalemia cause sporadic NDI
D. Pregnant women, in II or III trimester, may develop NDI due to excessive vasopressinase from placenta

Lithium, hypercalcemia and hypokalemia can cause sporadic NDI.

314. Gestational DI best relates to?

Harrison's 20th Ed. Chapter 49 Page 303

A. Leucine-rich proteins
B. Vasopressinase
C. Carnitine
D. Cryoglobulin

Gestational DI is a complication of late-term pregnancy in which there is increased activity of a circulating placental protease with "vasopressinase" activity leading to reduced circulating AVP & polyuria, often accompanied by hypernatremia. DDAVP is an effective therapy, given its resistance to the vasopressinase enzyme.

315. Major symptoms of hypernatremia are?

Harrison's 20th Ed. Chapter 49 Page 303

A. Cardiac
B. Neurologic
C. Respiratory
D. Gastroenterological

Major symptoms of hypernatremia are neurologic like altered mental status, weakness, neuromuscular irritability, focal neurologic deficits & coma or seizures.

316. Which of the following can occur in acute hypernatremia?

Harrison's 20th Ed. Chapter 49 Page 303

A. Parenchymal or subarachnoid hemorrhage
B. Subdural hematoma
C. Rhabdomyolysis
D. All of the above

317. Increasing plasma Na^+ by how much is considered as overcorrection?

Harrison's 20th Ed. Chapter 49 Page 303

A. > 2 mM/day
B. > 5 mM/day
C. > 8 mM/day
D. > 10 mM/day

318. Which of the following laboratory investigation is useful in a case of hypernatremia?

Harrison's 20th Ed. Chapter 49 Page 303

A. Serum osmolality
B. Urine osmolality
C. Urine electrolytes
D. All of the above

319. Which of the following indicate to an extrarenal source of water loss primarily responsible for hypernatremia?

Harrison's 20th Ed. Chapter 49 Page 303

A. Serum osmolality >295 mOsm/kg
B. Excretion of low volumes (<500 mL/day) of urine
C. Urine osmolality >800 mOsm/kg
D. All of the above

320. Which of the following is false about patients with baseline hypernatremia?

Harrison's 20th Ed. Chapter 49 Page 303

A. Hypertonicity
B. Adequate stimulus for AVP by posterior pituitary
C. Water deprivation test is unnecessary
D. None of the above

321. Which of the following is false about patients with nephrogenic diabetes insipidus (NDI)?

Harrison's 20th Ed. Chapter 49 Page 303

A. Will not to respond to DDAVP
B. DDAVP will not ↑ urine osmolality by <50% or <150 mOsm/kg
C. Normal or high circulating AVP level
D. None of the above

322. Which of the following is false about patients with central diabetes insipidus (CDI)?

Harrison's 20th Ed. Chapter 49 Page 303

A. Will respond to DDAVP
B. DDAVP will not ↑ urine osmolality by >50% but <800 mOsm/kg
C. Reduced circulating AVP
D. None of the above

323. After administering 'desmopressin', urine osmolality should increase by how much in CDI?

Harrison's 20th Ed. Chapter 49 Page 303

A. At least 10%
B. At least 25%
C. At least 35%
D. At least 50%

324. After administering 'desmopressin', urine osmolality should increase by how much in NDI?

Harrison's 20th Ed. Chapter 49 Page 303

A. At least 10%
B. At least 25%
C. At least 35%
D. None of the above

CDI & NDI can be distinguished by administering AVP analogue desmopressin (10 μg intranasally) after careful water restriction. Urine osmolality should increase by at least 50% in CDI & will not change in NDI.

325. Which of the following prevents degradation of placental vasopressinase?

Harrison's 20th Ed. Chapter 49 Page 303

A. Hydroxyproline
B. Tyrosinase
C. 1,10-phenanthroline
D. All of the above

In pregnant women, AVP assays should be drawn in tubes containing protease inhibitor 1,10-phenanthroline, to prevent in vitro degradation of AVP by placental vasopressinase.

326. In women, what percentage of body weight is total-body water (TBW)?

Harrison's 20th Ed. Chapter 49 Page 302 Table 49-3

A. 40%
B. 50%
C. 60%
D. 70%

327. In men, what percentage of body weight is total-body water (TBW)?

Harrison's 20th Ed. Chapter 49 Page 302 Table 49-3

A. 40%
B. 50%
C. 60%
D. 70%

50% of body weight in women and 60% in men is the estimated total-body water (TBW).

328. Which of the following is the correct formula to calculate free-water deficit?

Harrison's 20th Ed. Chapter 49 Page 302 Table 49-3

A. $[(Na^+ - 120)/140] \times TBW$
B. $[(Na^+ - 130)/140] \times TBW$
C. $[(Na^+ - 140)/140] \times TBW$
D. $[(Na^+ - 150)/140] \times TBW$

Free-water deficit is calculated by the formula $[(Na^+ - 140)/140] \times TBW$.

329. Which of the following variable is not included in the formula to calculate free-water clearance (C_eH_2O)?

Harrison's 20th Ed. Chapter 49 Page 302 Table 49-3

A. Urinary $[Na^+]$
B. Urinary $[K^+]$
C. Plasma $[Na^+]$
D. Plasma $[K^+]$

Formula to calculate free-water clearance (C_eH_2O) is Urinary volume × [1 - (urinary [Na+] + urinary [K+])/plasma [Na+]].

330. Normal insensible water loss is?

Harrison's 20th Ed. Chapter 49 Page 302 Table 49-3

A. ~ 2 mL/kg per day
B. ~ 5 mL/kg per day
C. ~ 10 mL/kg per day
D. ~ 15 mL/kg per day

331. It is imperative to correct hypernatremia 'slowly' to avoid?

Harrison's 20th Ed. Chapter 49 Page 304

A. Acute renal failure
B. Heart failure
C. Cerebral edema
D. All of the above

It is imperative to correct hypernatremia slowly to avoid cerebral edema.

332. In hypernatremia due to water loss, water deficit should be corrected in which of the following ways?

Harrison's 20th Ed. Chapter 49 Page 304

A. Rapidly
B. Over 12 to 24 hours
C. Over 24 to 36 hours
D. Slowly over at least 48 to 72 hours

In hypernatremia due to water loss, water deficit should be corrected slowly over 48–72 hours, raising plasma Na^+ concentration by no more than 10 mM/day except in patients with acute hypernatremia (<48 hours) due to sodium loading, who can safely be corrected rapidly at a rate of 1 mM/hour.

333. DDAVP can be administered through which of the following routes?

Harrison's 20th Ed. Chapter 49 Page 304

A. Intravenous
B. Intranasal
C. Oral
D. All of the above

Patients with central DI should respond to the administration of intravenous, intranasal or oral DDAVP.

334. Which of the following drugs is useful in NDI patients who have to take lithium?

Harrison's 20th Ed. Chapter 49 Page 304

A. Amiloride
B. Chlorpropamide
C. Clofibrate
D. Carbamazepine

Amiloride is useful NDI patients who have to take lithium. Nephrotoxicity of lithium requires it to be taken up into collecting duct cells via amiloride-sensitive Na^+ channel.

335. Which of the following is useful for 'chronic' management of polyuria from NDI?

Harrison's 20th Ed. Chapter 49 Page 304

A. Thiazides
B. Amiloride
C. NSAIDs
D. All of the above

336. Which of the following about diabetes insipidus is false?

Harrison's 20th Ed. Chapter 49 Page 303

A. CDI is characterized by impaired AVP secretion
B. NDI results from renal resistance to actions of AVP
C. Familial CDI is inherited as autosomal recessive
D. Familial CDI is due to mutation in propressophysin gene

Familial form of CDI is inherited as autosomal dominant and is attributed to mutations in propressophysin (AVP precursor) gene.

337. 'Solute excretion rate' is?

N Engl J Med. 2015; 372:2207-2216

A. Urine volume × Osmolality
B. Urine volume × Urine sodium
C. Urine volume × Urine potassium
D. Urine volume × Urine bicarbonate

The product of urine volume & osmolality is called solute excretion rate. Or, urinary volume in liters per day = Solute excretion in mOsm per day/urinary osmolality in mOsm per liter.

Hypokalemia

338. Potassium delivery to distal nephron approximates?

Harrison's 20th Ed. Chapter 49 Page 304

A. Dietary excess
B. Dietary intake
C. Dietary deficiency
D. Daily requirement

339. What percentage of daily intake of potassium is excreted in stool?

Harrison's 20th Ed. Chapter 49 Page 304

A. 1%
B. 5%
C. 10%
D. 15%

Entire daily intake of potassium is excreted, approximately 90% in urine & 10% in the stool. K^+ delivery to distal nephron [DCT + cortical collecting duct (CCD)] approximates dietary intake.

340. 98% of total-body potassium is intracellular, chiefly in?

Harrison's 20th Ed. Chapter 49 Page 304

A. Fat cells
B. Skin cells
C. Muscle cells
D. Liver cells

98% of total-body potassium is intracellular, chiefly in muscle. Most of the cellular K^+ in the body resides in the intracellular fluid (ICF) (~50 mEq/kg, 98%), largely in the skeletal muscles (3,000 mEq), red blood cells (300 mEq), and liver (200 mEq). Total K^+ content in the extracellular fluid (ECF) is very low (<1 mEq/kg, ~2%) and similar to the daily dietary intake and renal excretion of K^+.

341. All regulation of renal potassium excretion & total body potassium balance occurs in?

Harrison's 20th Ed. Chapter 49 Page 304

A. Proximal convoluted tubule
B. Loop of Henle
C. Distal nephron
D. All of the above

Virtually all regulation of renal K^+ excretion & total body K^+ balance occurs in distal nephron.

342. Normal plasma potassium concentration inside cells is about?

Pediatr Nephrol. 2011;26:377-384

A. 50 mmol/L
B. 100 mmol/L
C. 150 mmol/L
D. 200 mmol/L

Normal plasma K^+ concentration is 3.5 - 5.0 mmol/L, whereas that inside cells is about 150 mmol/L. <2% of total body K^+ content (2500–4500 mmol) is in ECF.

343. Normally, ratio of ICF to ECF K^+ concentration is about?

Electrolyte Blood Press. 2010;8(1):38-50

A. 28:1
B. 35:1
C. 48:1
D. 58:1

Normally, ratio of ICF to ECF K^+ concentration is ~ 35:1 due to resting membrane potential and is crucial for normal neuromuscular function.

344. What percentage of filtered potassium is reabsorbed in proximal tubule by diffusion and solvent drag?

Pediatr Nephrol. 2011;26:377-384

A. ~ 15–25%
B. ~ 25–45%
C. ~ 45–60%
D. ~ 60–75%

Approximately 60–75% of the filtered potassium is reabsorbed in the proximal tubule (PT) by diffusion and solvent drag, mainly coupled to Na^+ transport, mainly by the Na^+/H^+ antiporter.

345. What percentage of filtered potassium is reabsorbed in the thick ascending limb of the Loop of Henle (TALH)?

Pediatr Nephrol. 2011;26:377-384

A. ~ 15–20%
B. ~ 20–45%
C. ~ 45–60%
D. ~ 60–75%

~15-20% of the filtered potassium is reabsorbed in the thick ascending limb of the Loop of Henle (TALH), mainly by the Na-K-2Cl cotransporter (NKCC2). This cotransporter is inhibited by loop diuretics (furosemide).

346. Distal convoluted tubule (DCT) is the site of excretion of?

Pediatr Nephrol. 2011;26:377-384

A. Potassium
B. Calcium
C. Magnesium
D. All of the above

Distal convoluted tubule (DCT) is the site of the apical sodium chloride cotransporter (NCCT), which is blocked by thiazides. It modulates excretion of not only potassium but also calcium and magnesium.

347. The basolateral Na-K ATPase pump actively transports potassium in & sodium out of the cell in a ratio of?

Harrison's 20th Ed. Chapter 49 Page 304

A. 1:2
B. 2:3
C. 3:4
D. 4:5

The basolateral Na^+, K^+-ATPase pump actively transports K^+ in and Na^+ out of the cell in a 2:3 ratio, and the passive outward diffusion of K^+ is quantitatively the most important factor that generates the resting membrane potential. The main hormones that increase the activity of Na^+,K^+-ATPase include β2-adrenergic agonists, insulin, and thyroid hormone.

348. Renal adaptive mechanisms allow the kidneys to maintain potassium homeostasis until the GFR drops to?

Pediatr Nephrol. 2011;26:377-384

A. < 60 ml/min/1.73 m^2
B. < 45 ml/min/1.73 m^2
C. < 30 ml/min/1.73 m^2
D. < 15 ml/min/1.73 m^2

Renal adaptive mechanisms allow the kidneys to maintain potassium homeostasis until the glomerular filtration rate (GFR) drops to less than 15 ml/min/1.73 m^2.

349. K^+ intake in an average western diet is?

Pediatr Nephrol. 2011;26:377-384

A. 10–40 mmol/day
B. 40–120 mmol/day
C. 120–350 mmol/day
D. 350–550 mmol/day

K^+ intake in an average western diet is 40–120 mmol/day, or approximately 1 mmol/kg per day, 90% of which is absorbed by the gastrointestinal tract.

350. Which is the most important site of K^+ secretion in the kidney?
Harrison's 20th Ed. Chapter 49 Page 304

A. Proximal tubule
B. Thick ascending limb of loop of Henle
C. Distal tubule convolute
D. Cortical collecting duct

Although, K^+ is transported along the entire nephron, it is the principal cells of the connecting segment (CNT) and cortical collecting duct (CD) that play a dominant role in renal K^+ secretion.

351. Which of the following is a flow-sensitive channel for potassium secretion?
Harrison's 20th Ed. Chapter 49 Page 304

A. Renal outer medullary K^+ channel (ROMK)
B. "Big potassium" (BK) or maxi-K K^+ channel
C. ENaC channel
D. All of the above

The maxi-K^+ channel (also known as the large-conductance K^+ (BK) channel) is characterized by a large single channel conductance and quiescence in the basal state and activation under conditions of increased flow. In addition to increased delivery of Na^+ and dilution of luminal K^+ concentration, recruitment of maxi-K^+ channels contributes to flow-dependent increased K^+ secretion.

352. Which of the following mediates bulk of constitutive K^+ secretion?
Harrison's 20th Ed. Chapter 49 Page 304

A. Renal outer medullary K^+ channel (ROMK)
B. "Big potassium" (BK) or maxi-K K^+ channel
C. ENaC channel
D. All of the above

Two major K^+ channels mediate distal tubular K^+ secretion. They are secretory K^+ channel ROMK (renal outer medullary K^+ channel, also known as Kir1.1 or KcnJ1) and the flow-sensitive "big potassium" (BK) or maxi-K K^+ channel. ROMK mediates bulk of constitutive K^+ secretion.

353. Which of the following hormones has a major influence on potassium excretion?
Harrison's 20th Ed. Chapter 49 Page 304

A. Aldosterone
B. Renin
C. Angiotensin II
D. All of the above

Aldosterone has a major influence on potassium excretion. It increases the activity of ENaC channels to amplify the driving force for K^+ secretion across the luminal membrane of principal cells. Aldosterone as key regulator of renal potassium homeostasis binds to the nuclear mineralocorticoid receptor (MR) within the distal tubule and the principal cells in the CCD. It activates the basolateral Na^+/K^+-ATPase, thereby increasing Na^+ and water reabsorption into the blood and secretion of K^+ into the urine. Aldosterone also upregulates the amiloride sensitive sodium channels (ENaCs) in the apical membrane of CCD and stimulates H^+ secretion by intercalated CCD cells, thereby influencing acid/base balance.

354. Hypokalemia is defined as a plasma potassium concentration of?
Harrison's 20th Ed. Chapter 49 Page 304

A. < 3.5 mM
B. < 3.6 mM
C. < 3.7 mM
D. < 3.8 mM

Hypokalemia is defined as a plasma K^+ concentration <3.5 mM.

355. Which of the following can cause treatment-resistant hypokalemia?
Harrison's 20th Ed. Chapter 49 Page 304

A. Hypomagnesemia
B. Hypocalcemia
C. Hyponatremia
D. All of the above

Systemic hypomagnesemia can also cause treatment-resistant hypokalemia, due to a combination of reduced cellular uptake of K^+ and exaggerated renal secretion.

356. Spurious hypokalemia or "pseudohypokalemia" best relates to?
Harrison's 20th Ed. Chapter 49 Page 304

A. Erythrocytosis
B. Leukocytosis
C. Thrombocytosis
D. All of the above

Spurious hypokalemia or "pseudohypokalemia" can occasionally result from in vitro cellular uptake of K^+ after venipuncture due to profound leukocytosis in acute leukemia.

357. Which of the following promote Na^+/K^+-ATPase-mediated cellular uptake of K^+?
Harrison's 20th Ed. Chapter 49 Page 304

A. Insulin
B. β-adrenergic activity
C. Alkalosis
D. All of the above

Insulin, β-adrenergic activity, thyroid hormone and alkalosis promote Na^+/K^+-ATPase-mediated cellular uptake of K^+ leading to hypokalemia.

358. Inhibition of the passive efflux of K^+ occurs with?
Harrison's 20th Ed. Chapter 49 Page 304

A. Arsenic
B. Barium
C. Cobalt
D. All of the above

Inhibition of the passive efflux of K^+ can also cause hypokalemia. This typically occurs due to systemic inhibition of K^+ channels by toxic barium ions.

359. In malnourished patients given a carbohydrate load, stimulation of endogenous insulin can lead to?
Harrison's 20th Ed. Chapter 49 Page 304

A. Hypokalemia
B. Hypomagnesemia
C. Hypophosphatemia
D. All of the above

In malnourished patients given a carbohydrate load, stimulation of endogenous insulin can provoke hypokalemia, hypomagnesemia and/or hypophosphatemia.

360. Which of the following can cause hypokalemia?
Harrison's 20th Ed. Chapter 49 Page 304

A. Pseudoephedrine and ephedrine
B. Ritodrine
C. Theophylline
D. All of the above

β2 agonists, bronchodilators (salmeterol), tocolytics (ritodrine) and "hidden" sympathomimetics (pseudoephedrine & ephedrine), are powerful activators of cellular K^+ uptake may cause unexpected hypokalemia.

361. Thyrotoxic periodic paralysis (TPP) best relates to?

Harrison's 20th Ed. Chapter 49 Page 305

A. Kir1.6
B. Kir2.6
C. Kir3.6
D. Kir4.6

TPP is linked to genetic variation in Kir2.6, a muscle-specific, thyroid hormone responsive K^+ channel.

362. Patients with TPP typically develop paralytic episodes most frequently between?

Harrison's 20th Ed. Chapter 49 Page 305

A. 1 AM and 6 AM
B. 6 AM and 12 Noon
C. 12 Noon and 6 PM
D. 6 PM and 12 Midnight

Patients with TPP typically present with weakness of extremities & limb girdles, with paralytic episodes that occur most frequently between 1 & 6 AM. Signs & symptoms of hyperthyroidism are not invariably present.

363. Which of the following occurs in thyrotoxic periodic paralysis?

Harrison's 20th Ed. Chapter 49 Page 305

A. Hypokalemia
B. Hypophosphatemia
C. Hypomagnesemia
D. All of the above

In TPP, hypokalemia is usually profound and almost invariably accompanied by hypophosphatemia and hypomagnesemia.

364. Which of the following reverses hypokalemia, hypophosphatemia and paralysis in TPP?

Harrison's 20th Ed. Chapter 49 Page 305

A. Glucagon
B. Adrenaline
C. Propranolol
D. Amiodarone

Hypokalemia in TPP is attributed to both direct & indirect activation of the Na^+/K^+-ATPase, resulting in increased uptake of K^+ by muscle and other tissues. High-dose propranolol (3 mg/kg) rapidly reverses the associated hypokalemia, hypophosphatemia and paralysis.

365. Which of the following is the least likely cause of hypokalemia?

Harrison's 20th Ed. Chapter 49 Page 305

A. Ileostomy
B. Loss of gastric secretions
C. Chronic laxative abuse
D. Colonic pseudo-obstruction

K^+ concentration of gastric fluid is only 5–10 mmol/L and is a less likely cause of hypokalemia. Loss of gastric contents results in volume depletion & metabolic alkalosis, both promote kaliuresis. Celiac disease, ileostomy, villous adenomas, inflammatory bowel disease, colonic pseudo-obstruction (Ogilvie's syndrome), VIPomas and chronic laxative abuse can also cause significant hypokalemia.

366. Which of the following is false about acute colonic pseudo-obstruction (ACPO)?

World J Gastroenterol. 2017;23(30):5634-5644

A. Acute colonic dilatation
B. Absence of intrinsic mechanical obstruction
C. Absence of extrinsic inflammatory process
D. All of the above

Acute colonic pseudo-obstruction (ACPO) is characterised by acute colonic dilatation in the absence of intrinsic mechanical obstruction or extrinsic inflammatory process. "Sympathetic deprivation" of the colon as its mechanism was first postulated by Ogilvie. "Ogilvie's syndrome" has also been used to refer to ACPO, though this term is now discouraged due to ambiguity regarding its meaning.

367. Which of the following is a cause of decreased potassium intake?

Harrison's 20th Ed. Chapter 49 Page 305 Table 49-4

A. Ingestion of excess carbohydrates
B. Ingestion of excess proteins
C. Ingestion of excess fats
D. Ingestion of clay (geophagia)

Ingestion of clay (geophagia) is a cause of decreased K^+ intake as it binds dietary K^+ & iron.

368. Which of the following statements is false?

Harrison's 20th Ed. Chapter 49 Page 305

A. Thiazides cause more hypokalemia than loop diuretics
B. Thiazides cause hypocalciuria
C. Loop diuretics cause hypercalciuria
D. None of the above

Thiazides cause more hypokalemia than loop diuretics although they have lesser natriuretic effect. Diuretic effect of thiazides is due to inhibition of the Na^+-Cl^- cotransporter NCC in DCT cells that leads to increased delivery of luminal Na^+ to principal cells immediately downstream in CNT & cortical CD. This augments Na^+ entry via ENaC, increases lumen-negative potential difference and amplifies K^+ secretion. Thiazides cause hypokalemia also secondary to thiazide-associated hypocalciuria, versus hypercalciuria seen with loop diuretics. The increases in downstream luminal calcium in response to loop diuretics inhibit ENaC in principal cells, thus reducing the lumen-negative potential difference and attenuating distal K^+ excretion.

369. Which of the following drugs increase K^+ excretion by acting as nonreabsorbable anions in distal nephron?

Harrison's 20th Ed. Chapter 49 Page 305

A. Aminoglycosides
B. Amphotericin
C. Carbenicillin
D. Foscarnet

370. Which of the following drugs cause hypokalemia and hypomagnesemia?

Harrison's 20th Ed. Chapter 49 Page 305

A. Aminoglycosides
B. Amphotericin
C. Foscarnet
D. All of the above

High doses of penicillin-related antibiotics (nafcillin, dicloxacillin, ticarcillin, oxacillin and carbenicillin) can increase obligatory K^+ excretion by acting as nonreabsorbable anions in the distal nephron. Renal tubular toxins cause renal K^+ and magnesium wasting, leading to hypokalemia and hypomagnesemia. These include aminoglycosides, amphotericin, foscarnet, cisplatin & ifosfamide.

371. In congenital adrenal hyperplasia, hypertension & hypokalemia is due to increase in circulating?

Harrison's 20th Ed. Chapter 49 Page 305

A. 11-deoxycorticosterone
B. 12-deoxycorticosterone
C. 13-deoxycorticosterone
D. 14-deoxycorticosterone

Congenital adrenal hyperplasia is caused by defects in either steroid 11β-hydroxylase or steroid 17α-hydroxylase. Increase in circulating 11-deoxycorticosterone causes hypertension and hypokalemia.

372. Aldosterone is secreted by zona glomerulosa cells of adrenal cortex in response to?

Harrison's 20th Ed. Chapter 49 Page 305

A. High renin
B. High angiotensin II
C. Hyperkalemia
D. All of the above

Aldosterone is secreted by the zona glomerulosa cells of the adrenal cortex in response to high renin and angiotensin II or hyperkalemia.

373. Glucocorticoid-remediable hyperaldosteronism (GRA) is also called?

Harrison's 20th Ed. Chapter 49 Page 305

A. Familial hyperaldosteronism type I (FH-I)
B. Familial hyperaldosteronism type II (FH-II)
C. Familial hyperaldosteronism type III (FH-III)
D. Familial hyperaldosteronism type IV (FH-IV)

Familial hyperaldosteronism type I (FH-I) is also known as glucocorticoid-remediable hyperaldosteronism (GRA). FH-II and FH-III are forms of isolated primary genetic hyperaldosteronism in which aldosterone production is not repressible by exogenous glucocorticoids.

374. FH-I is caused by a chimeric gene duplication between?

Harrison's 20th Ed. Chapter 49 Page 305

A. CYP11B1 and CYP11B2
B. CYP11B1 and CYP11B3
C. CYP11B1 and CYP11B4
D. CYP11B1 and CYP11B5

FH-I is caused by a chimeric gene duplication between homologous 11β-hydroxylase (CYP11B1) and aldosterone synthase (CYP11B2) genes, fusing the adrenocorticotropic hormone (ACTH) responsive 11β-hydroxylase promoter to the coding region of aldosterone synthase. This chimeric gene is under the control of ACTH and thus repressible by glucocorticoids.

375. FH-III is caused by mutations in which of the following gene?

Harrison's 20th Ed. Chapter 49 Page 305

A. ABCB11
B. ATP8B1
C. UDPGT
D. KCNJ5

FH-III is caused by mutations in KCNJ5 gene, which encodes G-protein-activated inward rectifier K^+ channel 4 (GIRK4). These mutations lead to acquisition of sodium permeability in the mutant GIRK4 channels causing an exaggerated membrane depolarization in adrenal glomerulosa cells and activation of voltage-gated calcium channels. The resulting calcium influx is sufficient to produce aldosterone secretion & cell proliferation, leading to adrenal adenomas & hyper-aldosteronism.

376. Acquired causes of primary hyperaldosteronism include?

Harrison's 20th Ed. Chapter 49 Page 306

A. Aldosterone producing adenomas (APAs)
B. Primary or unilateral adrenal hyperplasia (PAH)
C. Idiopathic hyperaldosteronism (IHA)
D. All of the above

Acquired causes of primary hyperaldosteronism include aldosterone producing adenomas (APAs), primary or unilateral adrenal hyperplasia (PAH), idiopathic hyperaldosteronism (IHA) due to bilateral adrenal hyperplasia and adrenal carcinoma.

377. What value of plasma aldosterone : PRA ratio is suggestive of primary hyperaldosteronism?

Harrison's 20th Ed. Chapter 49 Page 306

A. > 20
B. > 30
C. > 40
D. > 50

Plasma aldosterone : PRA ratio of >50, due to suppression of circulating renin and an elevation of circulating aldosterone, is suggestive of primary hyperaldosteronism. However, hypokalemia and multiple antihypertensive drugs may alter aldosterone:PRA ratio.

378. Which of the following converts cortisol to cortisone?

Harrison's 20th Ed. Chapter 49 Page 306

A. 11β-hydroxysteroid dehydrogenase-1 (11βHSD-1)
B. 11β-hydroxysteroid dehydrogenase-2 (11βHSD-2)
C. 17α-hydroxylase
D. 11β-hydroxylase

The glucocorticoid cortisol has equal affinity for the mineralocorticoid receptor (MLR) to that of aldosterone, with resultant "mineralocorticoid-like" activity. However, cells in the aldosterone-sensitive distal nephron are protected from this "illicit" activation by the enzyme 11β-hydroxysteroid dehydrogenase-2 (11βHSD-2), which converts cortisol to cortisone; cortisone has minimal affinity for the MLR.

379. 'Syndrome of apparent mineralocorticoid excess' is due to deficiency of?

Harrison's 20th Ed. Chapter 49 Page 306

A. 11α-HSDH-2
B. 11β-HSDH-2
C. 12α-HSDH-2
D. 12β-HSDH-2

Cortisol is converted to cortisone by 11β-hydroxysteroid dehydrogenase 2 (11β-HSDH-2). 11β-HSDH-2 deficiency or suppression allows cortisol to bind to the aldosterone receptor & leads to syndrome of apparent mineralocorticoid excess (SAME).

380. Syndrome of apparent mineralocorticoid excess (SAME) is characterized by?

Harrison's 20th Ed. Chapter 49 Page 306

A. Hypertension
B. Hypokalemia
C. Hypercalciuria
D. All of the above

381. Syndrome of apparent mineralocorticoid excess (SAME) is characterized by?

Harrison's 20th Ed. Chapter 49 Page 306

A. Metabolic alkalosis
B. Suppressed PRA
C. Suppressed aldosterone
D. All of the above

Syndrome of apparent mineralocorticoid excess (SAME) is characterized by hypertension, hypokalemia, hypercalciuria and metabolic alkalosis with suppressed PRA and suppressed aldosterone.

382. Conditions that inhibit the activity of '11βHSD-2' include?

Harrison's 20th Ed. Chapter 49 Page 306

A. Glycyrrhetinic/glycyrrhizinic acid
B. Chewing tobacco
C. Carbenoxolone
D. All of the above

Glycyrrhetinic acid (in licorice), chewing tobacco & carbenoxolone inhibit activity of 11βHSD-2.

383. Which of the following is a cause of hypokalemia?

Harrison's 20th Ed. Chapter 49 Page 306

A. Metabolic alkalosis
B. Treatment of DKA with insulin
C. Uncontrolled hyperglycemia
D. All of the above

384. Which of the following is a cause of hypokalemia?

A. Patients of pernicious anemia treated with vitamin B12
B. Patients of neutropenia treated with GM-CSF
C. Massive transfusion with thawed washed RBCs
D. All of the above

Treatment of DKA with insulin causes hypokalemia due movement of K^+ inside the cells with glucose like anabolic states. Uncontrolled hyperglycemia causes K^+ depletion due to osmotic diuresis.

385. Primary hyperaldosteronism is due to dysregulated aldosterone secretion by?

A. Adrenal adenoma
B. Adrenal carcinoma
C. Adrenocortical hyperplasia
D. All of the above

Primary hyperaldosteronism is due to dysregulated aldosterone secretion by an adrenal adenoma (Conn's syndrome) or carcinoma or to adrenocortical hyperplasia.

386. Tumor that produce renin include?

A. Renal cell carcinoma
B. Ovarian carcinoma
C. Wilms' tumor
D. All of the above

Renin-secreting tumors of juxtaglomerular apparatus, renal cell carcinoma, ovarian carcinoma, and Wilms' tumor produce renin.

387. Which of the following is false about 'Liddle's syndrome'?

Harrison's 20th Ed. Chapter 49 Page 306

A. Autosomal dominant
B. Hypertension
C. Hypokalemic metabolic alkalosis
D. Excess renin and aldosterone secretion

Liddle's syndrome is an autosomal dominant gain-in-function mutations of ENaC subunits. The result is increased expression of activated ENaC channels at the plasma membrane of principal cells. It is characterized by hypertension, hypokalemic metabolic alkalosis, renal K^+ wasting & suppressed renin & aldosterone secretion.

388. Which of the following is false about 'Liddle's syndrome'?

Harrison's 20th Ed. Chapter 49 Page 306

A. Blunted aldosterone response to ACTH
B. Reduced urinary aldosterone excretion
C. Unresponsive to spironolactone yet sensitive to amiloride
D. None of the above

Patients with Liddle's syndrome classically manifest severe hypertension with hypokalemia, unresponsive to spironolactone yet sensitive to amiloride. Hypertension and hypokalemia are variable aspects of the Liddle's phenotype; more consistent features include a blunted aldosterone response to ACTH and reduced urinary aldosterone excretion.

389. Loss of transport functions of which nephron segment causes Bartter's syndrome (BS)?

Harrison's 20th Ed. Chapter 49 Page 306

A. PCT
B. TALH
C. DCT
D. All of the above

Loss of the transport functions of TALH nephron segment with reduction in renal concentrating ability causes Bartter's syndrome, a hereditary hypokalemic alkalosis.

390. Loss of transport functions of which nephron segment causes Gitelman's syndrome (GS)?

Harrison's 20th Ed. Chapter 49 Page 306

A. PCT
B. TALH
C. DCT
D. All of the above

Loss of the transport functions of in the thiazide-sensitive Na-Cl cotransporter of DCT nephron segment reduction in renal concentrating ability causes Gitelman's syndrome, a hereditary hypokalemic alkalosis.

391. Which of the following statements is false?

Harrison's 20th Ed. Chapter 49 Page 306

A. Bartter's syndrome relates to Na^+, K^+ & Cl^- transport of TALH
B. Gitelman's syndrome relates to thiazide-sensitive Na^+-Cl^- cotransporter of DCT
C. Urinary calcium excretion is a critical diagnostic test in BS/GS
D. None of the above

392. Bartter's syndrome is characterized by?

Harrison's 20th Ed. Chapter 49 Page 306

A. Hypokalemia
B. Metabolic alkalosis
C. Hyperreninemic hyperaldosteronism
D. All of the above

Bartter's syndrome is characterized by hypokalemia, metabolic alkalosis, hyperreninemic hyperaldosteronism secondary to ECF volume contraction, increase in urinary calcium excretion & juxtaglomerular apparatus hyperplasia.

393. Systemic symptoms of Bartter's syndrome are due to?

Harrison's 20th Ed. Chapter 49 Page 306

A. Increase in plasma renin
B. Increase in plasma aldosterone
C. Increase in renal prostaglandin
D. All of the above

In Bartter's syndrome, renal prostaglandin synthesis & excretion are significantly increased, accounting for much of the systemic symptoms.

394. Which of the following is a critical diagnostic test in Gitelman's syndrome (GS)?

Harrison's 20th Ed. Chapter 49 Page 306

A. Plasma renin activity (PRA)
B. Aldosterone
C. Urinary calcium excretion
D. Urinary magnesium excretion

395. Which of the following is a feature of Gitelman's syndrome?

Harrison's 20th Ed. Chapter 49 Page 306

A. Hypomagnesemia
B. Hypocalciuria
C. Chondrocalcinosis
D. All of the above

396. Which of the following statements is false?
Harrison's 20th Ed. Chapter 49 Page 306

A. GS is genetically homogeneous
B. Patients with GS are uniformly hypomagnesemic
C. Patients with GS exhibit marked hypocalciuria
D. None of the above

Hypomagnesemic patients are clinically refractory to K^+ replacement in the absence of Mg^{++} repletion.

397. Which of the following laboratory abnormalities is seen only in chronic renal failure?
Harrison's 20th Ed. Chapter 49 Page 306

A. Anemia
B. Hypocalcemia
C. Hyperphosphatemia
D. Radiographic evidence of renal osteodystrophy

398. Hypokalemia has prominent effects on which of the following?
Harrison's 20th Ed. Chapter 49 Page 306

A. Cardiac
B. Skeletal muscle cells
C. Intestinal muscle cells
D. All of the above

Hypokalemia has prominent effects on cardiac (precipitant of arrhythmia), skeletal (weakness, paralysis, skeletal myopathy, rhabdomyolysis) and intestinal muscle cells (intestinal ileus).

399. Electrocardiographic changes in hypokalemia include?
Harrison's 20th Ed. Chapter 49 Page 306

A. Broad flat T waves
B. ST depression
C. QT prolongation
D. All of the above

Electrocardiographic changes in hypokalemia include broad flat T waves, ST depression and QT prolongation.

400. Electrocardiographic changes in hypokalemia are most marked when serum K^+ is?
Harrison's 20th Ed. Chapter 49 Page 306

A. < 3.5 mmol/L
B. < 3.2 mmol/L
C. < 3.0 mmol/L
D. < 2.7 mmol/L

Electrocardiographic changes in hypokalemia are most marked when serum K^+ is <2.7 mmol/L.

401. Which of the following is false regarding ECG changes of hypokalemia?
Harrison's 20th Ed. Chapter 49 Page 306

A. Delayed ventricular repolarization
B. Do not correlate well with plasma K^+ levels
C. Prominent U wave
D. Shortened QU interval

ECG changes of hypokalemia are due to delayed ventricular repolarization and do not correlate well with the plasma K^+ concentration. Early changes include flattening or inversion of T wave, prominent U wave, ST-segment depression, and prolonged QU interval.

402. Which of the following ECG changes denote severe potassium depletion?
Harrison's 20th Ed. Chapter 49 Page 306

A. Prominent U wave
B. Inversion of T wave
C. Prolonged PR interval
D. Prolonged QU interval

Severe K^+ depletion may result in a prolonged PR interval, decreased voltage and widening of the QRS complex and ventricular arrhythmias.

403. Which of the following occurs in hypokalemia?
Harrison's 20th Ed. Chapter 49 Page 306

A. Phosphaturia
B. Hypocitraturia
C. Activation of renal ammoniagenesis
D. All of the above

The functional effects of hypokalemia on the kidney can include Na-Cl and HCO_3 retention, polyuria, phosphaturia, hypocitraturia and an activation of renal ammoniagenesis. Bicarbonate retention and other acid-base effects of hypokalemia can contribute to the generation of metabolic alkalosis.

404. Hypokalemia is associated frequently with?
Harrison's 20th Ed. Chapter 49 Page 306

A. Metabolic alkalosis
B. Respiratory acidosis
C. Respiratory alkalosis
D. All of the above

Metabolic alkalosis is associated with hypokalemia due to K^+ redistribution and excessive renal K^+ loss.

405. What value of a 24-h K^+ excretion is indicative of an extrarenal cause of hypokalemia?
Harrison's 20th Ed. Chapter 49 Page 307

A. < 15 mmol
B. < 30 mmol
C. < 45 mmol
D. < 60 mmol

A 24 hour K^+ excretion of <15 mmol is indicative of an extrarenal cause of hypokalemia. The etiology of hypokalemia can simply be divided into two groups: those with a low K^+ excretion rate and those with a high K^+ excretion rate.

406. Which of the following is a feature of hypokalemia due to renal K^+ wasting?
Electrolyte Blood Press. 2010;8(1):38-50

A. Chronic
B. Related to disorders with increased flow rate to the CCD
C. Related to disorders with increased K^+ in the CCD
D. None of the above

Hypokalemia due to renal K^+ wasting is chronic and usually related to disorders with either increased flow rate to the CCD or increased K^+ in the CCD (fast Na^+ or slow Cl^-).

407. Which of the following suggests hypokalemia due to gastrointestinal potassium loss?
Harrison's 20th Ed. Chapter 49 Page 307 Figure 49-7

A. Serum K^+ < 3.5 mmol/L
B. Urine K^+ < 15 mmol/day
C. Metabolic acidosis
D. All of the above

408. Which of the following suggests hypokalemia due to profuse sweating?

Harrison's 20th Ed. Chapter 49 Page 307 Figure 49-7

A. Serum $K^+ < 3.5$ mmol/L
B. Urine $K^+ < 15$ mmol/day
C. Normal acid-base status
D. All of the above

409. Which of the following suggests hypokalemia due to remote diuretic use?

Harrison's 20th Ed. Chapter 49 Page 307 Figure 49-7

A. Serum $K^+ < 3.5$ mmol/L
B. Urine $K^+ < 15$ mmol/day
C. Metabolic alkalosis
D. All of the above

410. Hypokalemia with minimal renal potassium excretion suggests that potassium loss is through?

Harrison's 20th Ed. Chapter 49 Page 307

A. Skin
B. Gastrointestinal tract
C. Diuretic use
D. All of the above

Hypokalemia with minimal renal K^+ excretion (<15 mmol/day of K^+ in urine) suggests that K^+ was lost via the skin or gastrointestinal tract or that there is a remote history of vomiting or diuretic use.

411. Plasma renin activity and aldosterone levels are high in patients with?

Electrolyte Blood Press. 2010;8(1):38-50

A. Renin-secreting tumor
B. Renal vascular stenosis
C. Malignant hypertension
D. All of the above

Plasma renin activity and aldosterone levels are high in patients with renin-secreting tumor, renal vascular stenosis, malignant hypertension, and pheochromocytoma.

412. High plasma aldosterone levels but low plasma renin activity indicates?

Harrison's 20th Ed. Chapter 49 Page 307 Figure 49-7

A. Cushing's syndrome
B. Malignant hypertension
C. Renal artery stenosis
D. Primary hyperaldosteronism

413. Primary hyperaldosteronism can be caused by?

Electrolyte Blood Press. 2010;8(1):38-50

A. Bilateral adrenal hyperplasia
B. Adrenal adenoma/carcinoma
C. Glucocorticoid-remediable aldosteronism (GRA)
D. All of the above

High plasma aldosterone levels but low plasma renin activity indicates primary hyperaldosteronism which can be caused by bilateral adrenal hyperplasia, adrenal adenoma/carcinoma, and glucocorticoid-remediable aldosteronism (GRA).

414. High plasma aldosterone levels but low plasma renin activity indicates?

Harrison's 20th Ed. Chapter 49 Page 307 Figure 49-7

A. Familial hyperaldosteronism type I (FH-I)
B. Familial hyperaldosteronism type II (FH-II)
C. Familial hyperaldosteronism type III (FH-III)
D. All of the above

415. Which of the following is false about Cushing's syndrome?

Harrison's 20th Ed. Chapter 49 Page 307 Figure 49-7

A. Urine $K^+ > 15$ mmol/day
B. TTKG < 2
C. Low aldosterone
D. High cortisol

416. Which of the following is false about Liddle's syndrome?

Harrison's 20th Ed. Chapter 49 Page 307 Figure 49-7

A. Urine $K^+ < 15$ mmol/day
B. TTKG > 4
C. Low aldosterone
D. Normal cortisol

417. Which of the following is false about renal artery stenosis?

Harrison's 20th Ed. Chapter 49 Page 307 Figure 49-7

A. Urine $K^+ < 15$ mmol/day
B. TTKG > 4
C. High aldosterone
D. High renin

418. Hypokalemia with acidosis is seen in?

Harrison's 20th Ed. Chapter 49 Page 307

A. Lower gastrointestinal losses
B. Diabetic ketoacidosis
C. Renal tubular acidosis
D. All of the above

419. Hypokalemia with alkalosis is seen in?

Harrison's 20th Ed. Chapter 49 Page 307

A. Diuretic use
B. Gitelman syndrome
C. Bartter syndrome
D. All of the above

420. Hypokalemia with potassium wasting is seen in?

Harrison's 20th Ed. Chapter 49 Page 307

A. Diabetic ketoacidosis
B. Renal tubular acidosis
C. Diuretic use
D. All of the above

421. Hypokalemia with potassium wasting is seen in all except ?

Harrison's 20th Ed. Chapter 49 Page 307

A. Vomiting
B. Gitelman syndrome
C. Bartter syndrome
D. Surreptitious vomiting (bulimia)

422. Secretion of K^+ in cortical & outer medullary collecting ducts is influenced by?

Indian J Pediatr. 2007;74(7):679-686

A. Aldosterone
B. Plasma K^+ concentration
C. Anion composition of the luminal fluid
D. All of the above

Secretion of K^+ in cortical & outer medullary collecting ducts accounts for the majority of its excretion in urine that is influenced by aldosterone, plasma K^+ concentration and anion composition of the luminal fluid.

423. Which of the following is a spot urine index of renal response to hypokalemia?

Electrolyte Blood Press. 2010;8(1):38-50

A. Fractional excretion of K^+
B. Urine K^+/creatinine ratio
C. Urine osmolality/creatinine
D. All of the above

Four spot urine indices of renal response to hypokalemia have been used: fractional excretion of K+, TTKG, urine K+/creatinine ratio and urine osmolality/creatinine.

424. Which of the following is the formula for calculating transtubular potassium gradient (TTKG)?

Harrison's 20th Ed. Chapter 49 Page 310

A. (Urine K^+ × serum osmolality) ÷ (Serum K^+ × urine osmolality)
B. (Serum K^+ × urine osmolality) ÷ (Urine K^+ × serum osmolality)
C. (Urine K^+ × urine osmolality) ÷ (Serum K^+ × serum osmolality)
D. (Serum K^+ × serum osmolality) ÷ (Urine K^+ × urine osmolality)

Formula to calculate TTKG is (urine/plasma $[K^+]$) ÷ (urine/plasma osmolality). The TTKG is an index of the gradient of K^+ in the distal tubular lumen and interstitial blood capillaries, independent of urine flow rate. TTKG provides an accurate estimate of aldosterone effect on late distal and cortical collecting tubules.

425. What value of transtubular K^+ concentration gradient (TTKG) is indicative of hypokalemia?

Harrison's 20th Ed. Chapter 49 Page 307

A. < 1
B. < 2
C. < 3
D. < 4

TTKG should be <3 in the presence of hypokaleemia. TTKG is the ratio of K^+ concentration in lumen of CCD ($[K^+]_{CCD}$) to that in peritubular capillaries or plasma ($[K^+]_p$). The TTKG in normal persons varies but is generally within the range of 6–12.

426. What value of urinary K^+ to creatinine ratio is compatible with excessive renal K^+ excretion?

Harrison's 20th Ed. Chapter 49 Page 307

A. > l0 mmol/gram creatinine
B. > l1 mmol/gram creatinine
C. > l2 mmol/gram creatinine
D. > l3 mmol/gram creatinine

Urinary K^+ to creatinine ratio of > l3 mmol/g creatinine (>1.5 mmol/mmol creatinine) is compatible with excessive renal K^+ excretion.

427. Hypokalemic patients with vomiting due to bulimia typically have a urinary Cl^- of?

Harrison's 20th Ed. Chapter 49 Page 307

A. < 10 mmol/L
B. < 20 mmol/L
C. < 30 mmol/L
D. < 40 mmol/L

Hypokalemic patients with vomiting due to bulimia typically have a urinary Cl^- <10 mmol/L.

428. Urine Na^+, K^+, and Cl^- Which of the following is persistently elevated in Gitelman's syndrome (GS)?

Harrison's 20th Ed. Chapter 49 Page 307

A. Urine Na^+
B. Urine K^+
C. Urine Cl^-
D. All of the above

Urine Na^+, K^+, and Cl^- are persistently elevated in Gitelman's syndrome (GS), due to loss of function in the thiazide-sensitive Na^+-Cl^- cotransporter.

429. Which of the following statements is false?

Harrison's 20th Ed. Chapter 49 Page 308

A. Patients with Liddle's syndrome respond to amiloride
B. Patients with Liddle's syndrome do not respond to spironolactone
C. Patients with SAME respond to spironolactone
D. None of the above

430. High-dose propranolol (3 mg/kg) should be considered in which of the following redistributive hypokalemia conditions?

Harrison's 20th Ed. Chapter 49 Page 308

A. Thyrotoxic periodic paralysis (TPP)
B. Theophylline overdose
C. Acute head injury
D. All of the above

In redistributive hypokalemia, as in TPP, theophylline overdose, and acute head injury, excessive activity of sympathetic nervous system plays a dominant role. High-dose propranolol (3 mg/kg) will correct hypokalemia without the risk of rebound hyperkalemia.

431. It is generally safer to correct hypokalemia via which route?

Harrison's 20th Ed. Chapter 49 Page 308

A. Oral
B. Peripheral vein
C. Central vein
D. Per rectum

It is generally safer to correct hypokalemia via the oral route.

432. Which is the preparation of choice for correction of hypokalemia with metabolic alkalosis?

Harrison's 20th Ed. Chapter 49 Page 308

A. Potassium chloride
B. Potassium bicarbonate
C. Potassium citrate
D. None of the above

Potassium chloride is preferred for more rapid correction of hypokalemia. Potassium phosphate, oral or IV, may be appropriate in patients with combined hypokalemia and hypophosphatemia. Potassium bicarbonate and citrate (metabolized to HCO_3^-) tend to alkalinize and is more appropriate for hypokalemia associated with chronic diarrhea or RTA. Hypomagnesemic patients are refractory to K^+ replacement alone.

433. Serum K^+ drops by about how much for every 100-mmol reduction in total-body stores?

Harrison's 20th Ed. Chapter 49 Page 308

A. 0.17 mM
B. 0.27 mM
C. 0.37 mM
D. 0.47 mM

In the absence of abnormal K^+ redistribution, the total deficit correlates with serum K^+, such that serum K^+ drops by approximately 0.27 mM for every 100-mmol reduction in total-body stores. Loss of 400-800 mmol of total-body K^+ results in a reduction in serum K^+ by approximately 2.0 mM.

434. A decrement of 1 mmol/L in plasma potassium concentration may represent a total body potassium deficit of?

Harrison's 20th Ed. Chapter 49 Page 308

A. 20 to 40 mmol
B. 50 to 100 mmol
C. 100 to 200 mmol
D. 200 to 400 mmol

A decrement of 1 mmol/L in plasma K^+ concentration reflects total body K^+ deficit of 200–400 mmol.

435. Plasma potassium levels of < 3 mmol/L require how much potassium to correct the deficit?

Harrison's 20th Ed. Chapter 49 Page 308

A. 100 mmol
B. 200 mmol
C. 400 mmol
D. 600 mmol

Patients with plasma levels <3.0 mmol/L require >600 mmol of K^+ to correct the deficit.

436. Rate of IV infusion of potassium in severe hypokalemia should not exceed?

Harrison's 20th Ed. Chapter 49 Page 308

A. 20 mmol/hour
B. 40 mmol/hour
C. 60 mmol/hour
D. 80 mmol/hour

Rate of K^+ infusion should not exceed 20 mmol/hour unless paralysis or malignant ventricular arrhythmias are present.

437. Through a peripheral vein, maximum concentration of administered K^+ should be no more than?

Harrison's 20th Ed. Chapter 49 Page 308

A. 20 mmol/L
B. 40 mmol/L
C. 60 mmol/L
D. 80 mmol/L

The maximum concentration of administered K^+ should be no more than 40 mmol/L via a peripheral vein or 60 mmol/L via a central vein.

438. Ideally, for infusion KCl should be mixed in?

Harrison's 20th Ed. Chapter 49 Page 308

A. Normal saline
B. Dextrose solutions
C. Ringer solutions
D. All of the above

Ideally, KCl is mixed in normal saline as dextrose solutions may initially exacerbate hypokalemia due to insulin-mediated movement of K^+ into cells.

Hyperkalemia

439. Hyperkalemia is defined as a plasma K^+ concentration of?

Harrison's 20th Ed. Chapter 49 Page 308

A. > 4.5 mM
B. > 5.0 mM
C. > 5.5 mM
D. > 6.0 mM

Hyperkalemia is defined as a plasma K^+ concentration of 5.5 mM. Levels >6.0 mM are called as severe hyperkalemia.

440. Which of the following is the most frequent underlying cause of hyperkalemia?

Harrison's 20th Ed. Chapter 49 Page 308

A. Redistribution
B. Reduced tissue uptake
C. Decrease in renal K^+ excretion
D. Excessive intake of K^+

A decrease in renal K^+ excretion is the most frequent underlying cause of hyperkalemia. Excessive intake of K^+ is a rare cause.

441. ↑ed dietary intake of K^+ can cause hyperkalemia in?

Harrison's 20th Ed. Chapter 49 Page 308

A. Diabetics with hyporeninemic hypoaldosteronism
B. Chronic kidney disease
C. Drugs that impact the renin-angiotensin-aldosterone axis
D. All of the above

Dietary intake can have a mäjor effect in susceptible patients like diabetics with hyporeninemic hypoaldosteronism and chronic kidney disease. Drugs that impact on the renin-angiotensin-aldosterone axis are also a major cause of hyperkalemia.

442. Pseudohyperkalemia or factitious hyperkalemia results from?

Harrison's 20th Ed. Chapter 49 Page 308

A. Prolonged use of tourniquet
B. Hemolysis
C. Marked leukocytosis
D. All of the above

Pseudohyperkalemia refers to an artificially elevated "plasma" K^+ concentration due to movement of K^+ out of cells on venipuncture in asymptomatic patient with no obvious underlying cause. Serum K^+ concentration is normal. Prolonged tourniquet use, cooling of blood following venipuncture, hemolysis & marked leukocytosis, erythrocytosis or thrombocytosis, acute anxiety with respiratory alkalosis contribute to its occurrence.

443. Hereditary pseudohyperkalemia is caused by increases in?

Harrison's 20th Ed. Chapter 49 Page 308

A. Passive K^+ permeability of erythrocytes
B. Active K^+ permeability of erythrocytes
C. Passive K^+ permeability of leucocytes
D. Active K^+ permeability of leucocytes

Hereditary pseudohyperkalemia is caused by increases in the passive K^+ permeability of erythrocytes. Causative mutations have been described in red cell anion exchanger (AE1, encoded by the SLC4A1 gene), leading to reduced red cell anion transport, hemolytic anemia, the acquisition of a novel AE1-mediated K^+ leak and pseudohyperkalemia.

444. Acidosis leading to hyperkalemia is seen in?
Harrison's 20th Ed. Chapter 49 Page 308

A. Non-anion gap causes of metabolic acidosis
B. Lactic acidosis
C. Ketoacidosis
D. All of the above

Acidosis leading to hyperkalemia is limited to non-anion gap causes of metabolic acidosis. Hyperkalemia due to an acidosis induced shift of potassium from the cells into ECF does not occur in the anion gap acidoses-lactic acidosis and ketoacidosis.

445. Hyperkalemia can occur due to?
Harrison's 20th Ed. Chapter 49 Page 308

A. Hypertonic mannitol
B. Hypertonic saline
C. Intravenous immune globulin
D. All of the above

Hyperkalemia due to hypertonic mannitol, hypertonic saline & intravenous immune globulin is attributed to a "solvent drag" effect as water moves out of cells along the osmotic gradient.

446. Hyperkalemia can occur due to?
Harrison's 20th Ed. Chapter 49 Page 308

A. Lysine
B. Arginine
C. Epsilon-aminocaproic acid
D. All of the above

Cationic amino acids like lysine, arginine and the structurally related drug epsilon-aminocaproic acid, cause efflux of K^+ and hyperkalemia through an effective cation-K^+ exchange.

447. Which of the following poisoning is typically associated with hyperkalemia?
Harrison's 20th Ed. Chapter 49 Page 308

A. Arsenic
B. Benzene
C. Fluoride
D. Mangnese

Fluoride poisoning is typically associated with hyperkalemia because fluoride ions inhibit Na^+/K^+-ATPase.

448. Which of the following drug can cause acute hyperkalemia?
Harrison's 20th Ed. Chapter 49 Page 308

A. Ethanol
B. Succinylcholine
C. Ketamine
D. Lidocaine

Succinylcholine depolarizes muscle cells, causing an efflux of K^+ through acetylcholine receptors (AChRs).

449. Hyperkalemia can result from?
Harrison's 20th Ed. Chapter 49 Page 308

A. Intravascular hemolysis
B. Tumor lysis syndrome
C. Rhabdomyolysis
D. All of the above

Intravascular hemolysis, tumor lysis syndrome, and rhabdomyolysis lead to K^+ release from cells as a result of tissue breakdown. Red cell transfusion is a well described cause of hyperkalemia, typically in the setting of massive transfusions.

450. Which of the following foods is rich in potassium?
Harrison's 20th Ed. Chapter 49 Page 308

A. Tomatoes
B. Bananas
C. Citrus fruits
D. All of the above

Foods rich in potassium include tomatoes, bananas and citrus fruits.

451. Which of the following is false about hyporeninemic hypoaldosteronism?
Harrison's 20th Ed. Chapter 49 Page 308

A. Suppressed PRA & aldosterone
B. Reduced renal excretion of NH_4^+
C. Positive urinary anion gap and urine pH <5.5
D. None of the above

Hyporeninemic hypoaldosteronism is a very common predisposing factor in several overlapping subsets of hyperkalemic patients: diabetics, the elderly and patients with renal insufficiency. Classically, patients should have suppressed PRA and aldosterone. About 50% have an associated acidosis, with a reduced renal excretion of NH_4^+, a positive urinary anion gap & urine pH <5.5. Most patients have secondary increases in circulating atrial natriuretic peptide (ANP) that inhibit both renal renin release and adrenal aldosterone release.

452. Hyporeninemic hypoaldosteronism is seen in?
Harrison's 20th Ed. Chapter 49 Page 308

A. Mild renal insufficiency
B. Diabetic nephropathy
C. Chronic tubulointerstitial disease
D. All of the above

Hyporeninemic hypoaldosteronism is seen in mild renal insufficiency, diabetic nephropathy or chronic tubulointerstitial disease.

453. Hyperkalemia out of proportion to GFR can also be seen in?
Harrison's 20th Ed. Chapter 49 Page 308

A. Sickle cell anemia
B. Interstitial nephritis
C. Obstructive uropathy
D. All of the above

Hyperkalemia out of proportion to GFR is seen in tubulointerstitial disease that affects the distal nephron like amyloidosis, sickle cell anemia, interstitial nephritis and obstructive uropathy.

454. Which of the following is also known as hereditary hypertension with hyperkalemia?
Harrison's 20th Ed. Chapter 49 Page 308

A. Autosomal recessive pseudohypoaldosteronism type 1
B. Autosomal dominant pseudohypoaldosteronism type 1
C. Pseudohypoaldosteronism type II
D. All of the above

Hereditary renal causes of hyperkalemia have overlapping clinical features with hypoaldosteronism are labeled as pseudohypoaldosteronism (PHA). PHA type II (PHA-II) is also known as hereditary hypertension with hyperkalemia.

455. Pseudohypoaldosteronism type II is also called?
Harrison's 20th Ed. Chapter 271 Page 1899 Table 271-4

A. Spragg's syndrome
B. Leopold's syndrome
C. Marcelo's syndrome
D. Gordon's syndrome

Gordon's syndrome is characterized by hyperkalemia, metabolic acidosis, normal GFR, volume-expansion with suppressed renin & aldosterone levels. It is refractory to kaliuretic effect of exogenous mineralocorticoids.

456. Autosomal dominant form of PHA type 1 is due to loss-of-function mutations in?
Harrison's 20th Ed. Chapter 49 Page 308

A. NCC
B. ENaC
C. MLR
D. WNKI

457. Autosomal recessive form of PHA type 1 is due to mutation in?
Harrison's 20th Ed. Chapter 49 Page 308

A. NCC
B. ENaC
C. MLR
D. WNKI

PHA type 1 (PHA-I) has both an autosomal recessive and an autosomal dominant form. Autosomal dominant form is due to loss-of-function mutations in MLR. Recessive form is caused by various combinations of mutations in the three subunits of ENaC, resulting in impaired Na^+ channel activity in principal cells and other tissues.

458. Autosomal recessive form of PHA type II is due to mutation in?
Harrison's 20th Ed. Chapter 49 Page 308

A. ENaC
B. MLR
C. WNK1
D. All of the above

459. Patients with recessive PHA-I present as?
Harrison's 20th Ed. Chapter 49 Page 308

A. Lifelong salt wasting
B. Hypotension
C. Hyperkalemia
D. All of the above

Patients with recessive PHA-I suffer from lifelong salt wasting, hypotension and hyperkalemia, whereas the phenotype of autosomal dominant PHA-1 due to MLR dysfunction improves in adulthood.

460. PHA type II is in every respect the mirror image of?
Harrison's 20th Ed. Chapter 49 Page 308

A. Liddle's syndrome
B. Bartter's syndrome
C. Gitelman's syndrome
D. Gordon's syndrome

PHA type II is in every respect the mirror image of GS. PHA-II behaves like a gain of function in NCC and treatment with thiazides results in resolution of the entire clinical phenotype. However, the NCC gene is not directly involved in PHA-II, which is caused by mutations in WNK1 & WNK4 serine-threonine kinases or the upstream Kelch-like 3 (KLHL3) and Cullin 3 (CUL3), two components of an E3 ubiquitin ligase complex that regulates these kinases. These proteins collectively regulate NCC activity, with PHA-II associated activation of the transporter.

461. Clinical features of PHA type II include?
Harrison's 20th Ed. Chapter 49 Page 308

A. Hypertension
B. Hyperkalemia
C. Hyperchloremic metabolic acidosis
D. All of the above

Clinical features of PHA type II include hypertension, hyperkalemia, hyperchloremic metabolic acidosis, suppressed PRA and aldosterone, hypercalciuria and reduced bone density.

462. Pseudohypoaldosteronism is characterized by all except?
Harrison's 20th Ed. Chapter 49 Page 308

A. High renin & aldosterone levels
B. End-organ resistance to aldosterone
C. Renal sodium wasting
D. Hypertension

463. Pseudohypoaldosteronism is characterized by all except ?
Harrison's 20th Ed. Chapter 49 Page 308

A. Hyperkalemia
B. Metabolic alkalosis
C. Renal sodium wasting
D. Hypotension

Pseudohypoaldosteronism (PHA) is characterized by hyperkalemia, metabolic acidosis, renal Na^+ wasting, hypotension, high renin and aldosterone levels, and end-organ resistance to aldosterone.

464. Which of the following cause hyperkalemia?
Harrison's 20th Ed. Chapter 49 Page 308

A. Renin inhibitors
B. MLRs
C. ACE inhibitors & angiotensin receptor blockers
D. All of the above

ACE inhibitors, angiotensin receptor blockers, renin inhibitors and MLRs are predictable and common causes of hyperkalemia.

465. Which of the following cause hyperkalemia?
Harrison's 20th Ed. Chapter 49 Page 308

A. Yasmin-28
B. Nafamostat
C. Pentamidine
D. All of the above

Yasmin-28 is an oral contraceptive agent that contains progestin drospirenon which inhibits the MLR and can cause hyperkalemia. Nafamostat is a protease inhibitor used for pancreatitis. It inhibits aldosterone induced renal proteases that activate ENaC by proteolytic cleavage.

466. Which of the following cause hyperkalemia?
Harrison's 20th Ed. Chapter 49 Page 308

A. Theophylline
B. Chloroquine
C. Tacrolimus
D. Licorice

Cyclosporine, tacrolimus, NSAIDs and cyclooxygenase 2 (COX2) inhibitors cause hyperkalemia by their the ability to cause hyporeninemic hypoaldosteronism.

467. Which of the following blocks the apical ENaC activity in the distal nephron?
Harrison's 20th Ed. Chapter 49 Page 308

A. Amiloride
B. Trimethoprim
C. Pentamidine
D. All of the above

Trimethoprim & pentamidine impair K^+ secretion by blocking distal nephron Na^+ reabsorption.

468. Which of the following medications affect aldosterone secretion?

Harrison's 20th Ed. Chapter 49 Page 308

A. Angiotensin-converting enzyme (ACE) inhibitors
B. Angiotensin II receptor blockers (ARBs)
C. Heparin
D. All of the above

469. Which of the following medications cause tubular resistance to the action of aldosterone?

Harrison's 20th Ed. Chapter 49 Page 308

A. Trimethoprim
B. Spironolactone
C. Pentamidine
D. Digoxin

Trimethoprim, an antibiotic similar to potassium-sparing diuretic amiloride, competitively inhibits luminal sodium transport channels, causing a reduction in negative luminal charge and decreased potassium secretion.

470. Which of the following medications cause transmembrane shifting of potassium?

Harrison's 20th Ed. Chapter 49 Page 308

A. Spironolactone
B. Nonsteroidal anti-inflammatory drugs
C. Nonselective beta blockers
D. Heparin

Catecholamine-stimulated renin release is inhibited by beta blockade and causes a decrease in the amount of aldosterone synthesis. To a greater extent, however, beta blockers decrease the function of Na+/K+-ATPase by decreasing the amount of cyclic adenosine monophosphate (cAMP) in the cells.

471. Cardiac arrhythmias associated with hyperkalemia include?

Harrison's 20th Ed. Chapter 49 Page 310

A. Slow idioventricular rhythms
B. Ventricular tachycardia
C. Ventricular fibrillation
D. All of the above

Cardiac arrhythmias associated with hyperkalemia include sinus bradycardia, sinus arrest, slow idioventricular rhythms, ventricular tachycardia, ventricular fibrillation and asystole.

472. The earliest ECG change in hyperkalemia is?

Harrison's 20th Ed. Chapter 49 Page 310

A. Increased T-wave amplitude
B. Prolonged PR interval
C. Prolonged QRS duration
D. Loss of P waves

473. sine wave pattern in ECG in hyperkalemia is seen when serum K^+ levels are more than?

Harrison's 20th Ed. Chapter 49 Page 310

A. 5.5 mM
B. 6.5 mM
C. 7.0 mM
D. 8.0 mM

Electrocardiographic manifestations in hyperkalemia progress from tall peaked T waves (5.5-6.5 mM), to a loss of P waves (6.5-7.5 mM) to a widened QRS complex (7.0-8.0 mM) and ultimately a sine wave pattern (>8.0 mM).

474. In ECG, hyperkalemia can cause which of the following?

Harrison's 20th Ed. Chapter 49 Page 310

A. Long QT syndrome
B. Torsade de pointis
C. Type 1 Brugada pattern
D. All of the above

475. Hyperkalemic Brugada's sign can be differentiated from genetic Brugada's syndrome by?

Harrison's 20th Ed. Chapter 49 Page 310

A. Absence of P waves
B. Marked QRS widening
C. Abnormal QRS axis
D. All of the above

Hyperkalemia can cause a type 1 Brugada pattern in the electrocardiogram (ECG), with a pseudo-right bundle branch block and persistent coved ST segment elevation in at least two precordial leads. Hyperkalemic Brugada's sign occurs in critically ill patients with severe hyperkalemia and can be differentiated from genetic Brugada's syndrome by an absence of P waves, marked QRS widening and an abnormal QRS axis. Most patients are male, and many are critically ill. There is absence of congenital sodium channel anomaly. This change is reversible and typically resolves with resolution of hyperkalemia.

476. Sine wave pattern seen in severe hyperkalemia is due to merging of?

Harrison's 20th Ed. Chapter 49 Page 310

A. P + QRS
B. QRS + T
C. P + QRS + T
D. All of the above

The earliest ECG changes in hyperkalemia include increased T-wave amplitude. More severe degrees result in prolonged PR interval and QRS duration, AV conduction delay and loss of P waves. Progressive widening of QRS complex and merging with T wave produces a sine wave pattern. The terminal event is ventricular fibrillation or asystole.

477. Which of the following cardiac structure is most sensitive to hyperkalemia?

Emergency Medicine Practice 2016;18(11):1-24

A. Atrial myocardium
B. Ventricular myocardium
C. SA node
D. HIS bundle

↑ed extracellular K^+ causes an increase in transmembrane permeability & influx of K^+ into cells leading to a decrease in magnitude of the resting potential, a decrease in velocity of phase 0 of action potential & delayed conduction between myocytes. Effects of these changes are dependent upon tissue affected, with atrial myocardium being the most sensitive & specialized tissue (SA node & HIS bundle) being the least sensitive.

478. Which of the following regarding secondary hyperkalemic paralysis is false?

Harrison's 20th Ed. Chapter 49 Page 310

A. Autosomal dominant disorder
B. Episodic weakness/paralysis precipitated by exercise
C. Due to mutation in gene for skeletal muscle Na^+ channel
D. None of the above

Secondary hyperkalemic paralysis is an autosomal dominant disorder characterized by episodic weakness or paralysis, precipitated by stimuli that normally lead to mild hyperkalemia (exercise). Genetic defect is due to mutation in gene for skeletal muscle Na^+ channel.

479. Which of the following parameter is not required in calculating TTKG?

Harrison's 20th Ed. Chapter 49 Page 310

A. Serum Osmolality
B. Urine Osmolality
C. pH
D. Serum K

To calculate following parameters are required : Serum Osmolality (mOsm/kg), Urine Osmolality (mOsm/kg), Serum K (mEq/L) and Urine K (mEq/L).

480. Formula for calculating Transtubular Potassium Gradient (TTKG) is?

Harrison's 20th Ed. Chapter 49 Page 310

A. $(K^+_{serum} \times K^+_{Urine})/(Osm_{serum} \times Osm_{Urine})$
B. $(Osm_{serum} \times K^+_{serum})/(K^+_{Urine} \times Osm_{Urine})$
C. $(K^+_{Urine} \times Osm_{serum})/(K^+_{serum} \times Osm_{Urine})$
D. $(K^+_{serum} \times Osm_{Urine})/(Osm_{serum} \times K^+_{Urine})$

Correct formula for TTKG is $(P_{Osm} \times U_{Potassium})/(P_{Potassium} \times U_{Osm})$. It is valid only when Uosm >300 & UNa >25.

481. TTKG in a normal person on a normal diet is?

Indian J Pediatr 2007;74(7):679-686

A. 2–6
B. 6–12
C. 12–20
D. 20–29

The TTKG in normal persons varies but is generally within 6–12 range. Hypokalemia from extrarenal causes results in renal K^+ conservation and a TTKG <2. A higher value suggests renal K^+ losses, as in hyperaldosteronism. During hyperkalemia, the expected TTKG is >10. An inappropriately low TTKG (< 8) in hyperkalemia suggests hypoaldosteronism or renal tubular resistance to aldosterone. Administration of mineralocorticoid fludrocortisone (0.05 mg) enables TTKG to rise to >7 in patients with hypoaldosteronism. When it does not increase after mineralocorticoid challenge, tubular resistance to aldosterone is suspected.

482. Which of the following statements is false?

Indian J Pediatr 2007;74(7):679-686

A. Hypokalemia should result in a TTKG < 3
B. Hyperkalemia should result in a TTKG > 7–8
C. Hypokalemia not resulting in a TTKG<2 suggests renal K^+ loss
D. Hyperkalemia not resulting in a TTKG>10 suggests type I renal tubular acidosis

Hyperkalemia not resulting in a TTKG>10 suggests type IV renal tubular acidosis.

483. Renal excretion of potassium is dependent on?

Emergency Medicine Practice 2016;18(11):1-24

A. Rate of flow in the distal nephron
B. Aldosterone
C. Secretory pathways of potassium
D. All of the above

Renal excretion of potassium is dependent upon the rate of flow in the distal nephron, aldosterone, and the secretory pathways of potassium.

484. Which of the following suggests tubular resistance as a cause of hyperkalemia?

Harrison's 20th Ed. Chapter 49 Page 311 Figure 49-8

A. ↓ed urinary K^+ excretion
B. TTKG < 5
C. TTKG < 8 after 9α Fludrocortisone challenge
D. All of the above

485. Which of the following suggests ACE inhibitors as a cause of hyperkalemia?

Harrison's 20th Ed. Chapter 49 Page 311 Figure 49-8

A. TTKG ≥ 8 after 9α Fludrocortisone challenge
B. Low aldosterone
C. High renin
D. All of the above

486. Which of the following suggests primary adrenal insufficiency as a cause of hyperkalemia?

Harrison's 20th Ed. Chapter 49 Page 311 Figure 49-8

A. TTKG ≥ 8 after 9α Fludrocortisone challenge
B. Low aldosterone
C. High renin
D. All of the above

487. Which of the following suggests advanced kidney failure as a cause of hyperkalemia?

Harrison's 20th Ed. Chapter 49 Page 311 Figure 49-8

A. ↓ed urinary K^+ excretion (< 40 mmol/day)
B. TTKG > 8
C. Reduced tubular flow
D. All of the above

488. Significant hyperkalemia is considered when plasma K^+ concentration is?

Harrison's 20th Ed. Chapter 49 Page 310

A. ≥ 4.5 mM
B. ≥ 5.5 mM
C. ≥ 6.5 mM
D. ≥ 7.5 mM

489. In hyperkalemia, calcium administration acts by?

Harrison's 20th Ed. Chapter 49 Page 310

A. Raising the action potential threshold
B. Reducing excitability
C. No change in the resting membrane potential
D. All of the above

Calcium raises the action potential threshold & reduces excitability, without changing the resting membrane potential. Thus, calcium reverses the depolarization blockade due to hyperkalemia.

490. In severe hyperkalemia, 10 mL of 10% calcium gluconate should be infused over?

Harrison's 20th Ed. Chapter 49 Page 310

A. Half to 1 minute
B. 1 to 2 minutes
C. 2 to 3 minutes
D. 5 to 10 minutes

IV Calcium gluconate decreases membrane excitability. Usual dose is 10 mL of a 10% solution infused over 2–3 minutes with cardiac monitoring. Its effect is short-lived (30-60 min). Dose can be repeated if no change in ECG is seen after 5–10 minutes.

491. Hypercalcemia potentiates the cardiac toxicity of?

Harrison's 20th Ed. Chapter 49 Page 310

A. Amiodarone
B. Beta blockers
C. Theophylline
D. Digoxin

Hypercalcemia potentiates the cardiac toxicity of digoxin.

492. Which of the following is true for insulin-glucose treatment in hyperkalemia?

Harrison's 20th Ed. Chapter 49 Page 310

A. 5 units of IV regular insulin + 25 grams of IV glucose
B. 10 units of IV regular insulin + 25 grams of IV glucose
C. 15 units of IV regular insulin + 25 grams of IV glucose
D. 20 units of IV regular insulin + 25 grams of IV glucose

In hyperkalemia, the recommended dose is 10 units of intravenous regular insulin followed immediately by 50 mL of 50% dextrose (D50W, 25 g of glucose total) with avoidance of hypoglycemia. The effect begins in 10-20 minutes, peaks at 30-60 minutes, and lasts for 4-6 hours. In hyperkalemic patients with glucose concentrations of ≥200-250 mg/dL, insulin should be administered without glucose.

493. In hyperkalemia, inhaled Albuterol should not be used without?

Harrison's 20th Ed. Chapter 49 Page 310

A. IV Calcium
B. IV Insulin
C. IV Bicarbonate
D. All of the above

Inhaled Albuterol and insulin with glucose have an additive effect on plasma K^+ concentration.

494. Which of the following has no role in the acute treatment of hyperkalemia?

Harrison's 20th Ed. Chapter 49 Page 311

A. Intravenous calcium
B. Insulin
C. Albuterol
D. Intravenous bicarbonate

495. Severity of hyperkalemia is determined by?

Harrison's 20th Ed. Chapter 49 Page 311

A. Symptoms
B. Plasma K^+ concentration
C. ECG abnormalities
D. All of the above

Severity of hyperkalemia is determined by symptoms, plasma K^+ & ECG abnormalities.

496. The appropriate renal response to hyperkalemia is to excrete how much of K^+ daily?

Harrison's 20th Ed. Chapter 49 Page 311

A. At least 50 mmol
B. At least 100 mmol
C. At least 200 mmol
D. At least 300 mmol

The appropriate renal response to hyperkalemia is to excrete at least 200 mmol of K^+ daily.

497. Potentially fatal hyperkalemia occurs when plasma potassium concentration exceeds?

Harrison's 20th Ed. Chapter 49 Page 311

A. 5.5 mmol/L
B. 6.5 mmol/L
C. 7.5 mmol/L
D. 8.5 mmol/L

Potentially fatal hyperkalemia rarely occurs unless plasma K^+ concentration exceeds 7.5 mmol/L.

498. Which of the following is used for lowering potassium levels in severe hyperkalemia?

Harrison's 20th Ed. Chapter 49 Page 311

A. Insulin-glucose infusion
B. Alkali therapy with IV $NaHCO_3$
C. β_2 adrenergic agonists
D. All of the above

499. Which of the following reduce plasma K^+ levels by shifting K^+ into cells?

Harrison's 20th Ed. Chapter 49 Page 311

A. Glucose–insulin therapy
B. Alkali therapy with IV $NaHCO_3$
C. β_2-adrenergic agonists
D. All of the above

Alkali therapy with IV $NaHCO_3$ shifts K^+ into cells. β_2-adrenergic agonists promote cellular uptake of K^+.

500. Which of the following is false regarding sodium polystyrene sulfonate (SPS)?

Harrison's 20th Ed. Chapter 49 Page 311

A. Exchanges Na^+ for K^+ in gastrointestinal tract
B. Increases fecal excretion of K^+
C. Always given in a premade suspension with 33% sorbitol
D. None of the above

501. Which of the following is false regarding sodium polystyrene sulfonate (SPS)?

Harrison's 20th Ed. Chapter 49 Page 311

A. Anion-exchange resin
B. One gram binds 1 mmol of K^+ & releases 2-3 mmol of Na^+
C. Usual dose is 25–50 gram orally
D. Can be administered as retention enema

Sodium polystyrene sulfonate is a cation-exchange resin that promotes the exchange of Na^+ for K^+ in the gastrointestinal tract. Each gram binds 1 mmol of K^+ and releases 2–3 mmol of Na^+. Usual dose is 25-50 grams in 100 mL of 20% sorbitol orally to prevent constipation. It can also be administered as a retention enema.

502. Which of the following is a complication of SPS?

Harrison's 20th Ed. Chapter 49 Page 311

A. Anaphylaxis
B. Hepatitis
C. Intestinal obstruction
D. Intestinal necrosis

Intestinal necrosis typically of the colon or ileum is a rare but usually fatal complication of SPS. Coadministration of SPS with sorbitol increases the risk of intestinal necrosis.

503. Patiromer binds K^+ in exchange for?

Harrison's 20th Ed. Chapter 49 Page 312

A. Na^+
B. Ca^{++}
C. H^+
D. NH_4^+

Patiromer (Veltassa®) is a nonabsorbed polymer which binds K^+ in exchange for Ca++ in the intestine. Its side-effect is hypomagnesemia.

504. Which of the following is used in the treatment of hyperkalemia?

Harrison's 20th Ed. Chapter 49 Page 312

A. ZS-8
B. ZS-9
C. ZS-10
D. ZS-11

ZS-9 (Sodium zirconium cyclosilicate) is an inorganic, nonabsorbable crystalline compound that exchanges both Na^+ and H^+ ions in exchange for K^+ and $NH4^+$ in the intestine.

505. The most rapid & effective way of lowering plasma potassium concentration is?

Harrison's 20th Ed. Chapter 49 Page 312

A. Insulin-glucose infusion
B. Calcium gluconate infusion
C. Peritoneal dialysis
D. Hemodialysis

The most rapid and effective way of lowering the plasma K^+ concentration is hemodialysis. Although dialysis removes 1 mmol/L of serum potassium in the first hour and 2 mmol/L by 3 hours, a rebound of serum potassium can be seen post dialysis. The magnitude of postdialysis serum K^+ rebound is proportional to the predialysis serum K^+ level, with 35% of the reduction equated by 1 hour post treatment. Peritoneal dialysis is only 15-20% as effective as hemodialysis.

Hypercalcemia and Hypocalcemia

506. What is the normal range of serum parathyroid hormone (intact)?

Harrison's 20th Ed. Chapter 50 Page 309

A. 1–8 pg/mL
B. 8–51 pg/mL
C. 51–95 pg/mL
D. 95–135 pg/mL

Normal range of serum parathyroid hormone (intact) is 8–51 pg/mL or 8–51 ng/L.

507. What is the normal range of serum phosphatase, alkaline?

Harrison's 19th Ed 2762

A. 1-33 U/L
B. 33-96 U/L
C. 96-146 U/L
D. 146-216 U/L

508. What is the normal range of serum magnesium?

Harrison's 19th Ed 2761

A. 0.5-1.2 mg/dL
B. 1.5-2.3 mg/dL
C. 2.8-4.3 mg/dL
D. 4.5-6.3 mg/dL

Normal range of serum magnesium is 1.5–2.3 mg/dL or 0.62–0.95 mmol/L.

509. What is the normal range of serum calcium?

Harrison's 19th Ed 2758

A. 5.7-8.2 mg/dL
B. 8.7-10.2 mg/dL
C. 10.7-13.2 mg/dL
D. 13.7-18.2 mg/dL

Normal range of serum calcium is 8.7–10.2 mg/dL or 2.2–2.6 mmol/L.

510. What is the normal range of serum vitamin D 1,25-dihydroxy, total?

Harrison's 19th Ed 2766

A. 5-15 pg/mL
B. 15-75 pg/mL
C. 75-125 pg/mL
D. 125-175 pg/mL

Normal range of serum calcium is 15–75 pg/mL or 36–180 pmol/L.

511. What is the normal range of plasma vitamin D 25-dihydroxy, total?

Harrison's 19th Ed 2766

A. 5-30 ng/mL
B. 30-100 ng/mL
C. 100-200 ng/mL
D. 230-400 ng/mL

Normal range of serum calcium is 30–100 ng/mL or 75–250 nmol/L.

512. Calcium ion regulates which of the following physiologic processes?

Harrison's 20th Ed. Chapter 50 Page 312

A. Neuromuscular signaling
B. Hormone secretion
C. Blood coagulation
D. All of the above

The calcium ion plays a critical role in normal cellular function and signaling, regulating neuromuscular signaling, cardiac contractility, hormone secretion and blood coagulation.

513. Feedback mechanisms for maintenance of extracellular calcium concentrations involve?

Harrison's 20th Ed. Chapter 50 Page 312

A. Parathyroid glands
B. Kidney
C. Intestine
D. All of the above

Extracellular calcium concentrations are maintained through feedback mechanisms involving parathyroid hormone (PTH) and active vitamin D metabolite 1,25-dihydroxyvitamin D [1,25(OH)$_2$D]. Feedback mechanisms are orchestrated by integrating signals between parathyroid glands, kidney, intestine & bone.

514. Decrease in serum calcium leads to?

Harrison's 20th Ed. Chapter 50 Page 312 Figure 50-1

A. Increase in parathyroid hormone (PTH)
B. Resorption of calcium from bone
C. Stimulates renal 1,25(OH)$_2$D production
D. All of the above

515. Which of the following is the action of PTH?

Harrison's 20th Ed. Chapter 50 Page 312 Figure 50-1

A. Increased tubular reabsorption of calcium by kidney
B. Resorption of calcium from bone
C. Stimulates renal 1,25(OH)$_2$D production
D. All of the above

A decrease in extracellular (ECF) calcium (Ca$^+$) triggers an increase in parathyroid hormone (PTH) secretion via the calcium sensor receptor on parathyroid cells. PTH causes increased tubular reabsorption of calcium by kidney and resorption of calcium from bone. PTH also stimulates renal 1,25(OH)$_2$D production. 1,25(OH)$_2$D then acts principally on intestine to increase calcium absorption.

516. Which of the following statements is false?

Harrison's 20th Ed. Chapter 50 Page 312 Figure 50-1

A. Normal serum calcium is 8.9-10.1 mg/dL (2.2-2.5 mM)
B. Ectopic PTH secretion by tumors is extremely rare
C. Hypercalcemia invariably leads to dehydration
D. None of the above

Normally, plasma PTH level varies inversely with plasma calcium level. Ectopic secretion of authentic PTH is a rare cause of hypercalcemia, having been well documented in only eight patients to date.

517. Excess PTH production not appropriately suppressed by increased serum calcium concentrations occurs in?

Harrison's 20th Ed. Chapter 50 Page 313

A. Hypercalcemia of malignancy
B. Parathyroid adenoma
C. Sarcoidosis
D. Hyperthyroidism

Excess PTH production not appropriately suppressed by increased serum calcium concentrations occurs in primary neoplastic disorders of parathyroid glands like parathyroid adenomas, hyperplasia, or carcinoma.

518. Which of the following is related to familial hypocalciuric hypercalcemia (FHH)?

Harrison's 20th Ed. Chapter 50 Page 313

A. PTH-related peptide (PTHrP)
B. $1,25(OH)_2D$
C. Calcium sensor receptor (CaSR) mutations
D. Exogenous calcium overload

Inappropriate PTH secretion for existing level of serum calcium occurs with heterozygous inactivating calcium sensor receptor (CaSR) mutations, which impair extracellular calcium sensing by parathyroid glands and kidneys, resulting in familial hypocalciuric hypercalcemia (FHH). Hypercalcemia is typically not treated in patients with familial hypocalciuric hypercalcemia, because the elevation in serum calcium is typically mild and produces few if any symptoms.

519. Calcium-sensing receptor (CaSR) is expressed in?

Am J Physiol Renal Physiol. 2010;298(3):F485-F499

A. Parathyroid hormone (PTH)-secreting parathyroid glands
B. Calcitonin (CT)-secreting thyroidal C cells
C. Kidney
D. All of the above

520. Which of the following determine how much Ca^{++} moves into or out of the body?

Am J Physiol Renal Physiol. 2010;298(3):F485-F499

A. Intestines
B. Bone
C. Kidney
D. All of the above

521. Ca^{++} fluxes are regulated by?

Am J Physiol Renal Physiol. 2010;298(3):F485-F499

A. Parathyroid hormone (PTH)
B. Calcitonin (CT)
C. 1,25-dihydroxyvitamin D3 [$1,25(OH)_2D3$]
D. All of the above

Key CaSR-expressing, homeostatic tissues include parathyroid hormone (PTH)-secreting parathyroid glands, calcitonin (CT)-secreting thyroidal C cells, intestines, bone, and kidney. The last three determine how much Ca^{++} moves into or out of the body (intestine and kidney, respectively) or how Ca^{++} moves between the extracellular fluids (ECF) and bone. These Ca^{++} fluxes are regulated by PTH and CT, PTHrP as well as by 1,25-dihydroxyvitamin D3 [$1,25(OH)_2D3$], whose renal synthesis is homeostatically regulated.

522. The CaSR belongs to?

Am J Physiol Renal Physiol. 2010;298(3):F485-F499

A. Family A of the G protein-coupled receptors
B. Family B of the G protein-coupled receptors
C. Family C of the G protein-coupled receptors
D. Family D of the G protein-coupled receptors

The CaSR belongs to family C of the G protein-coupled receptors. Family C also includes metabotropic glutamate receptors, $GABA_B$ receptors, receptors for taste and pheromones, and an amino acid- and divalent cation-sensing receptor called GPRC6A.

523. The biologically active cell surface CaSR, upon binding Ca^{++}, activates which of the following G proteins?

Am J Physiol Renal Physiol. 2010;298(3):F485-F499

A. Gq/11
B. Gi
C. G12/13
D. All of the above

The biologically active cell surface CaSR, upon binding Ca^{++}, activates G proteins Gq/11, Gi, and G12/13, which stimulate phospholipase C (PLC), thereby producing diacylglycerol & inositol 1,4,5-trisphosphate (IP3). The latter releases Ca^{++} from intracellular stores, inhibit adenylate cyclase, and activate Rho kinase, respectively.

524. CaSR controls which of the following parathyroid functions?

Am J Physiol Renal Physiol. 2010;298(3):F485-F499

A. PTH secretion
B. PTH synthesis
C. Parathyroid cellular proliferation
D. All of the above

The CaSR controls three important aspects of parathyroid function relevant to the kidney: PTH secretion, PTH synthesis, and parathyroid cellular proliferation. CaSR also controls expression of the PTH gene.

525. Which of the following is related to PTH-related peptide (PTHrP)?

Harrison's 20th Ed. Chapter 50 Page 313

A. Hypercalcemia of malignancy
B. Milk-alkali syndrome
C. Familial hypocalciuric hypercalcemia (FHH)
D. Sarcoidosis

Many solid tumors produce PTH-related peptide (PTHrP) which binds PTH receptor & mimicks effects of PTH on bone & kidney like PTHrP-mediated hypercalcemia of malignancy & suppression of PTH.

526. Enhanced conversion of 25(OH)D to $1,25(OH)_2D$ leading to hypercalcemia is related to?

Harrison's 20th Ed. Chapter 50 Page 313

A. Hypercalcemia of malignancy
B. Milk-alkali syndrome
C. Familial hypocalciuric hypercalcemia (FHH)
D. Sarcoidosis

Hypercalcemia in sarcoidosis or lymphomas is caused by enhanced conversion of 25(OH)D to potent $1,25(OH)_2D$ that enhances intestinal calcium absorption resulting in hypercalcemia & suppressed PTH.

527. Hypercalcemia with suppressed PTH secretion in hyperthyroidism is due to?

Harrison's 20th Ed. Chapter 50 Page 313

A. Enhanced intestinal calcium absorption
B. Increased calcium mobilization from bone
C. PTHrP-mediated hypercalcemia
D. Increased parathyroid cell mass

Hyperthyroidism or osteolytic metastases directly increase calcium mobilization from bone leading to hypercalcemia with suppressed PTH secretion.

528. Granulomatous disease that cause excessive $1,25(OH)_2D$ production is?

Harrison's 20th Ed. Chapter 50 Page 313 Table 50-1

A. Sarcoidosis
B. Tuberculosis
C. Silicosis
D. All of the above

Granulomatous diseases that cause excessive $1,25(OH)_2D$ production are Sarcoidosis, Tuberculosis and Silicosis.

529. Hypercalcemia due to excess secretion of 1,25(OH)$_2$ D occurs in which of the following?

N Engl J Med. 2005;352:373-9

A. Astrocytoma
B. Squamous-cell lung cancer
C. Ovarian cancer
D. Lymphoma

Some lymphomas secrete the active form of vitamin D, 1,25-dihydroxyvitamin D (1,25(OH)$_2$D), causing hypercalcemia as a result of the combination of enhanced osteoclastic bone resorption and enhanced intestinal absorption of calcium.

530. Endocrine disorder that causes hypercalcemia is?

Harrison's 20th Ed. Chapter 50 Page 313 Table 50-1

A. Adrenal insufficiency
B. Pheochromocytoma
C. VIPoma
D. All of the above

Endocrine disorders that can cause hypercalcemia are adrenal insufficiency, pheochromocytoma, VIPoma.

531. Medication that causes hypercalcemia is?

Harrison's 20th Ed. Chapter 50 Page 313 Table 50-1

A. Thiazides
B. Vitamin A
C. Antiestrogens
D. All of the above

532. Medication that may independently lead to hypercalcemia is?

N Engl J Med. 2005;352:373-9

A. Lithium
B. Vitamin D
C. Thiazides
D. All of the above

Medications that independently lead to hypercalcemia are lithium, calcitriol, vitamin D & thiazides.

533. Tertiary hyperparathyroidism refers to?

Harrison's 20th Ed. Chapter 50 Page 313 Table 50-1

A. Inactivating mutations in the CaSR or in G proteins
B. Long-term stimulation of PTH secretion in renal insufficiency
C. Overproduction of PTHrP
D. Lytic skeletal metastases

Tertiary hyperparathyroidism refers to long-term stimulation of PTH secretion in renal insufficiency.

534. Primary increase in bone resorptlon occurs in which of the following?

Harrison's 20th Ed. Chapter 50 Page 313 Table 50-1

A. Overproduction of PTHrP
B. Lytic skeletal metastases
C. Hyperthyroidism
D. All of the above

Primary increase in bone resorptlon occurs in hyperthyroidism and immobilization.

535. Type of hypercalcemia associated with cancer is?

N Engl J Med. 2005;352:373-9

A. Local osteolytic hypercalcemia
B. Humoral hypercalcemia of malignancy
C. 1,25(OH)$_2$D-secreting lymphomas
D. All of the above

In addition to the above three, ectopic hyperparathyroidism due to ectopic secretion of authentic PTH is a rare cause of hypercalcemia.

536. True hypercalcemia refers to?

N Engl J Med. 2005;352:373-9

A. Elevated serum level of total calcium
B. Elevated serum level of nonionized calcium
C. Elevated serum level of ionized calcium
D. All of the above

Elevated serum level of ionized calcium is true hypercalcemia.

537. Basic mechanism of true hypercalcemia is?

N Engl J Med. 2005;352:373-9

A. Enhanced osteoclastic bone resorption
B. Enhanced renal tubular reabsorption of calcium
C. Enhanced intestinal absorption of calcium
D. All of the above

True hypercalcemia is due to enhanced osteoclastic bone resorption (in local osteolytic hypercalcemia, humoral hypercalcemia of malignancy (HHM), 1,25(OH)$_2$D secreting lymphomas, & ectopic hyperparathyroidism), enhanced renal tubular reabsorption of calcium (in HHM & ectopic hyperparathyroidism), and enhanced intestinal absorption of calcium (in 1,25(OH)$_2$D-secreting lymphomas & ectopic hyperparathyroidism).

538. While treating hypercalcemia, serum phosphorus level should be kept in the range of?

N Engl J Med. 2005;352:373-9

A. 0.5–1.0 mg/dL
B. 1.0–2.0 mg/dL
C. 2.0–2.5 mg/dL
D. 2.5–3.0 mg/dL

539. While treating hypercalcemia, calcium - phosphorus product should be kept ideally below?

N Engl J Med. 2005;352:373-9

A. 5
B. 10
C. 20
D. 30

While treating hypercalcemia, serum phosphorus level should be kept in the range of 2.5–3.0 mg/dL and the calcium - phosphorus product below 40, ideally in the range of 30.

540. Serum levels of calcium in mild hypercalcemia are up to?

Harrison's 20th Ed. Chapter 50 Page 313

A. 7–8.5 mg/dL
B. 8–9.5 mg/dL
C. 9–10.5 mg/dL
D. 11–11.5 mg/dL

Serum levels of calcium in mild hypercalcemia is upto 11–11.5 mg/dL and is usually asymptomatic.

541. Serum levels of calcium in severe hypercalcemia is more than?

Harrison's 20th Ed. Chapter 50 Page 313

A. 11 mg/dL
B. 12 mg/dL
C. 13 mg/dL
D. 14 mg/dL

Serum levels of calcium in severe hypercalcemia is > 14.0 mg/dL. Patients with a serum calcium concentration >14 mg/dL (3.5 mmol/L) require treatment, regardless of symptoms.

542. Which of the following occurs in acute severe hypercalcemia (>12–13 mg/dL)?

Harrison's 20th Ed. Chapter 50 Page 313

A. Pancreatitis
B. Peptic ulcer disease
C. Nephrolithiasis
D. All of the above

Severe acute hypercalcemia (>12–13 mg/dL) may result in lethargy, stupor, coma or pancreatitis.

543. ECG changes in hypercalcemia include all except?

Harrison's 20th Ed. Chapter 50 Page 313

A. Bradycardia
B. AV block
C. Short QT interval
D. Prolonged PR interval

ECG changes in hypercalcemia include bradycardia, AV block & short QT interval.

544. Changes in serum calcium is preferably monitored by which of the following in ECG?

Harrison's 20th Ed. Chapter 50 Page 313

A. Heart rate
B. QRS amplitude
C. QT interval
D. ST segment

Changes in serum calcium can be monitored by following the QT interval.

545. What percentage of serum total calcium is ionized?

Harrison's 20th Ed. Chapter 50 Page 313

A. 10%
B. 25%
C. 50%
D. 80%

~50% of total calcium is ionized & rest is bound principally to albumin.

546. With a decrease in serum albumin of 1.0 g/dL, what quantity should be added to serum total calcium?

Harrison's 19th Ed 314

A. 0.2 mg/dL
B. 0.4 mg/dL
C. 0.6 mg/dL
D. 0.8 mg/dL

Serum albumin levels are determined to obtain "correct serum calcium". 0.8 mg/dL should be aded to total calcium for every decrement in serum albumin of 1.0 g/dL below the reference value of 4.1 g/dL for albumin, and conversely for elevations in serum albumin. In patients with hyperalbuminemia due to severe volume depletion and multiple myeloma, who have a calcium-binding paraprotein, have increased protein binding of calcium. This can cause an elevation in serum total calcium concentration without any rise in serum ionized calcium concentration. This phenomenon is called pseudohypercalcemia (or factitious hypercalcemia) since the patient has a normal ionized serum calcium concentration.

547. Chronic hypercalcemia is most commonly caused by?

Harrison's 20th Ed. Chapter 50 Page 313

A. Medication use
B. Primary hyperparathyroidism
C. Underlying malignancy
D. Sarcoidosis

Primary hyperparathyroidism is the most common cause of chronic hypercalcemia, followed by hypercalcemia due to an underlying malignancy.

548. Increases in PTH are often accompanied by?

Harrison's 20th Ed. Chapter 50 Page 313

A. Hypokalemia
B. Hyperphosphatemia
C. Hypophosphatemia
D. Hypernatremia

Increases in PTH are often accompanied by hypophosphatemia.

549. Lab findings in primary hyperparathyroidism include?

Harrison's 20th Ed. Chapter 50 Page 313

A. Elevated serum calcium
B. Low serum phosphorus
C. Increased PTH level
D. All of the above

If the PTH level is increased (or "inappropriately normal") in the setting of elevated calcium and low phosphorus, the diagnosis is almost always primary hyperparathyroidism.

550. Lab findings in hypercalcemia due to underlying malignancy include?

Harrison's 20th Ed. Chapter 50 Page 313

A. Hypercalcemia
B. Suppressed PTH level
C. Elevated PTHrP level
D. All of the above

551. In familial hypocalciuric hypercalcemia (FHH), calcium/creatinine clearance ratio is?

Harrison's 20th Ed. Chapter 50 Page 313

A. < 0.01
B. < 0.05
C. < 0.1
D. < 0.2

Calcium/creatinine clearance ratio (urine calcium/serum calcium divided by urine creatinine/serum creatinine) of <0.01 is suggestive of FHH.

552. Classic laboratory finding in milk alkali syndrome is?

N Engl J Med. 2008;358:1952-6

A. Hypercalcemia
B. Metabolic alkalosis
C. Impaired renal function
D. All of the above

Hypercalcemia, metabolic alkalosis & impaired renal function are classic laboratory findings in patients with milk alkali syndrome in those with excess oral intake of calcium and milk.

553. Effective treatments to reduce serum calcium is by?

Harrison's 20th Ed. Chapter 50 Page 313

A. Inhibiting bone resorption
B. Increasing urinary calcium excretion
C. Decreasing intestinal calcium absorption
D. All of the above

Effective treatments reduce serum calcium by inhibiting bone resorption, increasing urinary calcium excretion, or decreasing intestinal calcium absorption.

554. Initial therapy of significant hypercalcemia begins with?

Harrison's 20th Ed. Chapter 50 Page 313

A. Volume expansion with IV saline
B. Zoledronic acid
C. Calcitonin
D. Glucocorticoids

Initial therapy of significant hypercalcemia begins with volume expansion with saline (200–500 mL/hour, depending on patient's cardiovascular status & renal function) as hypercalcemia invariably leads to dehydration. Saline itself is calciuretic. Loop diuretics should not be administered until after full hydration has been achieved. Thiazide diuretics should not be used as they stimulate renal calcium reabsorption.

555. Bisphosphonate that is used for the treatment of hypercalcemia of malignancy in adults is?

Harrison's 20th Ed. Chapter 50 Page 313

A. Zoledronic acid
B. Pamidronate
C. Ibandronate
D. All of the above

Bisphosphonates that are commonly used for the treatment of hypercalcemia of malignancy in adults are Zoledronic acid, Pamidronate, clodronate, etidronate and Ibandronate. The bisphosphonates are nonhydrolyzable analogs of inorganic pyrophosphate that adsorb to the surface of bone hydroxyapatite and inhibit calcium release by interfering with osteoclast-mediated bone resorption.

556. Drug that inhibits bone resorption is?

Harrison's 20th Ed. Chapter 50 Page 314

A. Zoledronic acid
B. Pamidronate
C. Etidronate
D. All of the above

Intravenous bisphosphonates are the best studied, safest and most effective agents for use in patients with hypercalcemia associated with cancer. They work by blocking osteoclastic bone resorption. Ibandronate and Clodronate are the other two besides the above three.

557. Which of the following is an alternative to bisphosphonates in hypercalcemia?

Harrison's 20th Ed. Chapter 50 Page 314

A. Glucocorticoids
B. Gallium nitrate
C. Intravenous phosphate
D. Ketoconazole

An alternative to bisphosphonates is gallium nitrate (200 mg/m² IV daily for 5 days). It is effective, but has potential nephrotoxicity.

558. Which of the following is an alternative to bisphosphonates in hypercalcemia?

Harrison's 20th Ed. Chapter 50 Page 314

A. Glucocorticoids
B. Denosumab
C. Hydroxychloroquine
D. Ketoconazole

Denosumab (an antibody to RANKL) is a potent inhibitor of bone resorption, effective in treating hypercalcemia refractory to bisphosphonates. Its dose is 120 mg SC on days 1, 8, 15, and 29, and then every 4 weeks.

559. Salmon calcitonin is approved for the treatment of?

Harrison's 20th Ed. Chapter 405 Page 21962

A. Multiple myeloma
B. Paget's disease
C. Osteopetrosis
D. All of the above

The subcutaneous injectable form of salmon calcitonin is approved for the treatment of Paget's disease but is rarely used due to its low potency and should be reserved for patients who either do not tolerate bisphosphonates or have a contraindication to their use.

560. Which of the following is the preferred treatment in patients with $1,25(OH)_2D$-mediated hypercalcemia?

Harrison's 20th Ed. Chapter 50 Page 314

A. Zoledronic acid
B. Glucocorticoids
C. Gallium nitrate
D. All of the above

561. Glucocorticoids are the preferred therapy in hypercalcemia due to?

Harrison's 20th Ed. Chapter 50 Page 314

A. Malignancy
B. Severe hyperparathyroidism
C. Sarcoidosis
D. Familial hypocalciuric hypercalcemia (FHH)

In patients with $1,25(OH)_2D$-mediated hypercalcemia, glucocorticoids are the preferred therapy, as they decrease $1,25(OH)_2D$ production.

562. Pharmacologic therapy for hypercalcemia associated with cancer include?

N Engl J Med. 2005;352:373-9

A. Mithramycin
B. Calcitonin
C. Gallium nitrate
D. All of the above

563. Dose of Zoledronic acid is?

Harrison's 20th Ed. Chapter 50 Page 314

A. 2 mg IV infusion over 30-minutes
B. 4 mg IV infusion over 30-minutes
C. 6 mg IV infusion over 30-minutes
D. 8 mg IV infusion over 30-minutes

564. Drugs that decreases $1,25(OH)_2D$ production is?

Harrison's 20th Ed. Chapter 50 Page 314

A. Ketoconazole
B. Chloroquine
C. Hydroxychloroquine
D. All of the above

Other drugs, such as ketoconazole, chloroquine, and hydroxychloroquine, may decrease $1,25(OH)_2D$ production and are used occasionally.

565. Which of the following is the skeletal complication of severe form of primary hyperparathyroidism?

Harrison's 20th Ed. Chapter 50 Page 314

A. Osteomalacia
B. Osteitis fibrosa cystica
C. Hyperostosis
D. All of the above

Primary hyperparathyroidism often presents in its severe form with skeletal complications like osteitis fibrosa cystica. It is the distinctive bone manifestation of hyperparathyroidism.

566. Which of the following is a calcimimetic?

Harrison's 20th Ed. Chapter 381 Page 2748

A. Cinacalpet
B. Cinacalcet
C. Cinacalnet
D. Cinacalvet

Cinacalcet is a calcimimetic, which act via calcium-sensing receptor. It is used to treat primary hyperparathyroidism, in some patients when surgery is unsuccessful or contraindicated. Calcimimetics lower PTH secretion lower calcium but do not affect bone mass density (BMD).

Hypocalcemia

567. Main defense against hypocalcemia is?

Harrison's 20th Ed. Chapter 50 Page 314

A. Calcium
B. Vitamin D
C. PTH
D. PTH-related peptide (PTHrP)

PTH is the main defense against hypocalcemia.

568. Hypoparathyroidism is a cardinal feature of?

Harrison's 20th Ed. Chapter 50 Page 314

A. Autoimmune endocrinopathies
B. Hereditary endocrinopathies
C. Inflammatory endocrinopathies
D. All of the above

Hypoparathyroidism is a cardinal feature of autoimmune endocrinopathies (Isolated or part of APS-1, autoimmune polyendocrinopathy syndrome).

569. Which of the following syndromes is associated with hypoparathyroidism?

Harrison's 20th Ed. Chapter 50 Page 314

A. Sjogren's syndrome
B. Syndrome of apparent mineralocorticoid excess (SAME)
C. Immunodysregulation polyendocrinopathy enteropathy X-linked syndrome (IPEX)
D. DiGeorge's syndrome (CATCH-22)

A form of hypoparathyroidism associated with defective development of both the thymus and the parathyroid glands is termed the DiGeorge syndrome or the velocardiofacial syndrome. The chromosome 22 defect is now termed DSG1. A defect in chromosome 10p is also now recognized-and is called DSG2.

570. Which of the following syndromes is associated with hypoparathyroidism?

Harrison's 20th Ed. Chapter 403 Page 2937

A. Kenney-Caffey syndrome Type I
B. Sanjad-Sakati syndrome
C. Kearns-Sayre syndrome (KSS)
D. All of the above

571. Which of the following leads to reduced parathyroid function?

Harrison's 20th Ed. Chapter 50 Page 314

A. Iron deficiency
B. Hypomagnesemia
C. Hypokalemia
D. VIPoma

572. Pseudohypoparathyroidism best relates to?

Harrison's 20th Ed. Chapter 50 Page 314 Table 50-2

A. Vitamin D resistance
B. G protein mutations
C. Calcium chelators
D. PTH receptor mutations

573. Which of the following can lead to secondary hyperparathyroidism?

Harrison's 20th Ed. Chapter 50 Page 314 Table 50-2

A. Hungry bone syndrome
B. Osteoblastic metastasis of prostate cancer
C. Acute pancreatitis
D. All of the above

574. Which of the following drug can lead to secondary hyperparathyroidism?

Harrison's 20th Ed. Chapter 50 Page 314 Table 50-2

A. Plicamycin
B. Phenytoin
C. Ketoconazole
D. All of the above

575. Degree of hypocalcemia is most in which of these disorders?

Harrison's 20th Ed. Chapter 50 Page 314

A. Hypoparathyroidism
B. Vitamin D deficiency
C. Impaired 1,25$(OH)_2$D production
D. Vitamin D resistance

Degree of hypocalcemia is most in hypoparathyroidism.

576. Hypocalcemia may occur in?

Harrison's 20th Ed. Chapter 50 Page 314

A. Rhabdomyolysis
B. Tumor lysis
C. Pancreatitis
D. All of the above

Hypocalcemia may occur in severe tissue injury like burns, rhabdomyolysis, tumor lysis, or pancreatitis.

577. Paresthesias in moderate to severe hypocalcemia involve?
Harrison's 20th Ed. Chapter 50 Page 314

A. Fingers
B. Toes
C. Circumoral regions
D. All of the above

Moderate to severe hypocalcemia is associated with paresthesias, usually of the fingers, toes, and circumoral regions, and is caused by increased neuromuscular irritability.

578. Chvostek's sign is present in what percentage of normal individuals?
Harrison's 20th Ed. Chapter 50 Page 314

A. ~ 4%
B. ~ 6%
C. ~ 8%
D. ~ 10%

Chvostek's sign i.e. twitching of circumoral muscles in response to tapping of facial nerve just anterior to the ear is present in ~10% of normal individuals.

579. For eliciting Trousseau's sign, BP cuff is inflated how much above patient's systolic blood pressure?
Harrison's 20th Ed. Chapter 50 Page 314

A. 5 mm Hg
B. 10 mm Hg
C. 15 mm Hg
D. 20 mm Hg

Trousseau's sign refers to carpal spasm in hypocalcemia induced by inflation of a BP cuff to 20 mm Hg above patient's SBP for 3 minutes.

580. Which of the following is false about severe hypocalcemia?
Harrison's 20th Ed. Chapter 50 Page 314

A. Seizures
B. Bronchospasm
C. Laryngospasm
D. Short QT interval

Severe hypocalcemia can induce seizures, carpopedal spasm, bronchospasm, laryngospasm, and prolongation of the QT interval.

581. Nutritional vitamin D deficiency is best assessed by?
Harrison's 20th Ed. Chapter 50 Page 314

A. Serum 25-hydroxyvitamin D levels
B. Serum 1,25$(OH)_2$D levels
C. Serum calcium levels
D. Serum PTH levels

582. Vitamin D resistance is best assessed by?
Harrison's 20th Ed. Chapter 50 Page 314

A. Serum 25-hydroxyvitamin D levels
B. Serum 1,25$(OH)_2$D levels
C. Serum calcium levels
D. Serum PTH levels

Nutritional vitamin D deficiency is best assessed by obtaining serum 25-hydroxyvitamin D levels, which reflect vitamin D stores. In renal insufficiency or suspected vitamin D resistance, serum 1,25$(OH)_2$D levels are informative.

583. Acute, symptomatic hypocalcemia is initially managed with?
Harrison's 20th Ed. Chapter 50 Page 314

A. Vitamin D_2 or D_3
B. Magnesium sulphate
C. Calcium gluconate
D. All of the above

Acute, symptomatic hypocalcemia is initially managed with calcium gluconate, 10 mL of 10% (90 mg or 2.2 mmol) intravenously, diluted in 50 mL of 5% dextrose or 0.9% sodium chloride, given intravenously over 5 minutes.

584. Which of the following is used for the treatment of refractory hypoparathyroidism?
Harrison's 20th Ed. Chapter 50 Page 315

A. PTH (1-82)
B. PTH (1-83)
C. PTH (1-84)
D. PTH (1-85)

Recombinant parathyroid hormone rhPTH (1-84) has recently been approved by the FDA for the treatment of refractory hypoparathyroidism. N-terminal fragment of PTH is rhPTH (1-34).

Acidosis and Alkalosis

585. Systemic arterial pH is maintained between 7.35 & 7.45 by?
Harrison's 20th Ed. Chapter 51 Page 315

A. Central nervous system
B. Respiratory system
C. Kidney
D. All of the above

Control of arterial CO_2 tension ($PaCO_2$) by central nervous and respiratory systems & control of plasma bicarbonate by kidneys stabilize arterial pH by excretion or retention of acid or alkali maintains systemic arterial pH between 7.35 & 7.45.

586. Henderson-Hasselbalch equation is used to determine?
Harrison's 20th Ed. Chapter 51 Page 315

A. $PaCO_2$
B. PaO_2
C. Systemic pH
D. Anion gap

587. Which of the following is not a parameter in Henderson-Hasselbalch equation?
Harrison's 20th Ed. Chapter 51 Page 315

A. $PaCO_2$
B. PaO_2
C. pH
D. HCO_3^-

588. Henderson-Hasselbalch equation for systemic pH is?
Harrison's 20th Ed. Chapter 51 Page 315

A. $4.1 + \log (HCO_3^- / (PaCO_2 \times 0.0301))$
B. $5.1 + \log (HCO_3^- / (PaCO_2 \times 0.0301))$
C. $6.1 + \log (HCO_3^- / (PaCO_2 \times 0.0301))$
D. $7.1 + \log (HCO_3^- / (PaCO_2 \times 0.0301))$

Henderson-Hasselbalch equation includes metabolic & respiratory components that regulate systemic pH.

589. Increases or decreases in $PaCO_2$ represent derangements of?
Harrison's 20th Ed. Chapter 51 Page 315

A. Neural respiratory control
B. Compensatory response to alteration in plasma $[HCO_3^-]$
C. Both A and B
D. None of the above

590. Which of the following statements is false?
Harrison's 20th Ed. Chapter 51 Page 315

A. Usual steady-state $PaCO_2$ is 60 mm Hg
B. CO_2 underexcretion produces hypercapnia
C. CO_2 overexcretion causes hypocapnia
D. $PaCO_2$ regulated primarily by neural respiratory factors

Usual steady-state $PaCO_2$ is maintained at 40 mm Hg.

591. Which of the following statements is false?
Harrison's 20th Ed. Chapter 51 Page 315

A. Hypercapnia is the result of hypoventilation
B. Primary alteration of $PaCO_2$ evokes renal adaptation
C. $PaCO_2$ changes result from alteration in plasma $[HCO_3^-]$
D. None of the above

592. Which of the following conditions returns the pH to a normal value?
Harrison's 20th Ed. Chapter 51 Page 315

A. Metabolic acidosis
B. Metabolic alkalosis
C. Chronic respiratory alkalosis
D. Chronic metabolic alkalosis

Compensatory responses return pH toward, but not to, the normal value. Chronic respiratory alkalosis when prolonged is an exception to this rule and often returns the pH to a normal value.

593. Which of the following formula (Winter's) is correct?
Harrison's 20th Ed. Chapter 51 Page 315

A. $PaCO_2 = (1.3 \times [HCO_3^-]) + 8 \pm 2$
B $PaCO_2 = (1.4 \times [HCO_3^-]) + 8 \pm 2$
C. $PaCO_2 = (1.5 \times [HCO_3^-]) + 8 \pm 2$
D. $PaCO_2 = (1.6 \times [HCO_3^-]) + 8 \pm 2$

Winter's formula for expected CO_2 is $(1.5 \times \text{Bicarbonate}) + 8 \pm 2$

594. In simple metabolic acidosis, $PaCO_2$ would decrease by how much for each mmol/L decrease in $[HCO_3^-]$?
Harrison's 20th Ed. Chapter 51 Page 315 Table 51-1

A. 1.25 mm Hg
B. 1.50 mm Hg
C. 1.75 mm Hg
D. 2.00 mm Hg

Degree of respiratory compensation in simple metabolic acidosis is predicted by $PaCO_2 = (1.5 \times [HCO_3^-]) + 8 \pm 2$. Thus, $PaCO_2$ decreases by 1.25 mm Hg for each mmol/L decrease in $[HCO_3^-]$ or $PaCO_2 = [HCO_3^-] + 15$. Values for $PaCO_2$ <24 or >28 mm Hg define a mixed disturbance (metabolic acidosis and respiratory alkalosis or metabolic alkalosis and respiratory acidosis, respectively).

595. In simple metabolic alkalosis, $PaCO_2$ would increase by how much for each mmol/L increase in $[HCO_3^-]$?
Harrison's 20th Ed. Chapter 51 Page 315 Table 51-1

A. 0.25 mm Hg
B. 0.50 mm Hg
C. 0.75 mm Hg
D. 1.00 mm Hg

$PaCO_2$ increases by 0.75 mm Hg for each mmol/L increase in $[HCO_3^-]$ or $PaCO_2$ will increase by 6 mm Hg per 10 mmol/L increase in $[HCO_3^-]$.

596. In acute respiratory alkalosis, $[HCO_3^-]$ would decrease by how much for each mm Hg decrease in $PaCO_2$?
Harrison's 20th Ed. Chapter 51 Page 315 Table 51-1

A. 0.1 mmol/L
B. 0.2 mmol/L
C. 0.3 mmol/L
D. 0.4 mmol/L

597. In chronic respiratory alkalosis, [HCO_3^-] would decrease by how much for each mm Hg decrease in $PaCO_2$?

Harrison's 20th Ed. Chapter 51 Page 315 Table 51-1

A. 0.1 mmol/L
B. 0.2 mmol/L
C. 0.3 mmol/L
D. 0.4 mmol/L

598. In acute respiratory acidosis, [HCO_3^-] would increase by how much for each mm Hg increase in $PaCO_2$?

Harrison's 20th Ed. Chapter 51 Page 315 Table 51-1

A. 0.1 mmol/L
B. 0.2 mmol/L
C. 0.3 mmol/L
D. 0.4 mmol/L

599. In chronic respiratory acidosis, [HCO_3^-] would increase by how much for each mm Hg increase in $PaCO_2$?

Harrison's 20th Ed. Chapter 51 Page 315 Table 51-1

A. 0.1 mmol/L
B. 0.2 mmol/L
C. 0.3 mmol/L
D. 0.4 mmol/L

600. Acid-base nomogram is drawn between arterial blood pH and?

Harrison's 20th Ed. Chapter 51 Page 315 Table 51-1

A. Arterial plasma [HCO_3^-]
B. Arterial plasma $PaCO_2$
C. Arterial plasma PaO_2
D. Arterial blood [H^+]

601. Which of the following statements about mixed acid-base disorders is false?

Harrison's 20th Ed. Chapter 51 Page 316

A. Due to independently coexisting disorders
B. Relationship is not as compensatory responses
C. Can lead to dangerous extremes of pH
D. None of the above

Mixed acid-base disorders are due to independently coexisting disorders and not merely as compensatory responses. They can lead to dangerous extremes of pH.

602. Which of the following indicate metabolic acidosis - respiratory acidosis?

Harrison's 20th Ed. Chapter 51 Page 316 Table 51-2

A. Na^+ 140; K^+ 4.0; Cl^- 106; HCO_3^- 14; AG 20; $PaCO_2$ 24; pH 7.39
B. Na^+ 140; K^+ 4.0; Cl^- 102; HCO_3^- 18; AG 20; $PaCO_2$ 38; pH 7.30
C. Na^+ 140; K^+ 4.0; Cl^- 91; HCO_3^- 33; AG 16; $PaCO_2$ 38; pH 7.55
D. Na^+ 140; K^+ 3.5; Cl^- 88; HCO_3^- 42; AG 10; $PaCO_2$ 67; pH 7.42

603. Which of the following indicate metabolic acidosis - respiratory alkalosis?

Harrison's 20th Ed. Chapter 51 Page 316 Table 51-2

A. Na^+ 140; K^+ 4.0; Cl^- 106; HCO_3^- 14; AG 20; $PaCO_2$ 24; pH 7.39
B. Na^+ 140; K^+ 4.0; Cl^- 102; HCO_3^- 18; AG 20; $PaCO_2$ 38; pH 7.30
C. Na^+ 140; K^+ 4.0; Cl^- 91; HCO_3^- 33; AG 16; $PaCO_2$ 38; pH 7.55
D. Na^+ 140; K^+ 3.5; Cl^- 88; HCO_3^- 42; AG 10; $PaCO_2$ 67; pH 7.42

604. Which of the following indicate metabolic alkalosis - respiratory alkalosis?

Harrison's 20th Ed. Chapter 51 Page 316 Table 51-2

A. Na^+ 140; K^+ 4.0; Cl^- 106; HCO_3^- 14; AG 20; $PaCO_2$ 24; pH 7.39
B. Na^+ 140; K^+ 4.0; Cl^- 102; HCO_3^- 18; AG 20; $PaCO_2$ 38; pH 7.30
C. Na^+ 140; K^+ 4.0; Cl^- 91; HCO_3^- 33; AG 16; $PaCO_2$ 38; pH 7.55
D. Na^+ 140; K^+ 3.5; Cl^- 88; HCO_3^- 42; AG 10; $PaCO_2$ 67; pH 7.42

605. Which of the following indicate metabolic alkalosis - respiratory acidosis?

Harrison's 20th Ed. Chapter 51 Page 316 Table 51-2

A. Na^+ 140; K^+ 4.0; Cl^- 106; HCO_3^- 14; AG 20; $PaCO_2$ 24; pH 7.39
B. Na^+ 140; K^+ 4.0; Cl^- 102; HCO_3^- 18; AG 20; $PaCO_2$ 38; pH 7.30
C. Na^+ 140; K^+ 4.0; Cl^- 91; HCO_3^- 33; AG 16; $PaCO_2$ 38; pH 7.55
D. Na^+ 140; K^+ 3.5; Cl^- 88; HCO_3^- 42; AG 10; $PaCO_2$ 67; pH 7.42

606. Which of the following indicate metabolic acidosis - metabolic alkalosis?

Harrison's 20th Ed. Chapter 51 Page 316 Table 51-2

A. Na^+ 140; K^+ 4.0; Cl^- 106; HCO_3^- 14; AG 20; $PaCO_2$ 24; pH 7.39
B. Na^+ 140; K^+ 3.0; Cl^- 95; HCO_3^- 25; AG 20; $PaCO_2$ 40; pH 7.42
C. Na^+ 140; K^+ 4.0; Cl^- 91; HCO_3^- 33; AG 16; $PaCO_2$ 38; pH 7.55
D. Na^+ 140; K^+ 3.5; Cl^- 88; HCO_3^- 42; AG 10; $PaCO_2$ 67; pH 7.42

607. Which of the following indicate metabolic acidosis - metabolic acidosis?

Harrison's 20th Ed. Chapter 51 Page 316 Table 51-2

A. Na^+ 140; K^+ 4.0; Cl^- 106; HCO_3^- 14; AG 20; $PaCO_2$ 24; pH 7.39
B. Na^+ 140; K^+ 3.0; Cl^- 95; HCO_3^- 25; AG 20; $PaCO_2$ 40; pH 7.42
C. Na^+ 135; K^+ 3.0; Cl^- 110; HCO_3^- 10; AG 15; $PaCO_2$ 25; pH 7.20
D. Na^+ 140; K^+ 3.5; Cl^- 88; HCO_3^- 42; AG 10; $PaCO_2$ 67; pH 7.42

608. Which acid-base disorder is expected in lactic acidosis or sepsis in ICU?

Harrison's 20th Ed. Chapter 51 Page 316 Table 51-2

A. Metabolic acidosis–respiratory alkalosis
B. Metabolic acidosis–respiratory acidosis
C. Metabolic acidosis–metabolic alkalosis
D. Metabolic acidosis–metabolic acidosis

609. Which acid-base disorder is expected in severe pneumonia or pulmonary edema?

Harrison's 20th Ed. Chapter 51 Page 316 Table 51-2

A. Metabolic acidosis–respiratory alkalosis
B. Metabolic acidosis–respiratory acidosis
C. Metabolic acidosis–metabolic alkalosis
D. Metabolic acidosis–metabolic acidosis

610. Which acid-base disorder is expected in liver disease and diuretics?

Harrison's 20th Ed. Chapter 51 Page 316 Table 51-2

A. Metabolic acidosis–respiratory alkalosis
B. Metabolic acidosis–respiratory acidosis
C. Metabolic alkalosis–respiratory alkalosis
D. Metabolic acidosis–metabolic acidosis

611. Which acid-base disorder is expected in COPD on diuretics?

Harrison's 20th Ed. Chapter 51 Page 316 Table 51-2

A. Metabolic acidosis–respiratory alkalosis
B. Metabolic acidosis–respiratory acidosis
C. Metabolic alkalosis–respiratory alkalosis
D. Metabolic alkalosis–respiratory acidosis

612. Which acid-base disorder is expected in uremia with vomiting?

Harrison's 20th Ed. Chapter 51 Page 316 Table 51-2

A. Metabolic acidosis–respiratory alkalosis
B. Metabolic acidosis–respiratory acidosis
C. Metabolic acidosis–metabolic alkalosis
D. Metabolic acidosis–metabolic acidosis

613. Which acid-base disorder is expected in treatment of diabetic ketoacidosis?

Harrison's 20th Ed. Chapter 51 Page 316 Table 51-2

A. Metabolic acidosis–respiratory alkalosis
B. Metabolic acidosis–respiratory acidosis
C. Metabolic acidosis–metabolic alkalosis
D. Metabolic acidosis–metabolic acidosis

614. In clinical laboratory, which of the following is calculated from the Henderson-Hasselbalch equation?

Harrison's 20th Ed. Chapter 51 Page 316

A. pH
B. $PaCO_2$
C. $[HCO_3^-]$
D. All of the above

In clinical laboratory, pH and $PaCO_2$ are measured and $[HCO_3^-]$ is calculated from Henderson-Hasselbalch equation.

615. Which of the following is not used in the calculation of AG?

Harrison's 20th Ed. Chapter 51 Page 317

A. Na^+
B. K^+
C. Cl^-
D. HCO_3^-

616. Anionic gap (AG) is calculated by?

Harrison's 20th Ed. Chapter 51 Page 317

A. $AG = Na^+ + (Cl^- - HCO_3^-)$
B. $AG = Na^+ - (Cl^- - HCO_3^-)$
C. $AG = Na^+ + (Cl^- + HCO_3^-)$
D. $AG = Na^+ - (Cl^- + HCO_3^-)$

AG represents unmeasured anions in plasma (normal range is from 6 to 12 mmol/L, with an average of ~10 mmol/L) and is calculated as $AG = Na^+ - (Cl^- + HCO_3^-)$.

617. Anion gap represents "unmeasured" anions like?

Harrison's 20th Ed. Chapter 51 Page 317

A. Anionic proteins (Albumin)
B. Phosphate
C. Sulfate
D. All of the above

Unmeasured anions include anionic proteins, phosphate, sulfate, and organic anions. Unmeasured cations include calcium, magnesium & potassium.

618. Increase in AG is most often due to?

Harrison's 20th Ed. Chapter 51 Page 317

A. Increase in unmeasured anions
B. Increase in measured anions
C. Decrease in unmeasured cations
D. Decrease in measured cations

Increase in AG is most often due to increase in unmeasured anions and less commonly due to decrease in unmeasured cations (Ca^{++}, Mg^{++}, K^+).

619. Increase in AG is due to?

Harrison's 20th Ed. Chapter 51 Page 317

A. Increase in unmeasured anions
B. Increase in acid anions
C. Decrease in unmeasured cations
D. All of the above

Acetoacetate and lactate are acid anions. Lithium is an abnormal cation. Plasma cell dyscrasias produce cationic immunoglobulins.

620. A fall in serum albumin by 1 g/dL from the normal value (4.5 g/dL) decreases the anion gap by?

Harrison's 20th Ed. Chapter 51 Page 317

A. 1.5 mEq/L
B. 2.0 mEq/L
C. 2.5 mEq/L
D. 3.0 mEq/L

A fall in serum albumin by 1 g/dL from normal value (4.5 g/dL) decreases anion gap by 2.5 mEq/L.

621. Normal values of which of the following ensures the absence of an acid-base disturbance?

Harrison's 20th Ed. Chapter 51 Page 317

A. HCO_3^-
B. $PaCO_2$
C. pH
D. None of the above

Normal values for $[HCO_3^-]$, $PaCO_2$ and pH do not ensure the absence of an acid-base disturbance.

622. In cases of high-AG metabolic acidosis, increase in the AG (ΔAG) must be compared to?

Harrison's 20th Ed. Chapter 51 Page 317

A. Decline in $[HCO_3^-]$ (ΔHCO_3^-)
B. Decline in [pH] (ΔpH)
C. Rise in PCO_2
D. All of the above

In cases of high-AG metabolic acidosis it is valuable to compare the decline in $[HCO_3^-]$ (ΔHCO_3^- i.e. 25 – patient's $[HCO_3^-]$) with the increase in the AG (ΔAG: patient's AG – 10).

623. In acid-base disturbances, changes in $[Cl^-]$ must be compared to?

Harrison's 20th Ed. Chapter 51 Page 317 Table 51-3

A. $[Na^+]$
B. $[K^+]$
C. $[HCO_3^-]$
D. All of the above

624. Metabolic acidosis can occur because of?

Harrison's 20th Ed. Chapter 51 Page 317

A. Increase in endogenous acid production
B. Loss of bicarbonate
C. Accumulation of endogenous acids
D. All of the above

Metabolic acidosis occurs due to an increase in endogenous acid production (lactate & ketoacids), loss of bicarbonate (diarrhea), or accumulation of endogenous acids (renal failure).

625. Metabolic acidosis has profound effect on which of the following systems?

Harrison's 20th Ed. Chapter 51 Page 317

A. Respiratory
B. Cardiac
C. Nervous
D. All of the above

Metabolic acidosis has profound effects on the respiratory, cardiac, and nervous systems.

626. Fall in blood pH is accompanied by?

Harrison's 20th Ed. Chapter 51 Page 317

A. Increase in ventilation
B. Peripheral arterial vasodilation
C. Central venoconstriction
D. All of the above

Fall in blood pH is accompanied by increase in tidal volume (Kussmaul respiration), peripheral arterial vasodilation & central venoconstriction.

627. Non-AG metabolic acidosis is also called?

Harrison's 20th Ed. Chapter 51 Page 317

A. Hyperchloremic acidosis
B. Hypochloremic acidosis
C. Hyperkalemic acidosis
D. Hypokalemic acidosis

Clinical metabolic acidosis is of two types - high-AG and non-AG or hyperchloremic acidosis.

628. Increment (Δ) in AG (ΔAG) is estimated by?

Harrison's 20th Ed. Chapter 51 Page 317

A. Patient's AG × 10
B. Patient's AG + 10
C. Patient's AG – 10
D. Patient's AG ÷ 10

Potential [HCO_3^-] can be estimated from the increment (Δ) in the AG (ΔAG = patient's AG – 10).

629. Which of the following acid anion in plasma is metabolizable?

Harrison's 20th Ed. Chapter 51 Page 317

A. β-hydroxybutyrate
B. Acetoacetate
C. Lactate
D. All of the above

Metabolizable acid anion in plasma are β-hydroxybutyrate, acetoacetate & lactate.

630. Which of the following can cause ketoacidosis?

Harrison's 20th Ed. Chapter 51 Page 317 Table 51-4

A. Diabetes mellitus
B. Alcohol
C. Starvation
D. All of the above

631. Which of the following toxins can cause high-anion gap metabolic acidosis?

Harrison's 20th Ed. Chapter 51 Page 317 Table 51-4

A. Ethylene glycol
B. Methanol
C. Salicylates
D. All of the above

632. Which of the following toxins can cause high-anion gap metabolic acidosis?

Harrison's 20th Ed. Chapter 51 Page 317 Table 51-4

A. Propylene glycol
B. Pyroglutamic acid (5-oxoproline)
C. Salicylates
D. All of the above

633. Shohl's solution is?

Harrison's 20th Ed. Chapter 51 Page 317

A. Neutral
B. Acidic
C. Alkaline
D. All of the above

634. Sodium salt in Shohl's solution is?

Harrison's 20th Ed. Chapter 51 Page 320

A. Chloride
B. Citrate
C. Bicarbonate
D. Sulphate

635. In a pure AG severe metabolic acidosis, goal is to increase the [HCO_3^-] to?

Harrison's 20th Ed. Chapter 51 Page 317

A. 10 mEq/L
B. 15 mEq/L
C. 20 mEq/L
D. 25 mEq/L

636. In a pure AG severe metabolic acidosis, goal is to increase the pH to?

Harrison's 20th Ed. Chapter 51 Page 317

A. 7.20
B. 7.25
C. 7.35
D. 7.45

In severe acidosis i.e. pH < 7.20, goal is to increase [HCO_3^-] to 10 mEq/L and pH to 7.20 and not to increase these values to normal.

637. Which of the following can cause high anion-gap metabolic acidosis?

Harrison's 20th Ed. Chapter 51 Page 317

A. Lactic acidosis, ketoacidosis
B. Acute and chronic renal failure
C. Ingested toxins & their metabolites
D. All of the above

638. Which of the following 'toxins' can cause high-anion-gap metabolic acidosis?

Harrison's 20th Ed. Chapter 51 Page 318

A. Ethylene glycol
B. Methanol
C. Salicylates
D. All of the above

639. Which of the following 'ketoacidosis' producing states can cause high-anion-gap metabolic acidosis?

Harrison's 20th Ed. Chapter 51 Page 318

A. Diabetic ketoacidosis
B. Alcoholic ketoacidosis
C. Starvation ketoacidosis
D. All of the above

640. Normal serum lactate level is?

Harrison's 20th Ed. Chapter 51 Page 318

A. 0.5–1.7 mmol/L
B. 1.7–2.3 mmol/L
C. 2.5–3.7 mmol/L
D. 3.5–4.7 mmol/L

Normal serum lactate level is 0.5–1.7 mmol/L.

641. Type A lactic acidosis is due to all except?

Harrison's 20th Ed. Chapter 51 Page 318

A. Severe anemia
B. Mitochondrial enzyme defects
C. Diabetes mellitus
D. Shock

642. Type B lactic acidosis is due to all except?

Harrison's 20th Ed. Chapter 51 Page 318

A. Renal failure
B. Hepatic failure
C. Circulatory failure
D. Carbon monoxide poisoning

643. Which of the following can cause Type B lactic acidosis?

Harrison's 20th Ed. Chapter 51 Page 318

A. Biguanides
B. Ethanol
C. Methanol
D. All of the above

644. Which of the following can cause Type B lactic acidosis?

Harrison's 20th Ed. Chapter 51 Page 318

A. Isoniazid
B. AZT analogues
C. Fructose
D. All of the above

Increase in plasma L-lactate may be secondary to poor tissue perfusion (type A) - circulatory insufficiency (shock, cardiac failure), severe anemia, mitochondrial enzyme defects, and inhibitors (carbon monoxide, cyanide) or to aerobic disorders (type B) - malignancies, NRTI drugs, DM, renal or hepatic failure, thiamine deficiency, infections, seizures, or drugs/toxins (biguanides, ethanol, methanol, propylene glycol, isoniazid, and fructose).

645. Pyroglutamic acidemia best relates to?

Harrison's 20th Ed. Chapter 51 Page 318

A. Isoniazid
B. AZT analogues
C. Biguanides
D. Acetaminophen

Pyroglutamic acidemia is seen in critically ill patients receiving acetaminophen, which is associated with depletion of glutathione.

646. D-Lactic acid acidosis may be associated with?

Harrison's 20th Ed. Chapter 51 Page 318

A. Jejunoileal bypass
B. Short bowel syndrome
C. Intestinal obstruction
D. All of the above

D-Lactic acid acidosis, which may be associated with jejunoileal bypass, short bowel syndrome or intestinal obstruction, is due to formation of D-lactate by gut bacteria.

647. HCO_3^- stimulates which of the following?

Harrison's 20th Ed. Chapter 51 Page 318

A. Fructose-1,6-biphosphatase
B. Fructose-2,6-biphosphatase
C. Phosphofructokinase
D. Phosphoglycerate kinase

HCO_3^- stimulates phosphofructokinase. Therefore, $NaHCO_3$ therapy in L-lactic acid acidosis may paradoxically depress cardiac performance and exacerbate acidosis by enhancing lactate production.

648. In DKA, the relationship between ΔAG and ΔHCO_3^- is typically?

Harrison's 20th Ed. Chapter 51 Page 318

A. ~1:1
B. ~1:2
C. ~1:3
D. ~1:4

In DKA, the relationship between ΔAG and ΔHCO_3^- is typically ~1:1.

649. Which of the following develops during treatment of DKA?

Harrison's 20th Ed. Chapter 51 Page 318

A. Hyperchloremic acidosis
B. Hyperchloremic alkalosis
C. Hypochloremic acidosis
D. Hypochloremic alkalosis

Volume overexpansion with IV fluid administration contributes to the development of a hyperchloremic acidosis during treatment of DKA.

650. Which of the following is false about alcoholic ketoacidosis (AKA)?

Harrison's 20th Ed. Chapter 51 Page 318

A. Occurs when alcohol consumption is abruptly curtailed
B. Elevated ketones are predominantly β-hydroxybutyrate
C. Mixed acid-base disorders are common
D. None of the above

651. The nitroprusside ketone reaction can detect?

Harrison's 20th Ed. Chapter 51 Page 318

A. Acetoacetic acid
B. β-hydroxybutyrate
C. Both A and B
D. None of the above

Nitroprusside ketone reaction can detect acetoacetic acid but not β-hydroxybutyrate, so the degree of ketosis and ketonuria can be underestimated.

652. Which of the following about alcoholic ketoacidosis is false?

Harrison's 20th Ed. Chapter 51 Page 318

A. Occurs in chronic alcoholics when alcohol consumption is abruptly curtailed
B. Associated with binge drinking, vomiting, starvation and volume depletion
C. Glucagon levels are decreased
D. Increasingly (+) nitroprusside reaction as patient improves

653. Which of the following about alcoholic ketoacidosis is false?

Harrison's 20th Ed. Chapter 51 Page 318

A. Acidosis is because of elevated β-hydroxybutyrate
B. Nitroprusside ketone reaction does not detect β-hydroxybutyrate
C. Insulin levels are high
D. Triglyceride levels are increased

Chronic alcoholics can develop ketoacidosis when alcohol consumption is abruptly curtailed and nutrition is poor. AKA is usually associated with binge drinking, vomiting, abdominal pain, starvation and volume depletion. Typically, insulin levels are low, and triglyceride, cortisol, glucagon and growth hormone levels are increased.

654. Which of the following is exacerbated by glucose infusion for treatment of alcoholic ketoacidosis (AKA)?

Harrison's 20th Ed. Chapter 51 Page 318

A. Hypophosphatemia
B. Hypokalemia
C. Hypomagnesemia
D. All of the above

Hypophosphatemia usually emerges 12–24 hours after admission and may be exacerbated by glucose infusion. If severe, may induce rhabdomyolysis. Hypophosphatemia, hypokalemia and hypomagnesemia may coexist in AKA.

655. Which of the following is used in the treatment of salicylate induced acidosis?

Harrison's 20th Ed. Chapter 51 Page 318

A. Activated charcoal
B. Acetazolamide
C. Sodium bicarbonate
D. All of the above

656. Which of the following should be anticipated with vigorous bicarbonate therapy?

Harrison's 20th Ed. Chapter 51 Page 319

A. Hyperkalemia
B. Hypokalemia
C. Hypernatremia
D. Hyponatremia

Hypokalemia should be anticipated with vigorous bicarbonate therapy.

657. Kidneys regulate plasma [HCO_3^-] by?

Harrison's 20th Ed. Chapter 51 Page 319

A. Reabsorption of filtered HCO_3^-
B. Formation of titratable acid
C. Excretion of NH_4^+ in urine
D. All of the above

658. Kidneys excrete how much HCO_3^- ions per day?

Harrison's 20th Ed. Chapter 51 Page 319

A. About 2000 mmol
B. About 3000 mmol
C. About 4000 mmol
D. About 5000 mmol

659. Kidneys excrete how much H^+ ions per day?

Harrison's 20th Ed. Chapter 51 Page 319

A. About 2000 mmol
B. About 3000 mmol
C. About 4000 mmol
D. About 5000 mmol

Kidney filters ~4000 mmol of HCO_3^- per day and to reabsorb this filtered load of HCO_3^-, renal tubules must secrete 4000 mmol of hydrogen ions.

660. Which part of nephron reabsorbs most of HCO_3^- ions?

Harrison's 20th Ed. Chapter 51 Page 319

A. Proximal convoluted tubule
B. Loop of Henle
C. Distal convoluted tubule
D. Collecting ducts

80–90% of HCO_3^- is reabsorbed in the proximal convoluted tubule of kidney.

661. NH_4^+ production & excretion are impaired in?

Harrison's 20th Ed. Chapter 51 Page 319

A. Chronic renal failure
B. Hyperkalemia
C. Renal tubular acidosis
D. All of the above

NH_4^+ production & excretion are impaired in chronic renal failure, hyperkalemia & renal tubular acidosis.

662. Normally, what quantity of H^+ is secreted daily by distal nephron?

Harrison's 20th Ed. Chapter 51 Page 319

A. 40–60 mmol
B. 60–80 mmol
C. 80–100 mmol
D. 100–120 mmol

Distal nephron reabsorbs remainder of filtered HCO_3^- and secretes 40–60 mmol/day of H^+.

663. Secreted H^+ is represented in the urine as?

Harrison's 20th Ed. Chapter 51 Page 319

A. NH_4^+
B. Titratable acid
C. Titratable acid & NH_4^+
D. All of the above

Secreted H^+ is represented in urine as titratable acid and NH_4^+.

664. Under most physiologic conditions, osmotic pressure of blood is generated by?

Harrison's 20th Ed. Chapter 51 Page 319

A. Sodium
B. Urea
C. Glucose
D. All of the above

Under most physiologic conditions, sodium, urea and glucose generate osmotic pressure of blood.

665. Plasma osmolality (P_{osm}) is calculated by?

Harrison's 20th Ed. Chapter 51 Page 319

A. P_{osm} = $2Na^+$ + Glucose (mmol/L) + Urea (mmol/L)
B. P_{osm} = $2Na^+$ + Glucose (mmol/L) + BUN (mmol/L)
C. P_{osm} = $2Na^+$ + Glucose (mmol/L) + (3 × Albumin)
D. P_{osm} = $2Na^+$ + 3Glucose (mmol/L)

Plasma osmolality (P_{osm}) = $2Na^+$ + Glucose (mmol/L) + BUN (mmol/L), or P_{osm} = $2Na^+$ + Glucose (mg/dL)/18 + BUN (mg/dL)/2.8.

666. Osmolar gap is calculated by?

Harrison's 20th Ed. Chapter 51 Page 319

A. Calculated osmolality–measured osmolality
B. $2Na^+$ + Glucose (mmol/L) + (3 × Albumin)
C. $2Na^+$ + 3Glucose (mmol/L)
D. $2Na^+$ + Glucose (mmol/L) + Urea (mmol/L)

Difference between calculated osmolality and measured osmolality is called osmolar gap and is proportional to concentration of unmeasured solute.

667. Unit of osmolality is?

Harrison's 20th Ed. Chapter 51 Page 319

A. mOsm/kg/H_2O
B. mOsm/kg/Plasma
C. mOsm/kg/Serum
D. mOsm/kg/Blood

Unit of osmolality is mOsm/kg/H_2O.

668. Which of the following is an osmolyte?

Harrison's 20th Ed. Chapter 51 Page 319

A. Mannitol
B. Methanol
C. Acetone
D. All of the above

Osmolytes include mannitol, radiocontrast media, ethanol, isopropyl alcohol, ethylene glycol, propylene glycol, methanol and acetone.

669. Which of the following can cause an elevated osmolal gap?

Harrison's 20th Ed. Chapter 51 Page 319

A. Ethylene glycol
B. Methanol
C. Isopropyl alcohol
D. All of the above

Ethylene glycol, methanol and isopropyl alcohol cause an elevated osmolal gap. Ethylene glycol and methanol cause a high-AG acidosis.

670. Which of the following is a metabolite of ethylene glycol?

Harrison's 20th Ed. Chapter 51 Page 319

A. Lactic acid
B. Tricarboxylic acid
C. Oxalic acid
D. Hydrochloric acid

Ethylene glycol (used in antifreeze) causes metabolic acidosis and damage to CNS, heart, lungs and kidneys. Its metabolites are oxalic acid, glycolic acid, and other organic acids.

671. Which of the following is false about ethylene glycol toxicity?

Harrison's 20th Ed. Chapter 51 Page 319

A. Oxalate crystals in urine
B. Presence of an osmolar gap in serum
C. High-AG acidosis
D. None of the above

672. Which of the following is useful in the treatment of ethylene glycol toxicity?

Harrison's 20th Ed. Chapter 51 Page 319

A. Thiamine supplements
B. Pyridoxine supplements
C. Fomepizole
D. All of the above

673. The chemical name of Fomepizole is?

Harrison's 20th Ed. Chapter 51 Page 319

A. 2-methylpyrazole
B. 3-methylpyrazole
C. 4-methylpyrazole
D. 5-methylpyrazole

674. Fomepizole is a?

Harrison's 20th Ed. Chapter 51 Page 319

A. Aldehyde dehydrogenase inhibitor
B. Alcohol dehydrogenase inhibitor
C. Ketone dehydrogenase inhibitor
D. None of the above

Fomepizole or 4-methylpyrazole is an alcohol dehydrogenase inhibitor. It is used to treat ethylene glycol induced acidosis in an IV loading dose of 15 mg/kg.

675. In ethylene glycol intoxication, ethanol IV should be infused to achieve a blood level of?

Harrison's 20th Ed. Chapter 51 Page 319

A. 10 mg/dL
B. 50 mg/dL
C. 100 mg/dL
D. 150 mg/dL

Ethanol IV should be infused to achieve a blood level of 100 mg/dL (22 mmol/L).

676. In ethylene glycol intoxication, hemodialysis is indicated when osmolar gap exceeds?

Harrison's 20th Ed. Chapter 51 Page 319

A. 10 mOsm/kg
B. 20 mOsm/kg
C. 30 mOsm/kg
D. 40 mOsm/kg

Hemodialysis is indicated when the arterial pH is < 7.3 or the osmolar gap exceeds 20 mOsm/kg.

677. Which of the following about methanol is false?

Harrison's 20th Ed. Chapter 51 Page 319

A. Also called 'wood alcohol'
B. Has high molecular weight
C. Metabolites include formaldehyde and formic acid
D. Intoxication cause severe optic nerve & CNS damage

Methanol or wood alcohol causes metabolic acidosis. Its metabolites formaldehyde & formic acid cause optic nerve & CNS damage. It has a low molecular weight (32 Da).

678. Which of the following is metabolized by alcohol dehydrogenase?

Harrison's 20th Ed. Chapter 51 Page 319

A. Propylene glycol
B. Ethylene glycol
C. Methanol
D. All of the above

Propylene glycol, ethylene glycol and methanol are metabolized by alcohol dehydrogenase.

679. AG acidosis is not present in which of the following?

Harrison's 20th Ed. Chapter 51 Page 319

A. Ethylene glycol ingestion
B. Isopropyl alcohol ingestion
C. Methanol ingestion
D. Acetaminophen

680. Isopropyl alcohol is metabolized by alcohol dehydrogenase to?

Harrison's 20th Ed. Chapter 51 Page 319

A. Acetone
B. Acetoacetic acid
C. β-hydroxybutyric acid
D. All of the above

Isopropyl alcohol is metabolized by alcohol dehydrogenase to acetone. In Isopropyl alcohol ingestion, acidosis is not present because acetone is rapidly excreted.

681. Which of the following about acetaminophen-induced acidosis is false?

Harrison's 20th Ed. Chapter 51 Page 319

A. High-AG metabolic acidosis
B. 5-Oxoproline accumulation
C. No elevation of osmolar gap
D. None of the above

682. Which of the following about uremic acidosis is false?

Harrison's 20th Ed. Chapter 51 Page 319

A. Reduced rate of NH_4^+ production and excretion
B. $[HCO_3^-]$ levels rarely < 15 mmol/L
C. Anion gap (AG) rarely > 20 mmol/L
D. None of the above

Uremic acidosis is characterized by reduced rate of NH_4^+ production & excretion due to decreased renal mass. $[HCO_3^-]$ rarely falls to <15 mmol/L and AG is rarely >20 mmol/L.

683. Urine anion gap (UAG) is calculated by the formula?

Harrison's 20th Ed. Chapter 51 Page 320

A. $[Na^+ + K^+]_u/[Cl^-]_u$
B. $[Na^+ + K^+]_u \times [Cl^-]_u$
C. $[Na^+ + K^+]_u - [Cl^-]_u$
D. $[Na^+ + K^+]_u + [Cl^-]_u$

Urinary NH_4^+ levels are estimated by urine anion gap (UAG) i.e. $[Na^+ + K^+]_u - [Cl^-]_u$. Under normal circumstances, the UAG is positive due to the presence of dissolved anions. When $[Cl^-]_u > [Na^+ + K^+]$, the UAG is negative which indicates that urine ammonium level is appropriately increased, suggesting an extrarenal cause of the acidosis. When urine anion gap is positive, urine ammonium level is low, suggesting a renal cause of acidosis. Because urinary ammonia is not directly measured by the clinical laboratory, it is estimated by measuring UAG or urine osmolar gap. Both calculations only give a qualitative and not a quantitative measure of urinary ammonia. The usual UAG ranges from 20–90 mEq/L and NH_4^+ = 80 – UAG.

684. Which of the following is the correct Winter's formula for expected CO_2?

Clin J Am Soc Nephrol. 2012;7:1-8

A. (Bicarbonate × 1.3) + 8 ± 2
B. (Bicarbonate × 1.4) + 8 ± 2
C. (Bicarbonate × 1.5) + 8 ± 2
D. (Bicarbonate × 1.6) + 8 ± 2

Winter's formula for calculating expected CO_2 is (Bicarbonate × 1.5) + 8 ± 2.

685. Which of the following statements is false?

Clin J Am Soc Nephrol. 2012;7:1-8

A. Anion gaps of 25 or greater deserve a thorough evaluation
B. Winter's equation helps for appropriate respiratory response
C. Delta gap used to diagnose a "double" metabolic abnormality
D. None of the above

686. Which of the following about Delta gap is false?

Clin J Am Soc Nephrol. 2012;7:1-8

A. Delta gap is defined as rise in AG minus fall in bicarbonate
B. Delta gap = (change in anion gap)–(change in bicarbonate)
C. Delta gap = $(Na^+ - Cl^-)$–36
D. None of the above

687. Which of the following interpretations of generated delta ratio is false?

Clin J Am Soc Nephrol. 2012;7:1-8

A. –6 = Mixed high and normal anion gap acidosis
B. –6 to 6 = Only a high anion gap acidosis exists
C. > 6 = Mixed high anion gap acidosis and metabolic alkalosis
D. None of the above

Delta gap = Delta AG – Delta HCO_3 = (AG-12) – (24-bicarbonate) Or Delta Gap = Anion Gap - Baseline Gap. Delta HCO_3 = 25 - HCO_3, Delta Gradient = Delta Gap - Delta HCO_3. If Delta gap is < -6, then a NAGMA is present. If the gap is > 6, then an underlying metabolic alkalosis is present. If the gap is between -6 & 6, then only an anion gap acidosis exists.

688. Which of the following about Delta gap is false?
Clin J Am Soc Nephrol. 2012;7:1-8

A. Delta ratio = (Decrease in Anion Gap/Increase in bicarbonate)
B. Delta ratio = (change in anion gap)/(change in bicarbonate)
C. Delta gap is defined as rise in AG minus the fall in bicarbonate
D. The normal value for delta gap is zero

Delta ratio = (Increase in Anion Gap/Decrease in bicarbonate). The normal value for delta gap is zero, and it should remain zero as anion gap and bicarbonate change together (mole for mole, in opposite directions). If the bicarbonate is changing significantly less than the anion gap, the delta gap will become more and more positive, reflecting that an alkalosis is present. If the change in bicarbonate is significantly greater than the change in anion gap, there is clearly some acidosis present which is unrelated to the anion gap rise, and the delta gap will be very negative.

689. Which of the following values of delta ratio indicates purely due to a high anion gap metabolic acidosis?
Clin J Am Soc Nephrol. 2012;7:1-8

A. 0.4
B. 0.4–0.8
C. 0.8–1.0
D. > 2.0

Interpretation of the generated delta ratio is : 0.4 = normal anion gap metabolic acidosis, 0.4–0.8 = mixed high and normal anion gap acidosis exists, 0.8–1.0 = purely due to a high anion gap metabolic acidosis, 1.0–2.0 = still purely a high anion gap metabolic acidosis, Over 2.0 = high anion gap acidosis with pre-existing metabolic alkalosis.

690. Delta Gradient significantly > 0 usually indicates?
Clin J Am Soc Nephrol. 2012;7:1-8

A. A mixed high anion gap metabolic acidosis plus a primary metabolic alkalosis
B. A mixed high anion gap metabolic acidosis plus a chronic respiratory acidosis
C. A non-acidotic high anion gap state (excess penicillin)
D. All of the above

691. Delta Gradient significantly < 0 may result from?
Clin J Am Soc Nephrol. 2012;7:1-8

A. A mixed high anion gap metabolic acidosis plus a normal anion gap metabolic acidosis
B. A mixture of high anion gap metabolic acidosis plus chronic respiratory alkalosis plus hyperchloremia acidosis
C. A high anion gap acidosis with a pre-existing low anion gap state (hypoalbuminemia, para-proteinemia)
D. All of the above

A simple high anion gap metabolic acidosis produces a Delta Gradient around 0.

692. Which of the following statements is false?
Harrison's 20th Ed. Chapter 51 Page 320

A. Kidneys acidify urine by secreting NH_4^+
B. NH_4^+ is usually secreted coupled to Cl^-
C. Urinary Cl provides an indirect measurement of NH_4^+ secretion
D. None of the above

The kidneys acidify urine by secreting NH_4^+, which is usually secreted coupled to Cl^-. Therefore, urinary Cl^- provides an indirect measurement of NH_4^+ secretion.

693. Vomiting is a clue to which of the following acid-base disorder?
Harrison's 20th Ed. Chapter 51 Page 320

A. Metabolic acidosis
B. Metabolic alkalosis
C. Respiratory acidosis
D. Respiratory alkalosis

694. History of smoking/COPD is a clue to which of the following acid-base disorder?
Harrison's 20th Ed. Chapter 51 Page 320

A. Metabolic acidosis
B. Metabolic alkalosis
C. Respiratory acidosis
D. Respiratory alkalosis

695. History of liver disease is a clue to which of the following acid-base disorder?
Harrison's 20th Ed. Chapter 51 Page 320

A. Metabolic acidosis
B. Metabolic alkalosis
C. Respiratory acidosis
D. Respiratory alkalosis

696. Tachypnea is a clue to which of the following acid-base disorder?
Harrison's 20th Ed. Chapter 51 Page 320

A. Metabolic acidosis
B. Metabolic alkalosis
C. Respiratory acidosis
D. Respiratory alkalosis

697. In acidemia, which of the following looks like a laboratory error?
Harrison's 20th Ed. Chapter 51 Page 320

A. Low HCO_3^-, High PCO_2
B. Low HCO_3^-, Low PCO_2
C. High HCO_3^-, High PCO_2
D. High HCO_3^-, Low PCO_2

698. In acidemia, which of the following suggests predominant respiratory acidosis?
Harrison's 20th Ed. Chapter 51 Page 320

A. Low HCO_3^-, High PCO_2
B. Low HCO_3^-, Low PCO_2
C. High HCO_3^-, High PCO_2
D. High HCO_3^-, Low PCO_2

699. In acidemia, which of the following suggests predominant metabolic acidosis?
Harrison's 20th Ed. Chapter 51 Page 320

A. Low HCO_3^-, High PCO_2
B. Low HCO_3^-, Low PCO_2
C. High HCO_3^-, High PCO_2
D. High HCO_3^-, Low PCO_2

700. In acidemia, which of the following suggests mixed metabolic acidosis and respiratory acidosis?

Harrison's 20th Ed. Chapter 51 Page 320

A. Low HCO_3^-, High PCO_2
B. Low HCO_3^-, Low PCO_2
C. High HCO_3^-, High PCO_2
D. High HCO_3^-, Low PCO_2

701. In alkalemia, which of the following looks like a laboratory error?

Harrison's 20th Ed. Chapter 51 Page 320

A. Low HCO_3^-, High PCO_2
B. Low HCO_3^-, Low PCO_2
C. High HCO_3^-, High PCO_2
D. High HCO_3^-, Low PCO_2

702. In alkalemia, which of the following suggests predominant respiratory alkalosis?

Harrison's 20th Ed. Chapter 51 Page 320

A. Low HCO_3^-, High PCO_2
B. Low HCO_3^-, Low PCO_2
C. High HCO_3^-, High PCO_2
D. High HCO_3^-, Low PCO_2

703. In alkalemia, which of the following suggests predominant metabolic alkalosis?

Harrison's 20th Ed. Chapter 51 Page 320

A. Low HCO_3^-, High PCO_2
B. Low HCO_3^-, Low PCO_2
C. High HCO_3^-, High PCO_2
D. High HCO_3^-, Low PCO_2

704. In alkalemia, which of the following suggests mixed metabolic alkalosis and respiratory alkalosis?

Harrison's 20th Ed. Chapter 51 Page 320

A. Low HCO_3^-, High PCO_2
B. Low HCO_3^-, Low PCO_2
C. High HCO_3^-, High PCO_2
D. High HCO_3^-, Low PCO_2

705. Under normal conditions in individuals with a normal acid-base status, the average urinary pH is?

Harrison's 20th Ed. Chapter 51 Page 320

A. 3–4
B. 4–5
C. 5–6
D. 6–7

Under normal conditions in individuals with a normal acid-base status, the average urinary pH is 5–6. In patients with hyperchloremic metabolic acidosis & alkaline urine, considered as urine pH >5.5, RTA of some type is strongly suggested.

706. 'Extrarenal cause' of acidosis is suggested by?

Harrison's 20th Ed. Chapter 51 Page 320

A. Negative urine anion gap (UAG)
B. Positive urine anion gap
C. Zero urine anion gap
D. All of the above

707. Which of the following about renal tubular acidosis is false?

Harrison's 20th Ed. Chapter 51 Page 320

A. Can be inherited or acquired
B. Kidney's ability to reabsorb HCO_3^- or excreted NH_3 affected
C. Normal anionic gap (Hyperchloremic)
D. None of the above

In RTA, the capacity for normal urinary acidification is impaired, resulting in net acid retention and hyperchloremic metabolic acidosis. The defining feature of most cases of RTA is impaired renal acid-base buffering and the development of non-anion gap metabolic acidosis, renal performance is otherwise satisfactory.

708. Which of the following about renal tubular acidosis is false?

Harrison's 20th Ed. Chapter 51 Page 320

A. Limited urinary acid secretion is feature of Distal RTA
B. Restricted urinary HCO_3^- reabsorption is a feature of proximal RTA
C. Hypoaldosteronism hyperkalemic is feature of Type 4 RTA
D. None of the above

The 3 major forms of RTA are classified by their respective tubular transport defects, each of which produces persistent hyperchloremic metabolic acidosis. Distal RTA is characterized by limited urinary acid secretion, proximal RTA by restricted urinary bicarbonate reabsorption, and hyperkalemic RTA by hypoaldosteronism.

709. Fanconi syndrome is characterized by?

Harrison's 20th Ed. Chapter 51 Page 320

A. Glycosuria
B. Generalized aminoaciduria
C. Phosphaturia
D. All of the above

Fanconi syndrome refers to glycosuria, generalized aminoaciduria, and phosphaturia due to generalized proximal tubular dysfunction (type 2 RTA). Fanconi syndrome is a malabsorptive state of the proximal convoluted tubules, while proximal RTA refers only to the deficiency in HCO_3^- retention. Nutritional deficiencies typical of Fanconi syndrome include hypophosphatemia, hyponatremia, and rarely, hypoglycemia or hypoproteinemia.

710. Disorder associated with proximal RTA and Fanconi syndrome is?

Harrison's 20th Ed. Chapter 51 Page 320

A. Cystinosis
B. Lowe's syndrome
C. Wilson's disease
D. All of the above

Disorders that are associated with proximal RTA and Fanconi syndrome should be specifically screened for, including cystinosis, Lowe's syndrome, galactosemia and Wilson's disease.

711. Which of the following syndrome is associated with distal RTA?

Harrison's 20th Ed. Chapter 51 Page 320

A. Restless leg syndrome
B. Sjögren's syndrome
C. Hungry bone syndrome
D. Alport's syndrome

712. Which of the following about distal RTA (type 1 RTA) is false?

Harrison's 20th Ed. Chapter 51 Page 320

A. Lifelong disease
B. Frequent manifestation is nephrolithiasis during adolescence
C. Inability of kidneys to excrete hydrogen (H^+)
D. None of the above

713. Typical findings in classic distal RTA (type 1 RTA) include?
Harrison's 20th Ed. Chapter 51 Page 320

A. Hypokalemia
B. Low urinary NH_4^+ excretion
C. Urine pH > 5.5
D. All of the above

714. The typical findings in classic distal RTA (type 1 RTA) include all except?
Harrison's 20th Ed. Chapter 51 Page 320

A. Hyperkalemia
B. Non-AG metabolic acidosis
C. Low urinary NH_4^+ excretion
D. High urine pH

Typical findings of classic distal RTA (type 1 RTA) include hypokalemia, hyperchloremic acidosis or non-AG metabolic acidosis, low urinary NH_4^+ excretion (positive UAG, low urine $[NH_4^+]$), and high urine pH (pH > 5.5).

715. Hyperkalemia is indicative of which of the following RTA?
Harrison's 20th Ed. Chapter 51 Page 320

A. Distal RTA
B. Proximal RTA
C. Mixed RTA
D. Hypoaldosteronism RTA

Hypokalemia is characteristic of distal RTA & proximal RTA, while hyperkalemia is indicative of hyperkalemic RTA. The acidosis is thought to be induced by hyperkalemia that retards urinary NH_4^+ excretion.

716. Findings in classic distal RTA (type 1 RTA) include?
Harrison's 20th Ed. Chapter 51 Page 320

A. Nephrolithiasis
B. Nephrocalcinosis
C. Bone disease
D. All of the above

Most patients have hypocitraturia and hypercalciuria, so nephrolithiasis, nephrocalcinosis and bone disease are common.

717. Type 1 RTA may be associated with?
Harrison's 20th Ed. Chapter 51 Page 320

A. Systemic lupus erythematosus
B. Sjogren syndrome
C. Chronic hepatitis
D. All of the above

Type 1 RTA in older children may be associated with systemic lupus erythematosus, Sjogren syndrome or chronic hepatitis.

718. Which of the following renal tubular acidosis type is rare?
Harrison's 20th Ed. Chapter 51 Page 320

A. 1
B. 2
C. 3
D. 4

719. Serum anion gap is normal in which of the following renal tubular acidosis (RTA) type?
Harrison's 20th Ed. Chapter 51 Page 320

A. 1
B. 2
C. 4
D. All of the above

Inherited renal tubular acidosis presents as nonanion gap (hyperchloremic) metabolic acidosis from proximal tubular bicarbonate wasting or impaired distal net acid excretion.

720. Hereditary diseases that cause type 1 RTA include?
Harrison's 20th Ed. Chapter 51 Page 320

A. Ehler-Danlos syndrome
B. Fabry's disease
C. Wilson's disease
D. All of the above

721. Systemic disorder that cause type 1 RTA include?
Harrison's 20th Ed. Chapter 51 Page 320

A. Sjogren's syndrome
B. Chronic active hepatitis
C. Lupus
D. All of the above

722. Which of the following inherited disorders produce Type 2 (Proximal) RTA?
Harrison's 20th Ed. Chapter 51 Page 320

A. Wilson's disease
B. Cystinosis
C. Glycogen storage disease type I
D. All of the above

Inherited disorders that produce Type 2 (Proximal) RTA are Wilson's disease, cystinosis, tyrosinemia, galactosemia, hereditary fructose intolerance, glycogen storage disease type I, and Lowe's syndrome.

723. Serum potassium is high in which of the following RTA?
Harrison's 20th Ed. Chapter 51 Page 320

A. 1
B. 2
C. 4
D. All of the above

Type 4 RTA is acquired in association with moderate renal dysfunction & is characterized by hyperkalemia.

724. Drug-induced type 4 RTA is due to which of the following drugs?
Harrison's 20th Ed. Chapter 51 Page 320

A. NSAIDs
B. ACE inhibitors
C. Heparin
D. All of the above

725. Which of the following statements is false?
Harrison's 20th Ed. Chapter 51 Page 320

A. Type 1 RTA is due to impaired H^+ ion secretion or HCO_3^- reabsorption in distal nephron
B. Type 2 RTA is due to impaired HCO_3^- reabsorption in proximal tubule
C. Type 1 RTA may present as "marble-brain disease"
D. None of the above

726. Marble-brain disease consists of?

Journal of Molecular Biology 2004;342(2):619-633

A. Osteopetrosis
B. Short stature
C. Mental retardation
D. All of the above

727. Marble-brain disease is due to mutations in?

Journal of Molecular Biology 2004;342(2):619-633

A. CA2
B. SLC3A1
C. SLC6A19
D. CLCN5

Marble-brain disease consists of osteopetrosis, short stature, and mental retardation with dRTA. It is due to mutations in CA2 (carbonic anhydrase II).

728. Which of the following is not a feature of Type 1 (Distal) RTA?

Harrison's 20th Ed. Chapter 51 Page 320

A. Hypokalemia
B. Hypocitraturia
C. Hypocalciuria
D. Rickets or osteomalacia

Type 1 (Distal) RTA presents as hypokalemia, hypocitraturia, hypercalciuria, nephrocalcinosis, nephrolithiasis. Chronic untreated acidosis may lead to rickets or osteomalacia.

729. In Type 1 (Distal) RTA, patients fail to acidify urine to pH?

Harrison's 20th Ed. Chapter 51 Page 320

A. < 5.5
B. < 6.5
C. < 7.0
D. < 7.5

In Type 1 (Distal) RTA, patients fail to acidify urine to pH <5.5 even after acid loading with oral ammonium chloride or calcium chloride.

730. Which of the following stone is formed in Type 1 (Distal) RTA?

Harrison's 20th Ed. Chapter 51 Page 320

A. Uric acid
B. Cystine
C. Calcium oxalate
D. Calcium phosphate

Increased proximal citrate absorption leads to hypocitraturia and together with hypercalciuria predisposes to nephrocalcinosis & calcium phosphate stone formation.

731. Bicarbonate replacement dose in Type 1 (Distal) RTA is?

Harrison's 20th Ed. Chapter 51 Page 320

A. 0.2–1 mmol/kg/day
B. 1–3 mmol/kg/day
C. 3–5 mmol/kg/day
D. 5–10 mmol/kg/day

In Type 1 (Distal) RTA, bicarbonate replacement dose is 1–3 mmol/kg/day in divided doses. While, in Type 2 (proximal) RTA the dose is 5–15 mmol/kg/day along with supplemental potassium & vitamin D.

732. Renal glucosuria is due to mutations in which gene?

Harrison's 20th Ed. Chapter 51 Page 320

A. SLC6A19
B. SLC5A2
C. SLC3A1
D. SLC7A9

Renal isolated glucosuria with normal blood glucose concentration is due to mutations in SLC5A2 gene that encodes sodium-glucose co-transporter SGLT2 in the proximal renal tubule.

733. Low-molecular-weight proteinuria is a feature of?

Harrison's 20th Ed. Chapter 303 Page 2095

A. Renal glucosuria
B. Hartnup disease
C. Cystinuria
D. Dent's disease

Low-molecular-weight proteinuria, hypercalciuria, nephrocalcinosis and nephrolithiasis are features of Dent's disease.

734. Cerebellar ataxia & pellagra-like skin lesions are a feature of?

Harrison's 20th Ed. Chapter 414 Page 3023

A. Renal glucosuria
B. Hartnup disease
C. Cystinuria
D. Dent's disease

In Hartnup disease, tryptophan is retained in intestinal lumen & converted to indole compounds that are toxic to CNS. Consequent niacin deficiency leads to skin manifestations.

735. Inherited systemic disorders associated with Fanconi syndrome include?

Harrison's 20th Ed. Chapter 410 Page 3001

A. Wilson's disease
B. Galactosemia
C. Tyrosinemia
D. All of the above

736. Acquired disorders associated with Fanconi syndrome include?

Harrison's 20th Ed. Chapter 410 Page 3001

A. Multiple myeloma
B. Heavy metal toxicity
C. Chemotherapeutic drugs
D. All of the above

737. Which of the following RTA is principally associated with carbonic anhydrase II deficiency?

Harrison's 20th Ed. Chapter 51 Page 320

A. Distal RTA
B. Proximal RTA
C. Mixed RTA
D. Hypoaldosteronism RTA

Type 3 RTA is a mixed syndrome that has diagnostic findings characteristic of both distal & proximal RTA. Type 3 RTA manifests with debilitating congenital syndromes in children and is principally associated with carbonic anhydrase II deficiency.

738. Which of the following is type 4 renal tubular acidosis?

Harrison's 20th Ed. Chapter 51 Page 320

A. Distal RTA
B. Proximal RTA
C. Mixed RTA
D. Hypoaldosteronism RTA

Distal RTA is Type 1, Proximal RTA is Type 2, Mixed RTA is Type 3 (combined pRTA & dRTA), & Hypoaldosteronism RTA is Type 4.

739. Which of the following is false about hyperkalemic RTA?
Harrison's 20th Ed. Chapter 51 Page 320

A. Consequence of aldosterone deficiency or insensitivity
B. Occurs more frequently in adults than children
C. Usually an acquired rather than a heritable defect
D. None of the above

740. Clinical features that suggest RTA include all except?
Harrison's 20th Ed. Chapter 51 Page 320

A. Mental retardation
B. Polyuria
C. Polydipsia
D. Refractory rickets

Clinical features that suggest RTA include growth retardation, failure to thrive, polyuria, polydipsia, preference for savory foods and refractory rickets.

741. Mnemonic "MUDPILES" is to remember causes of?
Lancet. 2008;327 Issue 9642:892

A. Metabolic acidosis
B. Metabolic alkalosis
C. Respiratory acidosis
D. Respiratory alkalosis

Useful to memorize causes of anion gap metabolic acidemias. Letters in MUDPILES represent methanol, uremia, diabetic & alcoholic ketoacidosis, paraldehyde, iron or isoniazid (INH), lactic acidemia, ethylene glycol toxicity, and salicylates. Paraldehyde can be replaced with propylene glycol.

742. In mnemonic "KUSMALE" for metabolic acidosis, "M" stands for?
Lancet. 2008;327 Issue 9642:892

A. Methanol
B. Medication
C. Male
D. None of the above

Mnemonic KUSMALE for metabolic acidosis represents Ketoacidosis, Uremia, Salicylate poisoning, Methanol, Aldehyde (paraldehyde), Lactate, and Ethylene glycol.

743. In mnemonic "GOLD MARK" for metabolic acidosis, "O" stands for?
Lancet. 2008;327 Issue 9642:892

A. Oxyphenbutazone
B. Ofloxacin
C. Oxoproline
D. Omega 3 fatty acids

GOLD MARK mnemonic for anion-gap metabolic acidoses represents Glycols (ethylene and propylene), Oxoproline, L-lactate, D-lactate, Methanol, Aspirin, Renal failure, and Ketoacidosis.

744. In mnemonic "CAT MUDPILES" for anion gap metabolic acidosis differential, "C" stands for?
Lancet. 2008;327 Issue 9642:892

A. Carbon monoxide
B. Calcium
C. Cholesterol
D. Cancer

Mnemonic "CAT MUDPILES" for anion gap metabolic acidosis differential is Cyanide and carbon monoxide poisoning, Arsenic, Toluene, Methanol, Metformin, Uremia, DKA, Paraldehyde, Iron, INH, Lactate, Ethylene glycol, Salicylates.

745. In mnemonic "KULT IMPACT" for anion gap metabolic acidosis differential, "K" stands for?
Lancet. 2008;327 Issue 9642:892

A. Ketones
B. Kidney failure
C. Potassium
D. KIM-1

"KULT IMPACT", provides a practical and organized way of remembering the differential of metabolic acidosis. Ketones: diabetic ketoacidosis (DKA), alcoholic ketoacidosis, starvation ketoacidosis, Uremia, Lactate, Toxins, Iron, Isoniazid, Metformin, Phenformin, Paraldehyde, Aspirin, Acetaminophen, Alcohols (toxic), Cyanide, Carbon, Toluene

746. In mnemonic "KARMEL" for anion gap metabolic acidosis differential, "A" stands for?
Lancet. 2008;327 Issue 9642:892

A. Aspirin
B. Alcohol
C. Aldehyde
D. Acidoses

Mnemonic KARMEL stands for Ketoacidosis, Aspirin, Renal failure, Methanol, Ethylene glycol, Lactic acidosis.

747. In mnemonic "KUPIN" for anion gap metabolic acidosis differential, "I" stands for?
Lancet. 2008;327 Issue 9642:892

A. Iron
B. Isoniazid
C. Ingestion
D. Inhalation

Mnemonic KUPIN stands for Ketoacidosis (DKA, AKA), Uremia, Production (Lactic acidosis), Ingestion (Ethylene glycol, methanol), Need to Remember Drugs (aspirin, Metformin).

748. In mnemonic "DUMPSALE" for anion gap metabolic acidosis differential, "S" stands for?
Lancet. 2008;327 Issue 9642:892

A. Starvation
B. Salicylates
C. Salt
D. All of the above

Mnemonic DUMPSALE was proposed by of D. Robert Dufour. "I" of MUDPILES was omitted as "I" are exceedingly rare in clinical practice. DUMPSALE stands for Diabetic ketoacidosis, Uremia, Methanol, Paraldehyde, Salicylates, Alcoholic ketoacidosis, Lactic acidosis, Ethylene Glycol.

749. In mnemonic "ACE GIFT" for anion gap metabolic acidosis differential, "C" stands for?
Lancet. 2008;327 Issue 9642:892

A. Chronic renal failure
B. Cystatin C
C. Cyanide
D. Chloroform

Mnemonic for the toxins is ACE GIFTs: Aspirin, Cyanide, Ethanolic ketosis, Glycols (ethylene & propylene), Isoniazid, Ferrous iron, Toluene. Most of these cause a lactic acidosis.

750. Mnemonic "HARD POPS" is to remember causes of?

Lancet. 2008;327 Issue 9642:892

A. Anion gap metabolic acidosis
B. Non-anion gap metabolic acidosis
C. Respiratory acidosis
D. Respiratory alkalosis

Mnemonic "HARD POPS" stands for hyperalimentation (resulting from amino acid load in TPN), Amphotericin, Acetazolamide, Renal failure, RTA (type I, II, IV), diarrhea, Pancreatic fistula, Obstructive uropathy (RTA IV), PEE (ureteroenteric drain/ileal conduit), Saline.

751. Which condition does not cause anion gap acidosis?

Harrison's 20th Ed. Chapter 51 Page 320

A. Alcohol
B. Diabetic ketoacidosis
C. Lactic acid
D. Acetazolamide

Anion gap acidosis can be due to alcohol, methanol, diabetic ketoacidosis, iron, isoniazid, lactic acid, ethylene glycol, carbamazepine, aspirin, and toluene. Acetazolamide causes non-anion gap acidosis. Other causes of non-anion gap acidosis are hyperalimentation, renal tubular acidosis, diarrhea, spironolactone, and pancreatic fistula. Lactic acid is the most common cause of metabolic acidosis.

752. Which of the following does not cause a non-anion gap acidosis?

Harrison's 20th Ed. Chapter 51 Page 320

A. Total parenteral nutrition
B. Intense exercise
C. Acetazolamide
D. Pancreatic fistula

Diarrhea is the most common cause of non-anion gap acidosis. During exercise, there is a build up of lactate and the acidosis is that of anion gap. Other causes of non-anion gap acidosis include total parenteral nutrition, acetazolamide, and renal tubular acidosis. Enteric fistulas and pancreatico-duodenal fistulas are abdominal causes of non-anion gap acidosis.

753. Which of the following pairs is not correctly associated?

Harrison's 20th Ed. Chapter 51 Page 320

A. Metabolic alkalosis with mild dehydration
B. Non-anion gap metabolic acidosis and hypokalemia with hyperalimentation solutions
C. Hypokalemia and metabolic alkalosis with urinary chloride > 20 mEq/L
D. Metabolic alkalosis and urinary chloride < 20 mEq/L with infusion of normal saline

There are two types of non-anion gap metabolic acidosis. The first is due to a bicarbonate deficit and usually is associated with low serum potassium. This can occur with pancreatic fistulas, renal tubular acidosis, or diarrhea. The second is caused by an excess of chloride anion but serum potassium usually is normal. Common causes of this second type of non-anion gap metabolic acidosis include large volumes of normal saline for resuscitation and excess chloride salts in hyperalimentation solutions.

754. What type of metabolic acidosis is associated with diarrhea?

Harrison's 20th Ed. Chapter 51 Page 320

A. Normal anion gap
B. Anion gap of 20
C. Anion gap of 15
D. Anion gap of 25

A normal anion gap is usually seen with diarrhea causing metabolic acidosis. The anion gap is elevated if it is greater than 16. To calculate the anion gap the formula [Na]-[Cl]+[HCO_3] is used. The anions that aren't measure and create the gap are calcium, magnesium, gamma globulins, and potassium.

755. Which of the following electrolyte abnormalities is associated with metabolic acidosis?

Harrison's 20th Ed. Chapter 51 Page 320

A. Hypokalemia
B. Hyperkalemia
C. Hypercalcemia
D. Hypocalcemia

Acidosis results in the shift of potassium into the extracellular space. This results in hyperkalemia. This is seen in diabetic ketoacidosis. Administration of insulin to treat DKA causes the potassium to shift back into the cells and can create a state of hypokalemia.

756. Which of the following laboratory results is not consistent with a metabolic acidosis with respiratory compensation?

Harrison's 20th Ed. Chapter 51 Page 320

A. Arterial pH of 7.32
B. PCO_2 of 33 mm Hg
C. PO_2 of 110 mm Hg
D. Serum bicarbonate concentration of 20 mEq/L

An arterial pH of 7.32 indicates mild acidosis. A PCO_2 of 33 mm Hg indicates hypocapnia. The combination of acidosis with hypocapnia indicates that the hypocapnia is most likely compensatory and one would expect a lower PO_2. Serum bicarbonate of 20 is mildly elevated.

757. Which of the following findings is not present in metabolic acidosis?

Harrison's 20th Ed. Chapter 51 Page 320

A. pH of 7.25
B. PCO_2 of 30 mm Hg
C. PO_2 of 70 mm Hg
D. PCO_2 of 60 mm Hg

Metabolic acidosis is primarily noticed by reduced pH and increased HCO_3. This leads to compensatory hyperventilation and loss of PCO_2. A PCO_2 of 60 is not seen in such cases. The level of PCO_2 is actually expected to be lower.

758. A patient with pH=7.34, PCO_2 = 31, HCO_3 = 20 has what type of acid-base imbalance?

Harrison's 20th Ed. Chapter 51 Page 320

A. Compensated metabolic alkalosis
B. Compensated respiratory acidosis
C. Compensated respiratory alkalosis
D. Compensated metabolic acidosis

The correct interpretation is compensated metabolic acidosis. Normal PCO_2 is 35–45. The PCO_2 is decreased because the patient is compensating for the acidosis by breathing more quickly and reducing the amount of CO_2. Normal HCO_3 is 22–26. Bicarbonate is lost in the urine as a buffer during metabolic acidosis. Since the pH is normal, the acid-base balance is compensated.

759. Which of the following would explain an arterial blood gas with a pH of 7.36, PO_2 of 105, PCO_2 of 32 mm Hg, and bicarbonate of 17 mEq/L?

Harrison's 20th Ed. Chapter 51 Page 320

A. Respiratory and metabolic acidosis
B. Metabolic acidosis with respiratory compensation
C. Respiratory acidosis with metabolic compensation
D. Respiratory alkalosis with metabolic compensation

The low bicarbonate indicates metabolic acidosis. Bicarbonate is lost in the urine as a buffer during metabolic acidosis. The patient has been hyperventilating to reduce the PCO_2. Since the pH is a normal value, there is respiratory compensation.

760. A patient has the following laboratory values: sodium 135 mEq/L, potassium 2.7 mEq/L, HCO_3 9 mEq/L, chloride 116 mEq/L, BUN 18 mg/dL, creatinine 1.0 mg/dL. The arterial blood gas shows PO_2 = 80 mm Hg, PCO_2 = 24 mm Hg, pH = 7.29. The possibility is?

A. Non-anion gap metabolic acidosis
B. Respiratory acidosis with compensatory metabolic alkalosis
C. Anion gap metabolic acidosis
D. Metabolic alkalosis

The patient is acidotic with low PCO_2 ruling out respiratory acidosis. The anion gap is normal. There is a reduction in PCO_2 showing respiratory compensation.

761. A febrile patient presents to the emergency room with hypotension. Preliminary laboratory analysis reveals elevated lactic acid levels and evidence of metabolic acidosis. What is the major blood buffer which will help the patient counteract the acidosis?

A. Calcium carbonate
B. Water
C. Citric acid
D. Bicarbonate

The buffer present in blood plasma is composed of bicarbonate and carbonic acid. A buffer solution is composed of a weak acid and its conjugate base. Although a mixture of citric acid and sodium citrate can act as a buffer in the urine, it is not a major blood buffer. Bicarbonate combines with hydrogen ions forming carbonic acid. This becomes carbon dioxide and water. The carbon dioxide is removed by the lungs. This is called compensatory respiratory alkalosis.

762. What metabolic derangement is associated with shock?

Harrison's 20th Ed. Chapter 51 Page 320

A. Metabolic acidosis
B. Metabolic alkalosis
C. Respiratory acidosis
D. Respiratory alkalosis

Shock is associated with metabolic acidosis. Increasing lactate levels due to lack of tissue perfusion accounts for the metabolic acidosis. Other causes of metabolic acidosis include aspirin poisoning, diarrhea, diabetic ketoacidosis, and methanol poisoning.

763. Which chemical is increased in metabolic acidosis?

Harrison's 20th Ed. Chapter 51 Page 320

A. Sodium
B. BUN
C. Potassium
D. Albumin

Shock is the most common cause of metabolic acidosis. It results in an increase of lactic acid levels. There will be concern for hyperkalemia in acidotic states.

764. What electrolyte abnormality is most likely to be found in a patient with severe diarrhea?

Harrison's 20th Ed. Chapter 51 Page 320

A. Hyperkalemia
B. Hypercalcemia
C. Acidosis
D. Hypermagnesemia

Gastrointestinal tract secretions below the stomach are alkaline. Therefore, diarrhea tends to cause a metabolic acidosis. It is also usually associated with hypokalemia.

765. Which is consistent with metabolic acidosis?

Harrison's 20th Ed. Chapter 51 Page 320

A. High extracellular hydrogen ions
B. Low extracellular hydrogen ions
C. High extracellular sodium ions
D. Low extracellular sodium ions

Metabolic acidosis is associated with high extracellular hydrogen ions. Metabolic alkalosis is associated with low extracellular hydrogen ions. Hypernatremia is associated with high extracellular hydrogen ions. Hyponatremia is associated with low extracellular hydrogen ions.

766. A homeless patient presents with nausea, vomiting, and blurry vision. Laboratory results show serum pH 7.30, Na 145 mmol/L, Cl 100 mmol/L, and HCO_3 19 mmol/L. What is the likely diagnosis?

A. Methanol intoxication
B. Isopropyl alcohol intoxication
C. Ethylene glycol intoxication
D. Ethanol intoxication

The pH is < 7.35 and HCO_3 is less than normal range, therefore a metabolic acidosis is present. Anion gap is 21. An anion gap metabolic acidosis is present. Methanol is an alcohol found in windshield washer fluid. Classic findings are an anion gap metabolic acidosis in the setting of vision loss.

767. Hyporeninemic hypoaldosteronism can be seen in?

Harrison's 20th Ed. Chapter 51 Page 320

A. Diabetes mellitus
B. Tubulointerstitial disease
C. CKD
D. All of the above

Hyporeninemic hypoaldosteronism causes hyperchloremic or non-AG metabolic acidosis, in older adults with diabetes mellitus or tubulointerstitial disease and renal insufficiency (CKD).

768. Which of the following drugs can cause non-anionic gap acidosis?

Harrison's 20th Ed. Chapter 51 Page 320 Table 51-5

A. Cholestyramine
B. Acetazolamide
C. Topiramate
D. All of the above

769. Which of the following drugs can cause non-anionic gap acidosis?

Harrison's 20th Ed. Chapter 51 Page 320 Table 51-5

A. Amphotericin B
B. Ifosfamide
C. Calcium chloride
D. All of the above

Metabolic Alkalosis

770. Which of the following can induce metabolic alkalosis?

Harrison's 20th Ed. Chapter 51 Page 321

A. Intracellular shift, excessive GI/renal H^+ ion loss
B. Retention or addition of HCO_3^- ions
C. Volume contraction
D. All of the above

Metabolic alkalosis is a primary increase in serum HCO_3^- concentration as a result of loss of H^+ from body or a gain in HCO_3^- manifests as alkalemia (pH >7.40), usually compensated by alveolar hypoventilation with a rise in arterial carbon dioxide tension ($PaCO_2$) to decrease change in pH. Processes that drive hydrogen intracellularly include hypokalemia. HCO_3^- concentration >35 mEq/L is almost always caused by primary metabolic alkalosis. The serum HCO_3^- usually does not increase above 38 mmol/L.

771. Ability to eliminate bicarbonate is impaired due to?

Harrison's 20th Ed. Chapter 51 Page 321

A. Chloride depletion
B. Hypokalemia
C. Hyperaldosteronism
D. All of the above

Ability to eliminate bicarbonate is impaired due to hypovolemia, reduced effective arterial blood volume, chloride depletion, hypokalemia, reduced glomerular filtration rate, and/or hyperaldosteronism.

772. Metabolic alkalosis is manifested by all except?

Harrison's 20th Ed. Chapter 51 Page 321

A. Elevated arterial pH
B. Increase in serum $[HCO_3^-]$
C. Hyperchloremia
D. Increase in $PaCO_2$

773. Which of the following statements about metabolic alkalosis is false?

Harrison's 20th Ed. Chapter 51 Page 321

A. Loss of nonvolatile acid
B. Due to net gain of $[HCO_3^-]$
C. Kidneys retain, rather than excrete excess alkali
D. None of the above

Metabolic alkalosis manifests as elevated arterial pH, increased serum $[HCO_3^-]$ & increased $PaCO_2$ due to compensatory alveolar hypoventilation. It is often accompanied by hypochloremia & hypokalemia.

774. Metabolic alkalosis frequently occurs in association with?

Harrison's 20th Ed. Chapter 51 Page 321

A. Respiratory acidosis
B. Respiratory alkalosis
C. Metabolic acidosis
D. All of the above

Metabolic alkalosis frequently occurs as a mixed acid base disorder in association with other disorders such as respiratory acidosis or alkalosis or metabolic acidosis.

775. The $PaCO_2$ increases how much for each mmol/L increase in $[HCO_3^-]$ above normal?

Harrison's 20th Ed. Chapter 51 Page 315 Table 51-1

A. 0.25 mm Hg
B. 0.50 mm Hg
C. 0.75 mm Hg
D. 1.00 mm Hg

776. The $PaCO_2$ increases how much for each 10 mmol/L increase in $[HCO_3^-]$ above normal?

Harrison's 20th Ed. Chapter 51 Page 315 Table 51-1

A. 2 mm Hg
B. 4 mm Hg
C. 6 mm Hg
D. 8 mm Hg

777. Which of the following is high in metabolic alkalosis?

Harrison's 20th Ed. Chapter 51 Page 315 Table 51-1

A. pH
B. HCO_3^-
C. $PaCO_2$
D. All of the above

778. Which of the following formula is correct?

Harrison's 20th Ed. Chapter 51 Page 315 Table 51-1

A. $PaCO_2 = [HCO_3^-] + 12$
B. $PaCO_2 = [HCO_3^-] + 13$
C. $PaCO_2 = [HCO_3^-] + 14$
D. $PaCO_2 = [HCO_3^-] + 15$

779. In reduced GFR, kidneys will retain excess alkali and maintain alkalosis if there is?

Harrison's 20th Ed. Chapter 51 Page 321

A. Volume deficiency
B. Chloride deficiency
C. K^+ deficiency
D. All of the above

Kidneys will retain, rather than excrete, excess alkali & maintain alkalosis if volume deficiency, chloride deficiency, and K^+ deficiency exist in combination with a reduced GFR or hypokalemia exists because of autonomous hyperaldosteronism.

780. Assessment of which of the following is necessary to establish the cause of metabolic alkalosis?

Harrison's 20th Ed. Chapter 51 Page 321

A. Status of the extracellular fluid volume (ECFV)
B. Recumbent & upright blood pressure
C. Serum $[K^+]$
D. All of the above

781. Which of the following suggests primary mineralocorticoid excess?

Harrison's 20th Ed. Chapter 51 Page 321

A. Metabolic alkalosis
B. Low plasma renin activity
C. Normal values for urine $[Na^+]$ & $[Cl^-]$
D. All of the above

Metabolic alkalosis, low plasma renin activity and normal values for urine $[Na^+]$ and $[Cl^-]$, in a patient who is not taking diuretics, suggest primary mineralocorticoid excess.

782. Hypokalemia and alkalosis in a normotensive, nonedematous patient suggests?

Harrison's 20th Ed. Chapter 51 Page 321

A. Magnesium deficiency
B. Vomiting
C. Diuretic ingestion
D. All of the above

783. Hypokalemia and alkalosis in a normotensive, nonedematous patient suggests?

Harrison's 20th Ed. Chapter 51 Page 321

A. Bartter's syndrome
B. Gitelman's syndrome
C. Exogenous alkali
D. All of the above

Combination of hypokalemia & alkalosis in a normotensive, nonedematous patient can be due to Bartter's or Gitelman's syndrome, magnesium deficiency, vomiting, exogenous alkali, or diuretic ingestion.

784. Which of the following findings favor the diagnosis of metabolic alkalosis due to vomiting or alkali ingestion?

Harrison's 20th Ed. Chapter 51 Page 321

A. Alkaline urine
B. Elevated urine [Na^+] & [K^+]
C. Low urine [Cl^-]
D. All of the above

785. In metabolic alkalosis, acidic urine with low urine Na^+, K^+, and Cl^-, point towards the diagnosis of?

Harrison's 20th Ed. Chapter 51 Page 321

A. Prior vomiting
B. Posthypercapnic state
C. Prior diuretic ingestion
D. All of the above

786. In metabolic alkalosis, acidic urine with normal urine Na^+, K^+, and Cl^-, point towards the diagnosis of?

Harrison's 20th Ed. Chapter 51 Page 321

A. Magnesium deficiency
B. Bartter's or Gitelman's syndrome
C. Current diuretic ingestion
D. All of the above

787. In metabolic alkalosis, Bartter's or Gitelman's syndrome are mainly differentiated by?

Harrison's 20th Ed. Chapter 51 Page 321

A. Urine potassium
B. Urine magnesium
C. Urine calcium
D. Urine sodium

Hypocalciuria is a feature of Gitelman's syndrome.

788. Acetate load is increased resulting in alkalosis in patients receiving?

Harrison's 20th Ed. Chapter 51 Page 321

A. Parenteral hyperalimentation solutions
B. Transfusions
C. Antacids
D. All of the above

789. Citrate load is increased resulting in alkalosis in patients receiving?

Harrison's 20th Ed. Chapter 51 Page 321

A. Parenteral hyperalimentation solutions
B. Transfusions
C. Antacids
D. All of the above

790. Which of the following is true for urine in patients who are vomiting?

Harrison's 20th Ed. Chapter 51 Page 321

A. Acidic urine, elevated $[Na]_u$ and $[K]_u$, low $[Cl]_u$
B. Alkaline urine, low $[Na]_u$ and $[K]_u$, low $[Cl]_u$
C. Acidic urine, low $[Na]_u$ and $[K]_u$, low $[Cl]_u$
D. Alkaline urine, elevated $[Na]_u$ and $[K]_u$, low $[Cl]_u$

If urine is alkaline, with elevated [Na^+] & [K^+] but low [Cl^-], diagnosis is either vomiting or alkali ingestion.

791. High urine chloride metabolic alkalemia includes?

Disease-a-Month 2004;50:122-162

A. Bartter syndrome
B. Gitleman syndrome
C. Liddle's syndrome
D. All of the above

792. High urine chloride metabolic alkalemia with hypertension includes all except?

Disease-a-Month 2004;50:122-162

A. Conn's Syndrome
B. Cushing disease
C. Bartter's syndrome
D. Liddle's syndrome

793. High urine chloride metabolic alkalemia without hypertension includes all except?

Disease-a-Month 2004;50:122-162

A. Excess bicarbonate administration
B. Gitelman syndrome
C. Bartter's syndrome
D. Liddle's syndrome

794. Conn syndrome lead to?

Disease-a-Month 2004;50:122-162

A. Hypernatremia
B. Hypokalemia
C. Hydrogen ion loss in urine
D. All of the above

Metabolic alkalosis is split into 2 categories: Chloride responsive with urine chloride <10 mEq/L and chloride resistant with urine chloride >20 mEq/L. Chloride responsive etiologies include loss of H^+ via GI tract, congenital chloride diarrhea syndrome, contraction alkalosis, diuretic therapy, post-hypercapnia syndrome, cystic fibrosis, & exogenous alkalotic agent use. Chloride-resistant etiologies include retention of bicarbonate, shift of H^+ into intracellular spaces, hyperaldosteronism, Bartter syndrome, & Gitelman syndrome.

795. "Contraction alkalosis" best relates to?

Harrison's 20th Ed. Chapter 51 Page 322

A. Vomiting
B. Gastric aspiration
C. Diuretic use
D. All of the above

Diuretics or chloride diarrhea increase excretion of salt & acutely diminish ECFV without altering total body [HCO_3^-] content. Serum [HCO_3^-] increases because reduced ECFV "contracts" around [HCO_3^-] in plasma. This is called contraction alkalosis. Or, volume contraction around a constant amount of extracellular [HCO_3^-].

796. In chronic use of diuretics, metabolic alkalosis is maintained by persistence of?

Harrison's 20th Ed. Chapter 51 Page 322

A. Contraction of the ECFV
B. Secondary hyperaldosteronism
C. K^+ deficiency
D. All of the above

797. Which of the following statements is false?

Harrison's 20th Ed. Chapter 51 Page 322

A. Hypokalemia upregulates renal ammoniagenesis
B. Hypokalemia upregulates renal H^+, K^+-ATPase
C. Alkalosis due to severe K^+ depletion is salt resistant
D. None of the above

798. K^+ depletion occurs concomitant with Mg^{++} deficiency in?

Harrison's 20th Ed. Chapter 51 Page 322

A. Chronic administration of diuretics
B. Alcoholics with malnutrition
C. Transfusions of whole blood
D. Parenteral hyperalimentation

Potassium depletion often occurs concomitant with magnesium deficiency in alcoholics with malnutrition.

799. Lactate or ketones are metabolized to yield?

Harrison's 20th Ed. Chapter 51 Page 322

A. H^+
B. HCO_3^-
C. Cl^-
D. All of the above

Lactate or ketones are metabolized to yield an equivalent amount of HCO_3^-.

800. Which of the following is false about Liddle's syndrome?

Harrison's 20th Ed. Chapter 51 Page 322

A. Increased activity of collecting duct sodium channel
B. Hypertension due to volume expansion
C. Hypokalemic alkalosis
D. Elevated aldosterone levels

Liddle's syndrome results from increased activity of collecting duct Na^+ channel (ENaC) manifests as hypertension due to volume expansion leading to hypokalemic alkalosis & normal aldosterone levels.

801. Presentation of metabolic alkalosis is similar to?

Harrison's 20th Ed. Chapter 51 Page 322

A. Hypercalcemia
B. Hypocalcemia
C. Hyperkalemia
D. All of the above

Changes in central and peripheral nervous system function with metabolic alkalosis are similar to those of hypocalcemia.

802. Renal HCO_3^- loss can be accelerated by administration of?

Harrison's 20th Ed. Chapter 51 Page 322

A. Acetazolamide
B. Thiazide diuretics
C. Furosemide
D. Aluminum hydroxide

Renal HCO_3^- loss can be accelerated by administration of acetazolamide, a carbonic anhydrase inhibitor which is usually effective in patients with adequate renal function but can worsen K^+ losses.

Respiratory Acidosis

803. In acute respiratory acidosis, $[HCO_3^-]$ levels increase by how much for every 10 mm Hg increase in $PaCO_2$?

Harrison's 20th Ed. Chapter 51 Page 322

A. 1 mmol/L
B. 2 mmol/L
C. 3 mmol/L
D. 4 mmol/L

Carbon dioxide is the "respiratory acid" and is the only acid which can be controlled by respiration. When the PCO_2 is high, respiratory acidosis occurs.

804. In chronic respiratory acidosis, $[HCO_3^-]$ levels increase by how much for every 10 mm Hg increase in $PaCO_2$?

Harrison's 20th Ed. Chapter 51 Page 322

A. 1 mmol/L
B. 2 mmol/L
C. 3 mmol/L
D. 4 mmol/L

In acute respiratory acidosis, there is an increase of 1 mmol/L of HCO_3^- for every 10-mm Hg increase in $PaCO_2$. In chronic respiratory acidosis (>24 hours), the $[HCO_3^-]$ increases by 4 mmol/L for every 10-mmHg increase in $PaCO_2$.

805. In respiratory acidosis, serum HCO_3^- usually does not increase above?

Harrison's 20th Ed. Chapter 51 Page 322

A. 28 mmol/L
B. 38 mmol/L
C. 48 mmol/L
D. 58 mmol/L

In respiratory acidosis, serum HCO_3^- usually does not increase above 38 mmol/L.

806. In respiratory acidosis, papilledema is due to?

Harrison's 20th Ed. Chapter 51 Page 322

A. Vasoconstriction
B. Vasodilatation
C. Hyperviscosity
D. Renal failure

In respiratory acidosis, papilledema, abnormal reflexes and focal muscle weakness is due to vasoconstriction secondary to loss of the vasodilator effects of CO_2.

807. Diagnosis of respiratory acidosis requires measurement of?

Harrison's 20th Ed. Chapter 51 Page 323

A. $PaCO_2$
B. PaO_2
C. $[HCO_3^-]$
D. All of the above

Diagnosis of respiratory acidosis requires, by definition, measurement of $PaCO_2$ & arterial pH.

Respiratory Alkalosis

808. In chronic respiratory alkalosis a 1-mm Hg fall in $PaCO_2$ causes a drop in $[HCO_3^-]$ of?

Harrison's 20th Ed. Chapter 51 Page 324

A. 0.1–0.2 mmol/L
B. 0.2–0.3 mmol/L
C. 0.3–0.4 mmol/L
D. 0.4–0.5 mmol/L

In chronic respiratory alkalosis a 1 mm Hg fall in $PaCO_2$ causes a 0.4 to 0.5 mmol/L drop in $[HCO_3^-]$ and a 0.003 rise in pH.

809. $[HCO_3^-]$ falls by how much for each 10-mm Hg decrease in $PaCO_2$ in acute hypocapnia?

Harrison's 20th Ed. Chapter 51 Page 324

A. 2 mmol/L
B. 3 mmol/L
C. 4 mmol/L
D. 5 mmol/L

810. [HCO_3^-] falls by how much for each 10-mm Hg decrease in $PaCO_2$ in chronic hypocapnia?

Harrison's 20th Ed. Chapter 51 Page 324

A. 2 mmol/L
B. 3 mmol/L
C. 4 mmol/L
D. 5 mmol/L

In acute hypocapnia, [HCO_3^-] falls by 2 mmol/L and 4 mmol/L for each 10-mmHg decrease in $PaCO_2$ in acute and chronic hypocapnia respectively.

811. In pure respiratory alkalosis, plasma HCO_3^- is usually more than?

Harrison's 20th Ed. Chapter 51 Page 324

A. 12 mmol/L
B. 14 mmol/L
C. 16 mmol/L
D. 18 mmol/L

It is unusual to see a plasma HCO_3^- < 12 mmol/L due to pure respiratory alkalosis.

812. Which of the following shift inside the cell in acute respiratory alkalosis?

Harrison's 20th Ed. Chapter 51 Page 324

A. Na^+
B. K^+
C. PO_4^-
D. All of the above

Acute respiratory alkalosis causes intracellular shifts of Na^+, K^+, and PO_4^-. Hypocapnia-induced hypokalemia is usually minor.

813. Most common acid-base disturbance in critically ill patients is?

Harrison's 20th Ed. Chapter 51 Page 324

A. Acute respiratory acidosis
B. Acute respiratory alkalosis
C. Chronic respiratory acidosis
D. Chronic respiratory alkalosis

Chronic respiratory alkalosis is the most common acid-base disturbance in critically ill patients.

814. Most common cause of drug-induced respiratory alkalosis is by?

Harrison's 20th Ed. Chapter 51 Page 324

A. Salicylates
B. Theophylline
C. Progesterone
D. Aminophylline

Salicylates are the most common cause of drug-induced respiratory alkalosis as a result of direct stimulation of the medullary chemoreceptor. Methylxanthines, theophylline and aminophylline stimulate ventilation & increase ventilatory response to CO_2. Progesterone increases ventilation & lowers arterial $PaCO_2$. Chronic respiratory alkalosis is a common feature of pregnancy.

815. Which of the following is an early finding in gram-negative septicemia?

Harrison's 20th Ed. Chapter 51 Page 324

A. Fever
B. Hypoxemia
C. Respiratory alkalosis
D. Hypotension

Respiratory alkalosis is often an early finding in gram-negative septicemia, before fever, hypoxemia, or hypotension develops.

816. What is the anion gap in a patient if albumin is 2 g/dL, Na^+ is 140 mEq/L, Cl^- is 100 mEq/L, and HCO_3 is 20 mEq/L?

Harrison's 20th Ed. Chapter 51 Page 324

A. 15
B. 20
C. 25
D. 30

817. Which of the following is an ineffective osmole?

Harrison's 20th Ed. Chapter 51 Page 324

A. Inositol
B. Urea
C. Betaine
D. Glutamine

818. For each decrease in blood pH of 0.10, the plasma potassium rises by?

Harrison's 20th Ed. Chapter 51 Page 324

A. 0.5 mmol/L
B. 0.6 mmol/L
C. 0.7 mmol/L
D. 0.8 mmol/L

819. Normal range of urine ammonia is?

Harrison's 19th Ed. 2768

A. 10–30 mEq/day
B. 30–50 mEq/day
C. 50–100 mEq/day
D. 100–150 mEq/day

820. Normal range of urine creatinine is?

Harrison's 19th Ed. 2768

A. 1.0–1.6 g/day
B. 1.6–2.2 g/day
C. 2.2–2.6 g/day
D. 2.6–3.0 g/day

821. Normal range of urine potassium is?

Harrison's 19th Ed. 2769

A. 5–25 mEq/day
B. 25–100 mEq/day
C. 100–200 mEq/day
D. 200–300 mEq/day

822. Normal range of urine sodium is?

Harrison's 19th Ed. 2769

A. 10–60 mEq/day
B. 60–100 mEq/day
C. 100–260 mEq/day
D. 260–460 mEq/day

823. Normal range of urine uric acid is?

Harrison's 19th Ed. 2769

A. 50–250 mg/day
B. 250–800 mg/day
C. 800–1800 mg/day
D. 1800–3000 mg/day

824. Normal range of urine urea nitrogen is?

Harrison's 19th Ed. 2769

A. 6–17 g/day
B. 17–37 g/day
C. 37–57 g/day
D. 57–87 g/day

825. Normal range of urine osmolality is?

Harrison's 19th Ed. 2769

A. 50–100 mOsmol/kg
B. 100–800 mOsmol/kg
C. 800–1000 mOsmol/kg
D. 1000–1500 mOsmol/kg

Cellular and Molecular Biology of the Kidney

826. In kidneys, number of different cell types found is about?

Harrison's 20th Ed. Chapter 303 Page 2089

A. 10
B. 30
C. 50
D. 80

Kidney is one of the highly differentiated organs in body containing nearly 30 different cell types.

827. Which of the following is a function of kidneys?

Harrison's 20th Ed. Chapter 303 Page 2089

A. Endocrine function
B. Regulation of blood pressure
C. Solute and water transport
D. All of the above

Endocrine functions, the regulation of blood pressure and intraglomerular hemodynamics, solute and water transport, acid-base balance, and removal of drug metabolites are all accomplished by intricate mechanisms of renal response.

828. How many glomeruli does each kidney contain in a normal-birth-weight adult?

Harrison's 20th Ed. Chapter 303 Page 2089

A. ~ 100,000
B. ~ 400,000
C. ~ 900,000
D. ~ 1200,000

There are ~900,000 glomeruli in each kidney in normal-birth-weight adults. It is estimated that each kilogram in birth weight confers on average 260,000 more nephrons. Barker hypothesis proposes that adult disease has fetal origins and is based on epidemiologic studies showing a correlation between birth weight and the incidence of cardiovascular disease.

829. Which of the following is the first step in renal nephrogenesis?

Harrison's 20th Ed. Chapter 303 Page 2089 Figure 303-1

A. Comma-shaped bodies
B. Pretubular aggregation
C. S-shaped bodies
D. Ureteric bud induction and condensation

The various steps in renal nephrogenesis are : Ureteric bud induction and condensation, pretubular aggregation, Comma-shaped bodies, S-shaped bodies, Capillary loop and mature glomerulus. Human kidney development initiates around 4 weeks of gestation and ends around 34–37 weeks of gestation.

830. VEGF-A and angiopoietin-1 are secreted by?

Harrison's 20th Ed. Chapter 303 Page 2089

A. Bowman capsule
B. Podocytes
C. Mesangial cells
D. Juxtaglomerular cells

Glomeruli evolve as complex capillary filters with fenestrated endothelia under the guiding influence of VEGF-A & angiopoietin-1 secreted by adjacently developing podocytes. VEGF-A is a potent angiogenic factor related to normal and pathological angiogenesis. It is secreted by podocytes. Hypoxia is a key regulator of VEGF gene expression. It acts through tyrosine-kinase receptors, which are known as VEGF receptor 1 and 2 (VEGFR1 and 2), predominantly expressed in the glomerular capillaries. Two co-receptors called neuropilins 1 and 2 amplify the VEGFR2 signal. Angiopoietin is a growth factor.

831. Which of the following gene is involved in glomerulotubular development?

Harrison's 20th Ed. Chapter 303 Page 2089 Figure 303-1, Development. 2005;132(24):5437-49

A. Gdnf
B. Wt1
C. Flk1
D. All of the above

Kidney development is considered as the interaction of metanephric mesenchyme and ureteric bud to be the major inductive event that maintains tubular differentiation and branching morphogenesis. The mesenchyme produces Gdnf, which stimulates branching, and the ureteric bud stimulates continued growth of the mesenchyme and differentiation of nephrons from the induced mesenchyme. Null mutation of the Wt1 gene eliminates outgrowth of the ureteric bud, but Gdnf has been identified as a target of Pax2, but not of Wt1. Vegfa expression in mesenchyme is regulated by Wt1. Signaling through Flk1 is required to maintain expression of Pax2 in the mesenchyme of the early kidney, and for Pax2 to stimulate expression of Gdnf.

832. Contractile actin-myosin fibers are found in which of the following tissues of kidney?

Harrison's 20th Ed. Chapter 303 Page 2089

A. Glomeruli
B. Mesangial cells
C. Renal interstitium
D. All of the above

Glomerular capillaries are in the midst of a mesangial matrix and together form the Bowman's capsule. Mesangial cells contain contractile actin-myosin fibers to maintain structural integrity.

833. Vasa recta best relates to?

Harrison's 20th Ed. Chapter 303 Page 2089

A. Cortical nephrons
B. Juxtamedullary nephrons
C. Renal interstitium
D. Epithelial podocytes

Juxtamedullary nephrons have individual capillaries called vasa recta that run alongside the long loops of Henle. The peritubular capillaries surrounding cortical nephrons are shared among adjacent nephrons. Juxtamedullary nephron contains large glomeruli located near the corticomedullary border and a large network of vasa recta, more than cortical nephron. Consequently they have a high glomerular filtration rate. Afferent arterioles of cortical nephrons are larger than their respective efferent arterioles, while they are equal in juxtamedullary nephrons.

834. Pars Recta best relates to?

Harrison's 20th Ed. Chapter 303 Page 2089

A. Proximal tubule
B. Loop of Henle
C. Distal tubule
D. Collecting duct

Pars recta is the straight portion of the proximal tubule of the juxtamedullary nephron located in the outer stripe of the medulla (medullary rays).

835. Which of the following about kidney structure is false?

Harrison's 20th Ed. Chapter 303 Page 2089

A. Majority of nephrons are cortical
B. Majority of glomeruli located in mid-to-outer cortex
C. Cortical nephrons perform most of glomerular filtration
D. None of the above

836. Which of the following about kidney structure is false?

Harrison's 20th Ed. Chapter 303 Page 2089

A. Cortical nephrons have short loops of Henle
B. Juxtamedullary nephrons have long loops of Henle
C. Peritubular capillaries surrounding cortical nephrons are shared among adjacent nephrons
D. None of the above

Majority of nephrons are cortical, with glomeruli located in mid-to-outer cortex. Cortical nephrons have short loops of Henle, whereas juxtamedullary nephrons have long loops of Henle. Peritubular capillaries surrounding cortical nephrons are shared among adjacent nephrons. Juxtamedullary nephrons use separate capillaries called vasa recta. Cortical nephrons perform most of the glomerular filtration & their afferent arterioles are larger than their respective efferent arterioles. Juxtamedullary nephrons create a hyperosmolar gradient that allows for production of concentrated urine.

837. Juxtamedullary nephrons represent what percentage of the total number of nephrons?

Harrison's 20th Ed. Chapter 303 Page 2089

A. ~ 5%
B. ~ 10%
C. ~ 15%
D. ~ 20%

Juxtamedullary nephrons represent ~15% of the total number of nephrons. The main difference between cortical nephron & juxtamedullary nephron is that cortical nephron contains a short loop of Henle which only extends into outer region of renal medulla whereas juxtamedullary nephron have a large glomerulus, increasing the glomerular filtration rate of the nephron. longer loop of Henle which extends deeper into the inner medulla. Juxtamedullary nephrons have a vital role in concentrating urine or water conservation.

838. Slit-pore membrane formation is related to?

Harrison's 20th Ed. Chapter 303 Page 2089

A. Annexin-4
B. Podocin
C. Neph 1-3 proteins
D. All of the above

Podocytes attach to the basement membrane by special foot processes and share a slit-pore membrane with their neighbor. Slit-pore membrane forms a filter for plasma water & solute by synthetic interaction of nephrin, annexin-4, CD2AP, FAT, ZO-1, P-cadherin, podocin, TRPC6, PLCE1, and Neph 1-3 proteins.

839. Renal interstitium contains all of the following cells except?

Harrison's 20th Ed. Chapter 303 Page 2089

A. Fibroblasts
B. Osteoblasts
C. Dendritic cells
D. Lipid-laden macrophages

Renal interstitium is the functional space surrounding glomeruli & their downstream tubules. It is home to resident & trafficking cells like fibroblasts, dendritic cells, lymphocytes, and lipid-laden macrophages.

840. Renal blood flow normally drains what percentage of the cardiac output?

Harrison's 20th Ed. Chapter 303 Page 2090

A. ~ 5%
B. ~ 10%
C. ~ 15%
D. ~ 20%

Renal blood flow normally drains approximately 20% of the cardiac output or 1000 mL/minute.

841. Cortical nephron has how many capillary beds arranged in series?

Harrison's 20th Ed. Chapter 303 Page 2090

A. 1
B. 2
C. 3
D. 4

Cortical nephron has two capillary beds arranged in series separated by efferent arteriole that regulates hydrostatic pressure in both capillary beds.

842. Driving force for glomerular filtration at efferent arteriole is?

Harrison's 20th Ed. Chapter 303 Page 2090

A. Zero
B. 10
C. 20
D. 30

As the oncotic pressure rises along the length of the glomerular capillary, the driving force for filtration falls to zero before reaching the efferent arteriole.

843. What percentage of renal plasma flow is filtered into Bowman's space?

Harrison's 20th Ed. Chapter 303 Page 2090

A. ~ 20%
B. ~ 45%
C. ~ 60%
D. ~ 80%

~20% of the renal plasma flow is filtered into Bowman's space.

844. Autoregulation of glomerular filtration is the result of?

Harrison's 20th Ed. Chapter 303 Page 2090

A. Autonomous vasoreactive reflex in afferent arteriole
B. Tubuloglomerular feedback
C. Angiotensin II mediated vasoconstriction of efferent arteriole
D. All of the above

Autoregulation of glomerular filtration is the result of an autonomous vasoreactive (myogenic) reflex in the afferent arteriole, tubuloglomerular feedback, and angiotensin II mediated vasoconstriction of the efferent arteriole.

845. Which of the following is the first line of defense against fluctuations in renal blood flow in autoregulation of glomerular filtration?

Harrison's 20th Ed. Chapter 303 Page 2090

A. Myogenic reflex in afferent arteriole
B. Tubuloglomerular feedback
C. Angiotensin II mediated vasoconstriction of efferent arteriole
D. None of the above

Myogenic reflex is a first line of defense against fluctuations in renal blood flow.

846. Tubuloglomerular feedback changes the rate of filtration & tubular flow by reflex vasoconstriction or dilatation of?

Harrison's 20th Ed. Chapter 303 Page 2090

A. Afferent arteriole
B. Efferent arteriole
C. Vasa recta
D. All of the above

847. Tubuloglomerular feedback is mediated by?

Harrison's 20th Ed. Chapter 303 Page 2090

A. Juxtaglomerular apparatus
B. Macula densa
C. Granular cells in the wall of afferent arteriole
D. All of the above

848. Macula densa is located in which of the following?

Harrison's 20th Ed. Chapter 303 Page 2090

A. Proximal tubule
B. Thick ascending limb of the loop of Henle
C. Distal tubule
D. Collecting duct

Tubuloglomerular feedback is mediated by specialized cells in thick ascending limb of the loop of Henle called macula densa that act as sensors of solute concentration & flow of tubular fluid.

849. Which of the following blunts tubuloglomerular feedback?

Harrison's 20th Ed. Chapter 303 Page 2090

A. Angiotensin II
B. Reactive oxygen species
C. Nitric oxide
D. Adenosine

Angiotensin II & reactive oxygen species enhance, while nitric oxide blunts tubuloglomerular feedback.

850. Juxtaglomerular apparatus is located in?

Harrison's 20th Ed. Chapter 303 Page 2090

A. Afferent arteriole
B. Efferent arteriole
C. Distal tubule
D. Collecting duct

Juxtaglomerular apparatus is located within the wall of afferent arteriole near macula densa and its granular cells release renin.

851. Which of the following is a potent vasoconstrictor of the afferent arteriole?

Harrison's 20th Ed. Chapter 303 Page 2090

A. Adenosine
B. ATP
C. Angiotensin II
D. Nitric oxide (NO)

ATP is metabolized in the extracellular space to generate adenosine, a potent vasoconstrictor of the afferent arteriole.

852. Renin catalyzes the conversion of?

Harrison's 20th Ed. Chapter 303 Page 2090

A. Angiotensinogen to angiotensin I
B. Angiotensin I to angiotensin II
C. Angiotensin II to angiotensin III
D. All of the above

Renin is a proteolytic enzyme released from juxtaglomerular apparatus. It catalyzes conversion of angiotensinogen to angiotensin I.

853. Angiotensin-converting enzyme catalyzes conversion of?

Harrison's 20th Ed. Chapter 303 Page 2090

A. Angiotensinogen to angiotensin I
B. Angiotensin I to angiotensin II
C. Angiotensin II to angiotensin III
D. All of the above

Angiotensin I is converted to angiotensin II by angiotensin-converting enzyme (ACE).

854. Which of the following is false about angiotensin II?

Harrison's 20th Ed. Chapter 303 Page 2090

A. Enhances tubuloglomerular feedback
B. Evokes vasoconstriction of efferent arteriole
C. Inhibits renin secretion through a negative feedback loop
D. None of the above

855. Which of the following is false about angiotensin II?

Harrison's 20th Ed. Chapter 303 Page 2090

A. Renin & ACE activity eventually produce angiotensin II
B. Stimulation of proximal tubular Na^+/H^+ exchange by angiotensin II directly increases Na^+ reabsorption
C. Angiotensin II also promotes Na+ reabsorption along the collecting duct by stimulating aldosterone secretion
D. None of the above

856. Angiotensin II causes constriction of?

Harrison's 20th Ed. Chapter 303 Page 2090

A. Afferent glomerular arteriole
B. Efferent glomerular arteriole
C. Renal artery
D. All of the above

Constriction of the efferent glomerular arteriole by angiotensin II indirectly increases the filtration fraction and raises peritubular capillary oncotic pressure to promote tubular Na^+ reabsorption. Angiotensin II inhibits renin secretion through a negative feedback loop.

857. Which of the following about cells lining the various tubular segments is false?

Harrison's 20th Ed. Chapter 303 Page 2090

A. Apical membrane faces the tubular lumen
B. Basolateral membrane faces the interstitium
C. Renal epithelial cells are polarized
D. Membrane proteins have symmetric assignment

Membrane proteins of renal epithelial cells mediating transport processes have asymmetric assignment of proteins. This provides the machinery for directional movement of fluid & solutes by the nephron.

858. Which of the following is not a major tubular segment of the nephron?

Harrison's 20th Ed. Chapter 303 Page 2091 Figure 303-3

A. Proximal tubular cells
B. Thick ascending limb of the loop of Henle cells
C. Distal convoluted tubular & cortical collecting duct cells
D. Typical cell in the outer medullary collecting duct

The five major tubular segments are proximal tubular cells, typical cell in the thick ascending limb of the loop of Henle, distal convoluted tubular cell, cortical collecting duct cells and typical cell in the inner medullary collecting duct.

859. Epithelial cellular transport is mediated by?

Harrison's 20th Ed. Chapter 303 Page 2091

A. Transporters
B. Channels
C. Pumps
D. All of the above

Cell membranes are composed of hydrophobic lipids that repel water and aqueous solutes. Epithelial cellular transport i.e. movement of fluid & solutes "sequentially" across apical & basolateral cell membranes (or vice versa) is mediated by transporters, channels, or pumps.

860. Paracellular transport occurs through?
Harrison's 20th Ed. Chapter 303 Page 2091

A. Leaky junctions
B. Tight junctions
C. Perforated junctions
D. Slit junctions

Paracellular transport occurs through tight junctions.

861. Leaky epithelia is present in?
Harrison's 20th Ed. Chapter 303 Page 2091

A. Proximal convoluted tubule
B. Distal convoluted tubule
C. Collecting duct
D. All of the above

Proximal tubule contains leaky epithelia which are best suited for bulk fluid reabsorption. Distal nephron segments (distal convoluted tubule & collecting duct) contain tight epithelia with little water permeability and provide refined control & regulation of transport.

862. Facilitated diffusion occurs through which of the following?
Harrison's 20th Ed. Chapter 303 Page 2093

A. Pumps
B. Channels
C. Transporters
D. Co-transporters

863. Secondary active transport occurs through which of the following?
Harrison's 20th Ed. Chapter 303 Page 2093

A. Pumps
B. Channels
C. Transporters
D. Co-transporters

864. Passive transport occurs through which of the following?
Harrison's 20th Ed. Chapter 303 Page 2093

A. Pumps
B. Channels
C. Transporters
D. Co-transporters

865. Active transport occurs through which of the following?
Harrison's 20th Ed. Chapter 303 Page 2093

A. Pumps
B. Channels
C. Transporters
D. Co-transporters

Movement of solutes & water across cell membranes is made possible by pumps (active transport), channels (passive transport), transporters (facilitated diffusion), and co-transporters (secondary active transport).

866. Ion-translocating ATPases include?
Harrison's 20th Ed. Chapter 303 Page 2093

A. Na^+/K^+-ATPase
B. H^+-ATPase
C. Ca^{++}-ATPase
D. All of the above

Ion-translocating ATPases that mediate active transport ("pumps") are the ubiquitous Na^+/K^+-ATPase, the H^+-ATPases, and Ca^{++}-ATPases.

867. Which of the following is false about active transport pumps?
Harrison's 20th Ed. Chapter 303 Page 2094

A. Electrogenic
B. Ion-translocating ATPases
C. Establish a voltage or membrane potential
D. None of the above

868. Which of the following solute moves by simple diffusion or passive transport?
Harrison's 20th Ed. Chapter 303 Page 2094

A. K^+
B. Na^+
C. Cl^-
D. All of the above

In kidney, movement by simple diffusion or passive transport occurs of water, K^+, Na^+, and Cl^-.

869. Which of the following is a transporter?
Harrison's 20th Ed. Chapter 303 Page 2094

A. Carrier
B. Symporter
C. Antiporter
D. All of the above

870. GLUT2 is a?
Harrison's 20th Ed. Chapter 303 Page 2094

A. Pump
B. Channel
C. Transporter
D. Co-transporter

GLUT2 is a hexose transporter that mediates glucose transport by tubular cells.

871. Carriers or uniporters are related to?
Harrison's 20th Ed. Chapter 303 Page 2094

A. Active transport
B. Passive transport
C. Facilitated diffusion
D. Secondary active transport

872. Symporters or co-transporters, antiporters or exchangers are related to?
Harrison's 20th Ed. Chapter 303 Page 2094

A. Active transport
B. Passive transport
C. Facilitated diffusion
D. Secondary active transport

Facilitated diffusion is a specialized type of passive transport mediated by simple transporters called carriers or uniporters. Many transporters operate by translocating two or more ions/solutes either in the same direction (symporters or co-transporters) or in opposite directions (antiporters or exchangers) across the cell membrane.

873. Proximal tubule reabsorbs which of the following?

Harrison's 20th Ed. Chapter 303 Page 2095

A. NaCl and water
B. Bicarbonate
C. Glucose & amino acids
D. All of the above

874. Which of the following is "most" absorbed in proximal tubule?

Harrison's 20th Ed. Chapter 303 Page 2095

A. NaCl
B. Water
C. Bicarbonate
D. Glucose & amino acids

Proximal tubule is responsible for reabsorbing ~60% of filtered NaCl and water as well as ~90% of filtered bicarbonate, phosphate & most critical nutrients (glucose & amino acids) through cellular & paracellular transport mechanisms. Proximal tubular cells reclaim nearly all filtered bicarbonate by a mechanism dependent on carbonic anhydrases.

875. Which of the following is false about peritubular capillaries?

Harrison's 20th Ed. Chapter 303 Page 2095

A. Have high oncotic pressure
B. Have low hydrostatic pressure
C. Vasa recta are medullary peritubular capillaries
D. None of the above

876. Which of the following statements is false?

Harrison's 20th Ed. Chapter 303 Page 2095

A. Aquaporin-1 present on apical & basolateral membranes
B. Na^+/K^+-ATPase pump is on basolateral membranes
C. Filtered bicarbonate first titrated by protons
D. Carbonic acid diffuses into the cell

Carbonic acid is metabolized by brush border carbonic anhydrase to water and carbon dioxide. Dissolved CO_2 diffuses into the cell, whereby cytoplasmic carbonic anhydrase reforms carbonic acid which dissociates into H^+ and bicarbonate anions. Bicarbonate exits the cell through a basolateral Na^+/HCO_3^- co-transporter.

877. Which of the following about acetazolamide is false?

Harrison's 20th Ed. Chapter 303 Page 2095

A. Carbonic anhydrase inhibitor
B. Blocks proximal tubule bicarbonate reabsorption
C. Diuretic
D. Acidifies urine

Acetazolamide is a carbonic anhydrase inhibitor, a weak diuretic, blocks proximal tubule bicarbonate reabsorption and alkalinizes urine. Dorzolamide, methazolamide, brinzolamide and dichlorphenamide are also carbonic anhydrase inhibitors. The increased distal nephron sodium delivery caused by acetazolamide results in increased potassium secretion and thus carbonic anhydrase inhibitors typically result in moderate increases of urinary potassium excretion.

878. Renal NH_3 is produced in the proximal tubule by?

Harrison's 20th Ed. Chapter 303 Page 2095

A. Inositol metabolism
B. Glutamine metabolism
C. Taurine metabolism
D. Arginine metabolism

Renal NH_3 is produced by glutamine metabolism in the proximal tubule (ammoniagenesis), diffuses out of the proximal tubular cell and traps H^+, which is secreted by Na^+/H^+ exchange, to form ammonium ion ($NH4^+$).

879. Glutamine is synthesized in?

Harrison's 20th Ed. Chapter 303 Page 2095

A. Kidneys
B. Liver
C. Intestines
D. Cartilage

Glutamine is synthesized in the liver and transported via circulation to kidney proximal tubule, where it is taken up by specific transporters.

880. Which of the following is a urinary buffer?

Harrison's 20th Ed. Chapter 303 Page 2095

A. Phosphate buffer
B. Bicarbonate buffer
C. Ammonia buffer
D. All of the above

881. Which of the following about urinary buffer is false?

Harrison's 20th Ed. Chapter 303 Page 2095

A. Increases urine pH
B. Ammonia (NH_3) and phosphate are urinary buffers
C. Cellular K^+ levels inversely modulate proximal tubular ammoniagenesis
D. None of the above

For every H^+ which enters urine, one sodium ion is reabsorbed from urine into the blood and is conserved. For every H^+ ion excreted & every Na^+ ion conserved, one bicarbonate ion is also reabsorbed into the blood.

882. Which of the following about carbonic anhydrase is false?

Harrison's 20th Ed. Chapter 303 Page 2095

A. Carbonic anhydrase is present at brush border
B. Carbonic anhydrase is present in cytoplasm
C. Carbonic anhydrase inhibitors alkalinize the urine
D. None of the above

883. The kidneys regulate hydrogen ion concentration by?

Harrison's 20th Ed. Chapter 303 Page 2095

A. Reabsorption of filtered bicarbonate
B. Secretion of titratable acid
C. Secretion of ammonia
D. All of the above

The kidneys regulate hydrogen ion concentration by three mechanisms: reabsorption of filtered bicarbonate, secretion of titratable acid, and secretion of ammonia. The renal excretion of acid (H^+) is achieved by titratable acidity and ammonium (NH_4^+) excretion.

884. The urine has a physiological pH of?

Harrison's 20th Ed. Chapter 303 Page 2095

A. 2.8–5.5
B. 3.8–6.5
C. 4.8–7.5
D. 5.8–8.5

The urine has a physiological pH of 4.8–7.5 with a mean of ~6.

885. Titratable acid is defined as the amount of strong base needed to titrate the pH of the urine back to pH?

Harrison's 20th Ed. Chapter 303 Page 2095

A. 7.1
B. 7.2
C. 7.3
D. 7.4

Titratable acid is defined as the amount of strong base needed to titrate the pH of the urine back to pH 7.4. Titratable acid refers to the excretion of protons with urinary buffers. Under normal conditions, ~one-third to one-half of net acid excretion by the kidneys is in the form of titratable acid. The other one-half to two-thirds is the excretion of NH_4^+. ($H^+ + NH_3 \leftrightarrow NH_4^+$). Therefore, net acid excretion = titratable acid + ammonium - urinary HCO_3^-

886. The major titratable acid in the urine is?

Harrison's 20th Ed. Chapter 303 Page 2095

A. HPO_4^{--}
B. $H_2PO_4^-$
C. HCl
D. HNO_3

Filtered hydrogen phosphate ion (HPO_4^{--}) is titrated in proximal tubule by secreted H^+ to form $H_2PO_4^-$, and this reaction constitutes a major component of the urinary buffer referred to as titratable acid. Thus, the major titratable acid in the urine is the monovalent organic phosphate ($H_2PO_4^-$). Buffering by phosphate and, to a lesser extent, other buffers such as urate and creatinine is called titratable acidity.

887. Reabsorption of filtered phosphate ion is regulated by?

Harrison's 20th Ed. Chapter 303 Page 2095

A. Calcium
B. Calcitonin
C. Parathyroid hormone
D. All of the above

Most filtered phosphate ion (HPO_4^{--}) is reabsorbed by the proximal tubule through a sodium-coupled cotransport process that is regulated by parathyroid hormone (PTH).

888. Which of the following statements is false?

Harrison's 20th Ed. Chapter 303 Page 2095

A. H^+ requires combination with buffers for excretion
B. H^+ requires formation of ammonium for excretion
C. For each H^+ excreted as titratable acid, there is one new HCO_3^- transferred to blood
D. None of the above

For each H^+ excreted as titratable acid, there is one new HCO_3^- transferred to blood. For each H^+ excreted as NH_4^+, there is also one new HCO_3^- transferred to blood.

889. Which of the following statements is false?

Harrison's 20th Ed. Chapter 303 Page 2095

A. Renal tubular cells synthesize ammonia by enzymatic deamination of amino acids
B. Ammonia acts as an acceptor of hydrogen ions, forming $NH4^+$
C. Ammonium ion is lipid insoluble
D. None of the above

Renal tubular cells synthesize ammonia by enzymatic deamination of amino acids. Ammonia diffuses down its concentration gradient into the tubular fluid where it acts as an acceptor of hydrogen ions, forming ammonium ions. The ammonium ion is lipid insoluble; thus it is trapped in the tubule lumen and excreted in the urine.

890. Which of the following is relevant in the renal control of plasma HCO_3^-?

Harrison's 20th Ed. Chapter 303 Page 2095

A. Sodium-hydrogen exchanger NHE_3
B. Basolateral Na^+/K^+-ATPase
C. Apical H^+-ATPase
D. All of the above

The kidneys regulate the [HCO_3^-] by conserving or excreting the HCO_3^- present in the glomerular ultrafiltrate and by producing new HCO_3^- which enters the body fluids as the kidneys excrete ammonium salts and titratable acids (this sum is called net acid) in the urine.

891. H^+ secretion from cells across the luminal membrane is mostly in exchange for?

Harrison's 20th Ed. Chapter 303 Page 2095

A. Na^+ ions
B. K^+ ions
C. HCO_3^- ions
D. All of the above

892. Soluble carbonic anhydrase is also called?

Harrison's 20th Ed. Chapter 303 Page 2095

A. Type I
B. Type II
C. Type III
D. Type IV

H^+ secretion from cells across the luminal membrane is mostly in exchange for Na^+ ions. Secreted H^+ reacts with filtered HCO_3^- to form H_2CO_3. In the presence of carbonic anhydrase (type IV), luminal H_2CO_3 rapidly dehydrates to $CO_2 + H_2O$. Inside the cell, dissociation of H_2O into OH^- and H^+ is promoted by hydroxylation of CO_2 ($OH^- + CO_2 => HCO_3^-$) to generate bicarbonate, catalyzed by soluble (type II) carbonic anhydrase.

893. Bicarbonate exits the cell through the basolateral membrane in a cotransport ratio with Na^+ of?

Harrison's 20th Ed. Chapter 303 Page 2095

A. 1:1
B. 2:1
C. 3:1
D. 4:1

Bicarbonate exits the cell through the basolateral membrane in a 3:1 cotransport with Na^+. The net result is that $NaHCO_3$ disappears from the lumen and appears in the blood-side of the proximal tubule cells.

894. Proximal reabsorption HCO_3^- is stimulated by?

Harrison's 20th Ed. Chapter 303 Page 2095

A. Respiratory acidosis
B. Decreases in cellular K^+
C. High levels of Angiotensin II
D. All of the above

Proximal reabsorption HCO_3^- is stimulated by decreases in cell pH (due to metabolic acidosis, respiratory acidosis or to decreases in cell K^+) and high levels of Angiotensin II which stimulate Na-H exchange. The most potent stimulator of NH_4^+ generation and excretion is metabolic acidosis.

895. Which of the following inherited disorders involve the proximal tubule?

Harrison's 20th Ed. Chapter 303 Page 2095 Table 303-1

A. Fanconi-Bickel syndrome
B. Dent disease
C. Hartnup disorder
D. All of the above

Inherited disorders involving the proximal tubule are proximal renal tubular acidosis, Fanconi-Bickel syndrome, isolated renal glycosurla, cystinuria (type I and non type I), Lysinuric protein intolerance, Hartnup disorder, Hereditary hypophosphatemic rickets with hypercalcemia, renal hypouricemia (type 1 & 2), Dent disease, X-linked-recessive nephrolithiasis with renal failure, X-linked-recessive hypophosphatemic rickets.

896. Which of the following inherited disorders involve the loop of Henle?

Harrison's 20th Ed. Chapter 303 Page 2095 Table 303-1

A. Familial hypocalciuric hypercalcemia
B. Bartter syndrome
C. Primary hypomagnesemia
D. All of the above

Inherited disorders involving the loop of Henle are Bartter syndrome (type 1, 2 & 3), autosomal dominant hypocalcemia with Bartter-like syndrome, Familial hypocalciuric hypercalcemia, Primary hypomagnesemia and isolated renal magnesium loss.

897. Which of the following inherited disorders involve the distal tubule and collecting duct?

Harrison's 20th Ed. Chapter 303 Page 2095 Table 303-1

A. Gitelman syndrome
B. Pseudoaldosteronism (Liddle's syndrome)
C. Gordon's syndrome
D. All of the above

Inherited disorders involving the distal tubule and collecting duct are Gitelman syndrome, primary hypomagnesemia with secondary hypocalcemia, pseudoaldosteronism (Liddle's syndrome), recessive pseudohypoaldosteronism type 1, pseudohypoaldosteronism type 2 (Gordon's hyperkalemia-hypertension syndrome), X-linked nephrogenic diabetes insipidus, nephrogenic diabetes insipidus (autosomal), Distal renal tubular acidosis.

898. Which of the following is related to Glucose transporter, GLUT2 gene?

Harrison's 20th Ed. Chapter 303 Page 2095 Table 303-1

A. Hartnup disorder
B. Bartter's syndrome
C. Fanconi-Bickel syndrome
D. Liddle's syndrome

899. Chloride channel gene is affected in which of the following Bartter's syndrome?

Harrison's 20th Ed. Chapter 303 Page 2095 Table 303-1

A. Type I
B. Type II
C. Type III
D. All of the above

900. Which of the following gene is affected in autosomal dominant distal renal tubular acidosis?

Harrison's 20th Ed. Chapter 303 Page 2095 Table 303-1

A. Anion exchanger-1
B. Vasopressin V2 receptor
C. Sodium chloride cotransporter
D. Calcium-sensing receptor

901. Which of the following gene is affected in Hartnup disorder?

Harrison's 20th Ed. Chapter 303 Page 2095 Table 303-1

A. Urate-anion exchanger
B. Neutral amino acid transporter
C. Amino acid transporter
D. Sodium bicarbonate cotransporter

902. Which of the following drugs is not filtered at the glomerulus?

Harrison's 20th Ed. Chapter 303 Page 2095

A. Penicillins
B. Cephalosporins
C. Salicylates
D. All of the above

Protein-bound drugs like penicillins, cephalosporins, and salicylates are not filtered at the glomerulus and are secreted by proximal tubule by specific transporters.

903. Which of the following is a biogenic amine neurotransmitter?

Harrison's 20th Ed. Chapter 303 Page 2095

A. Dopamine
B. Acetylcholine
C. Epinephrine
D. All of the above

Organic cations secreted by the proximal tubule include various biogenic amine neurotransmitters (dopamine, acetylcholine, epinephrine, norepinephrine, and histamine) and creatinine.

904. Which of the following drugs is secreted by ATP-dependent transporter P-glycoprotein?

Harrison's 20th Ed. Chapter 303 Page 2095

A. Cyclosporine
B. Digoxin
C. Tacrolimus
D. All of the above

The ATP-dependent transporter P-glycoprotein is highly expressed in brush border membranes and secretes cyclosporine, digoxin, tacrolimus, and various cancer chemotherapeutic agents. P-glycoprotein (P-gp) is a plasma membrane ATP-binding cassette transporter, responsible for multidrug resistance in tumor cells.

905. Which of the following present in proximal tubular cell bioactivates circulating 25-hydroxy vitamin D?

Harrison's 20th Ed. Chapter 303 Page 2095

A. 1α-hydroxylase
B. 7α-hydroxylase
C. 17-α-hydroxylase
D. 21-hydroxylase

Circulating 25-hydroxy vitamin D (calcidiol) is bioactivated by proximal tubular 1α-hydroxylase to produce 1,25-di-hydroxy vitamin D (calcitriol) which is the most active form of the hormone, that acts on the small intestine to promote calcium absorption.

906. Which of the following statements about fibroblast growth factor (FGF) is false?

Harrison's 20th Ed. Chapter 303 Page 2095

A. Fibroblast growth factor 23 (FGF23) is produced in osteoblasts and osteocytes
B. Parathyroid hormone (PTH) and active vitamin D regulate FGF23 production
C. Klotho is the required co-factor of FGF23
D. None of the above

FGF23 requires Klotho protein as a coreceptor for high affinity binding to cognate FGF receptors (FGFRs).

907. Fibroblast growth factor 23 (FGF23) belongs to which of the following class of phosphate-regulating factors?

Kidney Int. 2004;65(1):1-14

A. Phosphataxin
B. Phosphatonin
C. Phosphatorin
D. Phosphatine

Phosphorus balance is primarily regulated by PTH but may also respond to fibroblast growth factor 23 (FGF-23) and its cofactor, klotho, which together and separately promote renal excretion of phosphorus.

908. Which of the following is a phosphatonin?

Clin Cases Miner Bone Metab. 2012;9(1):9-12

A. FGF-23
B. sFRP-4
C. MEPE
D. All of the above

FGF23, sFRP-4, MEPE, and FGF7 are phosphatonins.

909. Which of the following diseases has a high fibroblast growth factor (FGF)-23 level?

Kidney Int. 2004;65(1):1-14

A. X-linked hypophosphatemia (XLH)
B. Autosomal dominant hypophosphatemic rickets (ADHR)
C. Oncogenic osteomalacia (OOM)
D. All of the above

910. Which of the following is a feature of secondary hyperparathyroidism?

doi:10.4061/2011/364890 Kidney Int. 2004;65(1):1-14

A. Elevated serum phosphate
B. Low calcitriol
C. High PTH levels
D. All of the above

911. Proteins encoded by SLC3A1 and SLC7A9 genes transport which of the following amino acids?

Harrison's 20th Ed. Chapter 303 Page 2095

A. Cystine
B. Lysine
C. Arginine
D. All of the above

Cystine, lysine, arginine and ornithine are transported by a system comprising two proteins encoded by the SLC3A1 and SLC7A9 genes. Mutations in either of them impair reabsorption of these amino acids and cause cystinuria.

912. Absorptive endocytosis relates to the transport of?

Harrison's 20th Ed. Chapter 303 Page 2095

A. Amino acids
B. Peptide hormones
C. Biogenic amine neurotransmitters
D. Protein-bound drugs

Peptide hormones like insulin and growth hormone, β_2-microglobulin, albumin are taken up by the proximal tubule through a process of absorptive endocytosis and are degraded in acidified endocytic lysosomes.

913. Which of the following is not a major segment of loop of Henle?

Harrison's 20th Ed. Chapter 303 Page 2095

A. Descending thin limb
B. Descending thick limb
C. Ascending thin limb
D. Ascending thick limb

Loop of Henle consists of 3 major segments - descending & ascending thin limb & ascending thick limb.

914. Major segments of Loop of Henle are based on?

Harrison's 20th Ed. Chapter 303 Page 2095

A. Cellular morphology
B. Anatomic location
C. Specialization of function
D. All of the above

915. Site of action of loop diuretics is?

Harrison's 20th Ed. Chapter 303 Page 2095

A. Proximal convoluted tubule
B. Loop of Henle
C. Distal convoluted tubule
D. Collecting duct

Site of action of loop diuretics is loop of Henle.

916. Water-permeability is highest in?

Harrison's 20th Ed. Chapter 303 Page 2095

A. Descending thin limb
B. Ascending thin limb
C. Ascending thick limb
D. Proximal convoluted tubule

Descending thin limb of loop of Henle is highly water-permeable due to dense expression of aquaporin-1 water channels. Water permeability is negligible in the ascending limb.

917. Which of the following is false about countercurrent multiplication?

Harrison's 20th Ed. Chapter 303 Page 2095

A. Uses Na^+ transporters in TALH
B. Descending thin limb of LOH is permeable to water
C. TALH is not permeable to water
D. None of the above

Epithelium of the ascending thin and thick limb of Henle's loop is impermeable to water and there are no lymphatics in the inner medulla and few in the outer medulla. Any water added to the interstitium must be removed by ascending vasa recta (AVR).

918. "Countercurrent multiplication" leads to?

Harrison's 20th Ed. Chapter 303 Page 2095

A. Hypotonic medullary interstitium
B. Hypertonic medullary interstitium
C. Isotonic medullary interstitium
D. All of the above

Loop of Henle and vasa recta establishes a hypertonic medullary interstitium by phenomenon called countercurrent multiplication.

919. Which of the following is a capillary network in a nephron?

Harrison's 20th Ed. Chapter 303 Page 2095

A. Glomerular capillaries
B. Peritubular capillaries
C. Vasa recta
D. All of the above

920. Which of the following statements is false?

Am J Physiol Regul Integr Comp Physiol. 2003;284:R1153-R1175

A. Ratio of ascending to descending vasa recta is 2:1
B. Endothelium of ascending vasa recta (AVR) is fenestrated
C. Endothelium of descending vasa recta (DVR) is continuous
D. None of the above

921. Which of the following occurs in medullary interstitium as blood flows from corticomedullary junction toward the papillary tip?

Am J Physiol Regul Integr Comp Physiol. 2003;284:R1153-R1175

A. Rising interstitial concentrations of NaCl from PCT
B. Rising interstitial concentrations of urea from collecting duct
C. Water flows via AQP1 channels from DVR lumen to medullary interstitium
D. All of the above

922. Water is supplied to the medullary interstitium by reabsorption from?

Harrison's 20th Ed. Chapter 303 Page 2095

A. Pars recta of proximal tubule in outer medulla
B. Descending thin limb of Henle's loop in the inner medulla
C. Collecting duct
D. All of the above

A small difference in osmotic pressure (the single effect) is multiplied by countercurrent flow in adjacent channels of the limbs of Henle's loop to produce a large axial difference in osmotic pressure between the renal cortex and the tip of the renal papilla. This multiplier generates a hypertonic renal medulla. Countercurrent exchange preserves medullary hypertonicity rather than create it.

923. Which of the following about countercurrent multiplication (CCM) is false?

Harrison's 20th Ed. Chapter 303 Page 2095

A. Exchange occurs between capillary & interstitium of the medulla rather than between two adjacent capillary loops
B. Solute diffuses from medullary interstitium to blood flowing down the descending vas rectum
C. As blood returns in the ascending vas rectum, solute diffuses into the interstitium
D. None of the above

Exchange occurs between capillary and interstitium of the medulla rather than between two adjacent capillary loops. Solute diffuses from the medullary interstitium to the blood flowing down the descending vas rectum. As blood returns in the ascending vas rectum, the solute concentration difference is reversed and solute diffuses into the interstitium. This effectively "traps" solute in the interstitium by recycling between ascending and descending capillary. In this way, blood circulates through the renal medulla without "washing out" its hypertonicity. The greater the solute permeability of the capillary, the more complete the exchange.

924. Which of the following is false about loop of Henle?

Harrison's 20th Ed. Chapter 303 Page 2095

A. Site of action for loop diuretics
B. Contributes to reabsorption of calcium ions
C. Contributes to reabsorption of magnesium ions
D. None of the above

925. Which of the following is the primary target for loop diuretics?

Harrison's 20th Ed. Chapter 303 Page 2095

A. Na^+/Cl^- co-transporter
B. $Na^+/K^+/2Cl^-$ co-transporter
C. Na^+/K^+-ATPase
D. Apical Ca^{++}-selective channels (TRPV5)

In the thick ascending limb, high level of secondary active NaCl transport is enabled by $Na^+/K^+/2Cl^-$ cotransporter on the apical membrane in series with basolateral Cl^- channels & Na^+/K^+-ATPase The $Na^+/K^+/2Cl^-$ co-transporter is the primary target for loop diuretics.

926. Tubular concentration of K^+ is?

Harrison's 20th Ed. Chapter 303 Page 2096

A. ~ 2 mEq/L
B. ~ 4 mEq/L
C. ~ 6 mEq/L
D. ~ 8 mEq/L

Tubular concentration of K^+ is similar to plasma i.e. about 4 mEq/L.

927. Which of the following is an inherited disorder of the thick ascending limb?

Harrison's 20th Ed. Chapter 303 Page 2096

A. Gitelman's syndrome
B. Bartter's syndrome
C. Gordon's syndrome
D. Liddle's syndrome

Bartter's syndrome is an inherited disorder of thick ascending limb. It leads to a salt-wasting renal disease with hypokalemia & metabolic alkalosis.

928. Loss-of-function mutations in which of the following can cause Bartter's syndrome?

Harrison's 20th Ed. Chapter 303 Page 2096

A. NKCC2
B. KCNJ1
C. CLCNKB
D. All of the above

Loss-of-function mutations in one of five distinct genes encoding components of the $Na^+/K^+/2Cl^-$ cotransporter (NKCC2), apical K^+ channel (KCNJ1), basolateral Cl^- channel (CLCNKB, BSND), or calcium-sensing receptor (CASR) can cause Bartter's syndrome.

929. Positive electrostatic charge in the lumen relative to interstitium is caused by?

Harrison's 20th Ed. Chapter 303 Page 2096

A. Mg^{2+} reabsorption
B. Ca^{2+} reabsorption
C. Potassium recycling
D. All of the above

Potassium recycling contributes to a positive electrostatic charge in lumen relative to the interstitium.

930. Which of the following is a transmembrane protein located within the tight junction complex?

Harrison's 20th Ed. Chapter 303 Page 2096

A. Hensin
B. Paracellin-1
C. Nedd4-2
D. All of the above

Mutations in CLDN16 encoding paracellin-1, a transmembrane protein located within the tight junction complex, leads to familial hypomagnesemia with hypercalcuria and nephrocalcinosis.

931. Which of the following about TRPV5 is true?

Harrison's 20th Ed. Chapter 303 Page 2096

A. Basolateral Na^+/K^+-ATPase and Cl^- channels
B. Apical K^+ channels
C. Ca^+ selective channel
D. Thiazide-sensitive Na^+/Cl^- cotransporter

TRPV5 stands for Transient Receptor Potential Cation Channel Subfamily V Member 5. Diseases associated with TRPV5 include Hypervitaminosis D and Idiopathic Hypercalciuria.

932. Which of the following about TRPV5 is false?

Harrison's 20th Ed. Chapter 303 Page 2096

A. Apical Ca^{++}-selective channel
B. Promotes active renal calcium reabsorption
C. Localized to distal convoluted tubule and collecting tubule
D. None of the above

TRPV5 is a transient receptor potential channel involved in calcium reabsorption. The renal handling of calcium is similar to active intestinal absorption, but uses TRPV5 instead of TRPV6. Phosphatidylinositol 4,5-bisphosphate (PI(4,5)P2) and calmodulin (CaM) directly bind to TRPV5 and activate or inactivate the channel, respectively. PI(4,5)P2 is found in the inner leaflet of the plasma membrane.

933. Which of the following about calmodulin (CaM) is false?
N Engl J Med. 1986; 314:1164-1170

A. Calcium sensing protein
B. Endogenous inactivator of TRPV5
C. Calmodulin's structure is similar to that of troponin C
D. None of the above

Calmodulin (CaM) is an abbreviation for calcium-modulated protein.

934. A molecular complex of which of the following proteins is critical for Mg^{2+} reabsorption in thick ascending limb of Henle?
Harrison's 20th Ed. Chapter 303 Page 2096

A. TRPM1 and TRPM2
B. TRPM3 and TRPM4
C. TRPM5 and TRPM6
D. TRPM6 and TRPM7

A molecular complex of TRPM6 and TRPM7 proteins is critical for Mg^{2+} reabsorption in the thick ascending limb of Henle.

935. Loss-of-function mutations of SLC12A3 encoding the apical Na^+/Cl^- co-transporter cause?
Harrison's 20th Ed. Chapter 303 Page 2096

A. Gitelman's syndrome
B. Bartter's syndrome
C. Gordon's syndrome
D. Liddle's syndrome

Loss-of-function mutations of SLC12A3 encoding the apical Na^+/Cl^- co-transporter cause Gitelman's syndrome - a salt-wasting disorder associated with hypokalemic alkalosis and hypocalciuria.

936. Mutations in genes encoding WNK kinases, WNK-1 & WNK-4 cause?
Harrison's 20th Ed. Chapter 303 Page 2096

A. Gitelman's syndrome
B. Bartter's syndrome
C. Gordon's syndrome
D. Liddle's syndrome

Mutations in genes encoding WNK kinases, WNK-1 and WNK-4 cause pseudohypoaldosteronism type II or Gordon's syndrome characterized by familial hypertension with hyperkalemia.

937. Which of the following modulates the final composition of the urine?
Harrison's 20th Ed. Chapter 303 Page 2096

A. Proximal convoluted tubule
B. Loop of Henle
C. Distal convoluted tubule
D. Collecting duct

The collecting duct modulates the final composition of urine. Its two major divisions are cortical collecting duct and inner medullary collecting duct.

938. Which of the following about principal cells of cortical collecting duct is false?
Harrison's 20th Ed. Chapter 303 Page 2096

A. Main Na^+ reabsorbing cells
B. Site of action of aldosterone
C. Site of action of K^+-sparing diuretics
D. None of the above

Principal cells are the main water and Na^+ reabsorbing & K^+ secreting cells and the site of action of aldosterone, K^+-sparing diuretics, and mineralocorticoid receptor antagonists such as spironolactone and eplerenone.

939. Which of the following is true for type A intercalated cells of cortical collecting duct?
Harrison's 20th Ed. Chapter 303 Page 2096

A. Acid secretion & bicarbonate reabsorption
B. Bicarbonate secretion & acid reabsorption
C. Acid & bicarbonate secretion
D. Acid & bicarbonate reabsorption

940. Which of the following is true for type B intercalated cells of cortical collecting duct?
Harrison's 20th Ed. Chapter 303 Page 2096

A. Acid secretion & bicarbonate reabsorption
B. Bicarbonate secretion & acid reabsorption
C. Acid & bicarbonate secretion
D. Acid & bicarbonate reabsorption

Type A intercalated cells of cortical collecting duct mediate acid secretion and bicarbonate reabsorption. Type B intercalated cells mediate bicarbonate secretion and acid reabsorption.

941. Activating mutations occur in which of the following channels in Liddle's syndrome?
Harrison's 20th Ed. Chapter 303 Page 2096

A. Na^+
B. K^+
C. Cl^-
D. HCO_3^-

942. Epithelial Na^+ channel (ENaC) are sensitive to?
Harrison's 20th Ed. Chapter 303 Page 2096

A. Amiloride
B. Aldosterone
C. Spironolactone
D. Eplerenone

In principal cells, passive apical Na^+ entry occurs through an amiloride-sensitive, epithelial Na^+ channel (ENaC) with basolateral exit mediated by the Na^+/K^+-ATPase.

943. In principal cells of cortical collecting ducts, sodium reabsorptive process is tightly regulated by?
Harrison's 20th Ed. Chapter 303 Page 2096

A. Renin
B. Angiotensin II
C. Aldosterone
D. All of the above

In principal cells of cortical collecting ducts, sodium reabsorptive process is tightly regulated by aldosterone which enters the cell across basolateral membrane, binds to cytoplasmic mineralocorticoid receptor, and translocates into nucleus, where it modulates gene transcription, resulting in increased Na^+ reabsorption and K^+ secretion.

944. All of the following are features of Liddle's syndrome except?
Harrison's 20th Ed. Chapter 303 Page 2096

A. Hypokalemia
B. Hypernatremia
C. Hypertension
D. Metabolic alkalosis

In Liddle's syndrome, activating mutations occur in epithelial Na^+ channel (ENaC) causing increase in Na^+ reclamation that produces hypokalemia, hypertension, and metabolic alkalosis.

945. Which of the following block ENaC?

Harrison's 20th Ed. Chapter 303 Page 2096

A. Trimethoprim
B. Pentamidine
C. Triamterene
D. All of the above

K^+-sparing diuretics amiloride & triamterene block ENaC, causing reduced Na^+ reabsorption. Trimethoprim & pentamidine, block ENaCs and predispose to hyperkalemia.

946. Which of the following statements about intercalated cells is false?

Harrison's 20th Ed. Chapter 303 Page 2097

A. Intercalated cells do not participate in Na^+ reabsorption
B. Intercalated cells mediate acid-base secretion
C. Type A intercalated cells have Cl^-/HCO_3^- exchanger on the apical membrane
D. Type B intercalated cells have Cl^-/HCO_3^- exchanger on the apical membrane

Type A intercalated cells have an apical proton pump (H^+-ATPase) that mediates acid secretion and a basolateral Cl^-/HCO_3^- anion exchanger for bicarbonate reabsorption. Type B intercalated cells have the Cl^-/HCO_3^- exchanger on the apical membrane to mediate bicarbonate secretion while the proton pump resides on the basolateral membrane to enable acid reabsorption.

947. Extracellular protein hensin is best related to?

Harrison's 20th Ed. Chapter 303 Page 2097

A. Principal cells
B. Intercalated cells
C. Podocytes
D. Mesangial cells

In acidemia, kidneys uses type A intercalated cells to secrete excess H^+ & generate more HCO_3^-. In bicarbonate excess with alkalemia type B intercalated cells predominate. Extracellular protein 'hensin' mediates this adaptation.

948. Atrial natriuretic peptide or renal natriuretic peptide (urodilatin) acts on?

Harrison's 20th Ed. Chapter 303 Page 2097

A. Cortical collecting duct
B. Inner medullary collecting duct
C. Distal convoluted tubule
D. All of the above

The two major divisions of collecting duct are the cortical collecting duct and inner medullary collecting duct. Natriuretic peptides like atrial natriuretic peptide or renal natriuretic peptide (urodilatin) interact with either apical (urodilatin) or basolateral (atrial natriuretic peptides) receptors on inner medullary collecting duct cells.

949. Which of the following is false about renal natriuretic peptide (urodilatin)?

Harrison's 20th Ed. Chapter 303 Page 2097

A. Secreted by renal tubular epithelia
B. Interacts with apical receptors on inner medullary collecting duct cells
C. Attenuates net Na^+ reabsorption
D. None of the above

950. Urodilatin resembles which of the following?

Harrison's 20th Ed. Chapter 303 Page 2097

A. Atrial natriuretic peptide
B. Aldosterone
C. Renin
D. PGE_2

951. Routine surrogate marker for assessing clinical tonicity is the concentration of?

Harrison's 20th Ed. Chapter 303 Page 2098 Figure 303-4

A. Na^+
B. K^+
C. Cl^-
D. All of the above

Routine surrogate marker for assessing clinical tonicity is the concentration of serum Na^+.

952. Which of the following water channels "aquaporin" is not present in inner medullary collecting duct cells?

Harrison's 20th Ed. Chapter 303 Page 2098

A. Aquaporin-1
B. Aquaporin-2
C. Aquaporin-3
D. Aquaporin-4

Inner medullary collecting duct cells have vasopressin-regulated water channels (aquaporin-2 on apical & aquaporin-3 & 4 on basolateral membrane). Aquaporin-1 water channels are densely expressed in descending thin limb of loop of Henle.

953. Which of the following aquaporin is not regulated by vasopressin in the collecting duct?

Harrison's 20th Ed. Chapter 303 Page 2098

A. Aquaporin 1
B. Aquaporin 2
C. Aquaporin 3
D. Aquaporin 4

Aquaporin 1 is active in all water-permeable segments of proximal & distal tubules, while aquaporins 2, 3, and 4 are regulated by vasopressin in the collecting duct.

954. Which of the folowing TRPV channels is osmoreceptive?

Harrison's 20th Ed. Chapter 303 Page 2098

A. $TRPV1^+$
B. $TRPV2^+$
C. $TRPV3^+$
D. $TRPV4^+$

Vanilloid receptors Transient receptor potential (TRPV) channels respond to changes in tonicity. $TRPV4^+$ neuronal cells connected to supraoptic and paraventricular nuclei in hypothalamus are osmoreceptive. They modulate release of vasopressin by posterior lobe of the pituitary gland.

955. Aldosterone leads to which of the following in principal cells of the collecting duct?

Harrison's 20th Ed. Chapter 303 Page 2098

A. Increase activity of apical membrane Na^+ channel
B. Increase activity of apical membrane K^+ channel
C. Increase activity of basolateral Na^+/K^+-ATPase
D. All of the above

Aldosterone binds to cytoplasmic mineralocorticoid receptors in principal cells of collecting duct & increases activity of apical membrane Na^+ channel, apical membrane K^+ channel & basolateral Na^+/K^+-ATPase.

956. Aldosterone mediates its effects by which of the following genes?

Harrison's 20th Ed. Chapter 303 Page 2098

A. SLC2A2
B. CLCN5
C. SGK1
D. CASR

Aldosterone mediates its effects in part by serum/glucocorticoid-induced kinase 1 (SGK1).

957. Which of the following is false about aldosterone escape?

Harrison's 20th Ed. Chapter 303 Page 2098

A. Chronic exposure to aldosterone
B. Decreased proximal tubular Na^+ reabsorption
C. Facilitated by atrial natriuretic peptides
D. None of the above

958. Who proposed the "Hyperfiltration hypothesis"?

Kidney International. 1996; 49:1774-1777

A. JL Olson
B. Timothy W. Meyer
C. HG Rennke
D. Barry Brenner

Barry Brenner in his hyperfiltration hypothesis in 1982 demonstrated that alterations in glomerular hemodynamics associated with renal ablation are accompanied by structural lesions and suggest that sustained single nephron hyperfiltration (SNGFR) may have maladaptive consequences by damaging remnant glomeruli.

959. Nephrons are not generated after how many weeks of gestation?

Mol Cell Pediatr. 2017;4:12

A. 30–32
B. 32–34
C. 34–36
D. 36–40

Nephrons are not generated after 34–36 weeks of gestation or after birth.

960. Reduced nephron numbers at birth may be due to?

Mol Cell Pediatr. 2017;4:12

A. Developmental abnormalities
B. Genetic predisposition
C. Malnutrition
D. All of the above

Reduced nephron numbers at birth may be due to developmental abnormalities, genetic predisposition and environmental factors such as malnutrition.

961. Which of the following is a CAKUT disorder?

Harrison's 20th Ed. Chapter 309 Page 2156

A. Kidney agenesis
B. Ureteropelvic junction obstruction
C. Vesicoureteral reflux
D. All of the above

Congenital abnormalities of the kidney and urinary tract (CAKUT) disorders include kidney hypoplasia, kidney agenesis, ureteropelvic junction obstruction, and vesicoureteral reflux.

962. Which of the following can be caused by prenatal exposure of ACE inhibitors or angiotensin receptor blockers?

Harrison's 20th Ed. Chapter 309 Page 2156

A. Kidney dysgenesis
B. Ureteropelvic junction obstruction
C. Vesicoureteral reflux
D. All of the above

963. Which of the following is a syndromic forms of CAKUT?

Harrison's 20th Ed. Chapter 309 Page 2156

A. Hepatorenal syndrome
B. Branchio-oto-renal syndrome
C. Pulmonary-renal syndrome
D. All of the above

Branchio-oto-renal (BOR) syndrome and autosomal dominant renal coloboma syndrome are syndromic forms of CAKUT. BOR is characterized by developmental abnormalities in neck, ears, and kidney, and is caused by mutations in EYA1 & SIX1 genes. Mutations in the PAX2 transcription factor gene causes the autosomal dominant renal coloboma syndrome.

964. Time of most rapid nephrogenesis is?

Mol Cell Pediatr. 2017;4:12

A. Early gestation
B. Mid gestation
C. Late gestation
D. All of the above

Mid gestation is the time of most rapid nephrogenesis.

965. Deficiency of which of the following predisposes to abnormal kidney development?

Mol Cell Pediatr. 2017;4:12

A. Vitamin A
B. Sodium
C. Zinc
D. All of the above

966. Which of the following medications taken by mother influences kidney development?

Mol Cell Pediatr. 2017;4:12

A. Dexamethasone
B. Angiotensin converting enzyme inhibitors
C. Gentamicin
D. All of the above

Factors implicated as predisposing to abnormal kidney development include deficiency in vitamin A, sodium, zinc or iron, and medications like dexamethasone, Gentamicin, Nonsteroidal anti-inflammatory drugs, angiotensin converting enzyme inhibitors and angiotensin receptor antagonists.

967. Who was the first to describe association between low birth weight & later cardiovascular death?

Indian Pediatrics 2009;46:S48-S54

A. Barry Brenner
B. Timothy W. Meyer
C. David Barker
D. Neal Bricker

Barker fetal origins hypothesis proposed that intrauterine growth retardation, low birth weight, and premature birth have a causal relationship to the origins of hypertension, coronary heart disease, and non-insulin-dependent diabetes, in middle age.

968. Nephrons of which of the followng can regenerate?

J Am Soc Nephrol. 2006;17:2390-2401

A. Duck
B. Bat
C. Fish
D. Dog

Nephrons of mammals, in contrast to those of fish, cannot regenerate.

969. Which of the following participates in compensatory renal growth after nephron loss?

Pediatr Endocrinol Rev. 2012;10(1):152-63

A. Hepatocyte growth factor
B. Glucose transporters
C. Insulin-like growth factor
D. All of the above

970. Whose name is associated with intact nephron hypothesis?

Nephrol Dial Transplant 2015;30:1602–1604

A. Herbert Lubowitz
B. Neil Bricker
C. Doris Rolf
D. Fred Weisser

An exposition of the Intact Nephron Hypothesis was published by Bricker et. al. in American Journal of Medicine (1960). Dr. Bricker defined the "intact nephron hypothesis" that the number of functioning nephrons is reduced in chronic renal disease and that the remaining nephrons undergo adaptations that maintain renal homeostasis.

971. Bricker's trade-off hypothesis best relates to?

Nutrients. 2017;9(5):427

A. Calcium
B. Phosphorus
C. PTH
D. All of the above

Slatopolsky and Bricker's trade-off hypothesis in 1972 is based on the effects of uremia on the balance between calcium, phosphorus & PTH levels. Elevations in PTH that occur in CKD restore calcium & phosphorus levels but lead to hyperplasia of parathyroid gland & secondary hyperparathyroidism (trade-off).

972. Urine specific gravity of 1.010 equals how many mOsmol/L of urine osmolality?

Harrison's 18th Ed 2291

A. 300
B. 325
C. 350
D. 375

Urine specific gravity of 1.010 equals ~350 mOsmol/L of urine osmolality.

973. Delta metabolic acidosis occurs when GFR falls below?

Harrison's 18th Ed 2292

A. 25 mL/minute
B. 40 mL/minute
C. 60 mL/minute
D. 75 mL/minute

When GFR falls below 25 mL/minute, organic acids accumulate producing a delta metabolic acidosis.

Acute Kidney Injury

974. Which of the following about acute kidney injury (AKI) is false?
Harrison's 20th Ed. Chapter 304 Page 2099

A. Clinical rather than a structural diagnosis
B. Increase in serum creatinine (SCr) concentration
C. Often associated with a reduction in urine volume
D. None of the above

975. Which of the following is not a cause of community-acquired acute kidney injury (AKI)?
Harrison's 20th Ed. Chapter 304 Page 2099

A. Volume depletion
B. Nephrotoxic medication administration
C. Obstruction of the urinary tract
D. Malignancy

AKI may be community-acquired or hospital-acquired. Common causes of community-acquired AKI include volume depletion, heart failure, adverse effects of medications, obstruction of the urinary tract, or malignancy. Most common clinical settings for hospital-acquired AKI are sepsis, major surgical procedures, critical illness involving heart or liver failure, and nephrotoxic medication administration.

976. Which of the following is the cause of AKI?
Harrison's 20th Ed. Chapter 304 Page 2099

A. Prerenal azotemia
B. Intrinsic renal parenchymal disease
C. Postrenal obstruction
D. All of the above

Causes of AKI have traditionally been divided into three broad categories : prerenal azotemia, intrinsic renal parenchymal disease and postrenal obstruction. Prerenal azotemia is the most common form of AKI.

977. Which of the following is a cause of prerenal AKI?
Harrison's 20th Ed. Chapter 304 Page 2099 Figure 304-1

A. Congestive heart failure
B. Liver failure
C. Hypovolemia
D. All of the above

978. Which of the following is not a cause of intrinsic AKI?
Harrison's 20th Ed. Chapter 304 Page 2099 Figure 304-1

A. Sepsis
B. Ischemia
C. Hemolysis
D. Congestive heart failure

979. Which of the following is a cause of intrinsic AKI?
Harrison's 20th Ed. Chapter 304 Page 2099 Figure 304-1

A. Malignant hypertension
B. TTP-HUS
C. Acute glomerulonephritis
D. All of the above

980. Which of the following is an endogenous nephrotoxin?
Harrison's 20th Ed. Chapter 304 Page 2099 Figure 304-1

A. Rhabdomyolysis
B. Myeloma
C. Hemolysis
D. All of the above

981. "Azo" means?
Harrison's 20th Ed. Chapter 304 Page 2099

A. Urea
B. Ammonia
C. Nitrogen
D. Waste

Word azotemia is derived from "azo" meaning nitrogen.

982. Term azotemia is used mostly for?
Harrison's 20th Ed. Chapter 304 Page 2099

A. Prerenal ARF
B. Intrinsic ARF
C. Postrenal ARF
D. All of the above

Prerenal acute renal failure is also called azotemia.

983. Acute tubular necrosis (ATN) best relates to?
Harrison's 20th Ed. Chapter 304 Page 2099

A. Sepsis
B. Ischemic injury
C. Vasculitis
D. Nephrotoxin

Prolonged periods of prerenal azotemia may lead to ischemic injury. This is termed as acute tubular necrosis (ATN).

984. Which of the following about acute renal failure is false?
Lancet 2005;365:417-430

A. Abrupt & sustained decrease in renal function with retention of nitrogenous and non-nitrogenous waste products
B. Acute & sustained increase in serum creatinine of 0.5 mg/dL, if the baseline is < 2.5 mg/dL
C. Increase in serum creatinine of > 20% if the baseline is > 2.5 mg/dL
D. None of the above

985. RIFLE system is used to classify?
Lancet 2005;365:417-430

A. Acute renal failure
B. Chronic renal failure
C. Glomerulonephritis
D. Nephrotic syndrome

RIFLE = Risk-Injury-Failure-Loss-End-stage kidney disease (ESKD). RIFLE classification was established by the Acute Dialysis Quality Initiative (ADQI) group in order to supply the obligation for uniform definition, early detection, and grading of AKI. After this, the AKIN criteria were created by the Acute Kidney Injury Network (AKIN) for further refinement of the definition of AKI.

986. Which of the following about prerenal azotemia is false?
Lancet 2005;365:417-430

A Integrity of renal tissue is disturbed
B. Appropriate physiological response to renal hypoperfusion
C. Certain drugs can provoke acute prerenal failure
D. Persistent renal hypoperfusion leads to ischemic ATN

By definition, no parenchymal damage to the kidney occurs in prerenal azotemia. It is rapidly reversible once parenchymal blood flow and intraglomerular hemodynamics are restored.

987. Typical histological features of human acute tubular necrosis include?
Lancet 2005;365:417-430

A. Loss of brush border in proximal tubular cells
B. Sloughing of tubular cells into the lumen
C. Interstitial oedema
D. All of the above

988. In kidneys, most of the blood supply is directed to?
Lancet 2005;365:417-430

A. Renal cortex
B. Outer medulla
C. Medullary rays
D. None of the above

989. In established acute tubular necrosis, selective reduction in blood supply occurs in?
Lancet 2005;365:417-430

A. Renal cortex
B. Outer medulla
C. Medullary rays
D. None of the above

990. Vasoconstrictors implicated in reduced renal blood flow in acute tubular necrosis are?
Lancet 2005;365:417-430

A. Angiotensin II
B. Thromboxane A_2
C. Prostaglandin H_2
D. All of the above

991. Vasoconstrictors implicated in the reduced renal blood flow in acute tubular necrosis are?
Lancet 2005;365:417-430

A. Leukotrienes C4 and D4
B. Endothelin 1
C. Adenosine
D. All of the above

992. Which of the following about urine findings in pre-renal ARF is false?
Lancet 2005;365:417-430

A. Specific gravity about 1.020
B. Urine osmolality > 500
C. Fractional excretion of sodium (%) < 1
D. Fractional excretion of urea (%) > 35

993. Which of the following about urine findings in pre-renal ARF is false?
Lancet 2005;365:417-430

A. Urine sodium < 10 mmol/L
B. Urine osmolality > 500
C. Fractional excretion of sodium (%) > 2
D. Fractional excretion of urea (%) < 35

994. Which of the following about urine findings in pre-renal ARF is false?
Lancet 2005;365:417-430

A. Fractional excretion of uric acid (%) < 7
B. Fractional excretion of Lithium (%) < 7
C. Low brush border enzyme levels
D. None of the above

995. Which of the following about urine findings in renal ARF is false?
Lancet 2005;365:417-430

A. Specific gravity about 1.010
B. Urine osmolality > 300
C. Fractional excretion of sodium (%) > 2
D. Fractional excretion of urea (%) < 35

996. Which of the following about urine findings in renal ARF is false?
Lancet 2005;365:417-430

A. Urine sodium > 20 mmol/kg
B. Urine osmolality > 300
C. Fractional excretion of sodium (%) < 1
D. Fractional excretion of urea (%) > 35

997. Which of the following about urine findings in renal ARF is false?
Lancet 2005;365:417-430

A. Fractional excretion of uric acid (%) > 15
B. Fractional excretion of Lithium (%) > 20
C. High brush border enzyme levels
D. None of the above

998. Biomarkers proposed for the early diagnosis of acute renal failure include?
Lancet 2005;365:417-430

A. Urinary interleukin 18
B. Intestinal form of alkaline phosphatase
C. N-acetyl-β-glucosaminidase & alanine aminopeptidase
D. All of the above

999. Biomarkers specifically higher in ischaemic ATN is?
Lancet 2005;365:417-430

A. Urinary interleukin 18
B. Kidney injury molecule 1
C. N-acetyl-β-glucosaminidase
D. Alanine aminopeptidase

1000. Normal GFR is maintained by?

Harrison's 20th Ed. Chapter 304 Page 2099

A. Renal blood flow
B. Afferent renal arteriole resistance
C. Efferent renal arteriole resistance
D. All of the above

Normal GFR is maintained by renal blood flow and the relative resistances of afferent and efferent renal arterioles, which determine the glomerular plasma flow rate and the transcapillary hydraulic pressure gradient that drive glomerular ultrafiltration.

1001. Which of the following is a mediator of homeostatic response to decreased effective circulating volume or cardiac output?

Harrison's 20th Ed. Chapter 304 Page 2099

A. Angiotensin II
B. Norepinephrine
C. Vasopressin (antidiuretic hormone)
D. All of the above

1002. Glomerular filtration is maintained despite reduced renal blood flow by?

Harrison's 20th Ed. Chapter 304 Page 2099

A. Angiotensin II
B. Norepinephrine
C. Vasopressin (antidiuretic hormone)
D. All of the above

Glomerular filtration is maintained despite reduced renal blood flow by angiotensin II–mediated renal efferent vasoconstriction, which maintains glomerular capillary hydrostatic pressure closer to normal, if renal blood flow reduction is not excessive.

1003. Which of the following occur in response to low renal perfusion pressure?

Harrison's 20th Ed. Chapter 304 Page 2100

A. Increased intrarenal biosynthesis of prostaglandins
B. Increased intrarenal biosynthesis of kallikrein and kinins
C. Increased intrarenal biosynthesis of nitric oxide (NO)
D. All of the above

1004. Myogenic reflex relates best to?

Harrison's 20th Ed. Chapter 304 Page 2100

A. Afferent arteriole
B. Efferent arteriole
C. Glomerular capillaries
D. All of the above

In a low perfusion pressure situation, a myogenic reflex within the afferent arteriole leads to dilation, thereby maintaining glomerular perfusion.

1005. Agents that impair autoregulation of renal blood flow include?

Lancet 2005;365:417-430

A. NSAIDs
B. ACE inhibitors
C. Angiotensin-II-receptor blockers
D. All of the above

1006. Which of the following about prerenal azotemia is false?

Harrison's 20th Ed. Chapter 304 Page 2099

A. Related to intraglomerular hemodynamics
B. No parenchymal damage to the kidney
C. May lead to ischemic injury–acute tubular necrosis (ATN)
D. None of the above

1007. Acute tubular necrosis (ATN) relates best with?

Harrison's 20th Ed. Chapter 304 Page 2099

A. Prerenal ARF
B. Intrinsic ARF
C. Postrenal ARF
D. All of the above

More severe or prolonged prerenal ARF (renal hypoperfusion) may lead to ischemic injury of kidneys leading to acute tubular necrosis (ATN).

1008. Prerenal ARF can result from which of the following?

Harrison's 20th Ed. Chapter 304 Page 2099

A. Low cardiac output
B. Systemic vasodilatation
C. Selective intrarenal vasoconstriction
D. All of the above

Prerenal ARF can complicate any disease that induces hypovolemia, low cardiac output, systemic vasodilatation or selective intrarenal vasoconstriction.

1009. Which of the following is an action of Angiotensin II?

Harrison's 20th Ed. Chapter 304 Page 2099

A. Increased biosynthesis of Prostaglandin E_2
B. Increased biosynthesis of prostacyclin
C. Preferential constriction of efferent arterioles
D. All of the above

Angiotensin II increases biosynthesis of vasodilator prostaglandins (Pg E_2 & prostacyclin) resulting in afferent arteriolar vasodilation. Angiotensin II also induces preferential constriction of efferent arterioles.

1010. Which of the following drugs cause impairment of renal autoregulatory responses?

Harrison's 20th Ed. Chapter 304 Page 2099

A. Nonsteroidal anti-inflammatory drugs
B. Angiotensin-converting enzyme inhibitors
C. Angiotensin II receptor blockers
D. All of the above

Impairment of renal autoregulatory responses is caused by COX inhibitors (NSAID's), ACE inhibitors & angiotensin II receptor blockers. The combined use of NSAIDs with ACE inhibitors or ARBs poses a higher risk for developing prerenal azotemia.

1011. Autoregulation by tubuloglomerular feedback mechanism is mediated by?

Harrison's 20th Ed. Chapter 304 Page 2100

A. Prostaglandins
B. Kallikrein
C. Nitric oxide (NO)
D. All of the above

Autoregulation by tubuloglomerular feedback mechanism, in which decreases in solute delivery to macula densa elicit dilation of juxtaposed afferent arteriole in order to maintain glomerular perfusion, is mediated, in part, by nitric oxide (NO).

1012. Renal autoregulation fails when systolic blood pressure falls below?

Harrison's 20th Ed. Chapter 304 Page 2100

A. 100 mm Hg
B. 90 mm Hg
C. 80 mm Hg
D. 70 mm Hg

Even in healthy adults, renal autoregulation usually fails once the systolic blood pressure falls below 80 mm Hg.

1013. Hepatorenal syndrome (HRS) is a form of?

Harrison's 20th Ed. Chapter 304 Page 2101

A. Prerenal ARF
B. Intrinsic ARF
C. Intratubular obstruction
D. Postrenal ARF

Hepatorenal syndrome (HRS) is a unique form of prerenal ARF.

1014. Which of the following is false about hepatorenal syndrome?

Harrison's 20th Ed. Chapter 304 Page 2101

A. Kidneys are structurally normal
B. Kidneys fail due to intense renal vasoconstriction
C. Type I HRS is the more aggressive form
D. None of the above

1015. Which of the following is a cause of intrinsic AKI?

Harrison's 20th Ed. Chapter 304 Page 2101

A. Sepsis
B. Ischemia
C. Endogenous and exogenous nephrotoxins
D. All of the above

1016. Which of the following leads to intrinsic ARF?

Harrison's 20th Ed. Chapter 304 Page 2101

A. Ischemic or nephrotoxic tubular injury
B. Tubulointerstitial diseases
C. Diseases of renal microcirculation & glomeruli
D. All of the above

Intrinsic causes of ARF can be ischemic or nephrotoxic tubular injury, tubulointerstitial diseases, diseases of renal microcirculation & glomeruli and diseases of larger renal vessels. Prerenal azotemia and ischemia-associated AKI represent a continuum of manifestations of renal hypoperfusion.

1017. In AKI associated with sepsis, which of the following is most affected?

Harrison's 20th Ed. Chapter 304 Page 2102

A. Glomeruli
B. Tubulointerstitium
C. Vessels
D. All of the above

1018. Which of the following play a role in the pathophysiology of sepsis-induced AKI?

Harrison's 20th Ed. Chapter 304 Page 2102

A. Inflammation
B. Mitochondrial dysfunction
C. Interstitial edema
D. All of the above

1019. Activation of which of the following leads to renal vasoconstriction?

Harrison's 20th Ed. Chapter 304 Page 2102

A. Renin-angiotensin-aldosterone system
B. Vasopressin
C. Endothelin
D. All of the above

Renal vasoconstriction occurs from activation of sympathetic nervous system, renin-angiotensin-aldosterone system, vasopressin, and endothelin.

1020. Hypovolemia leads to activation of?

Harrison's 20th Ed. Chapter 304 Page 2102

A. Sympathetic nervous system
B. Renin-angiotensin-aldosterone system
C. Release of arginine vasopressin
D. All of the above

Hypovolemia triggers neurohormonal responses that include activation of the sympathetic nervous system and renin-angiotensin-aldosterone system, and release of arginine vasopressin.

1021. Which of the following about healthy human kidneys is false?

Harrison's 20th Ed. Chapter 304 Page 2102

A. Receive 20% of the cardiac output
B. Consume 10% of resting oxygen
C. Constitute 0.5% of the human body mass
D. None of the above

Healthy kidneys receive 20% of the cardiac output and consume 10% of resting oxygen, despite constituting only 0.5% of the human body mass.

1022. Which of the following is the site of the most hypoxic region in the body?

Harrison's 20th Ed. Chapter 304 Page 2102

A. Pituitary
B. Hypothalamus
C. Renal medulla
D. Retina

Kidneys are the site of most hypoxic regions in the body, the renal medulla, outer medulla is particular.

1023. Ischemic renal injury is most prominent in?

Harrison's 20th Ed. Chapter 304 Page 2102

A. S_1 segment of proximal tubule
B. S_2 segment of proximal tubule
C. S_3 segment of proximal tubule
D. Cortical thick ascending limb of loop of Henle

Ischemic renal injury is most prominent in metabolically very active S_3 segment of PCT and in medullary portion of the thick ascending limb of the loop of Henle.

1024. Which of the following cause vasoconstriction of glomerular and medullary microvasculature?

Harrison's 20th Ed. Chapter 304 Page 2102 Figure 304-4

A. Endothelin
B. Thromboxane A2
C. Adenosine
D. All of the above

1025. Which of the following cause vasodilation of glomerular and medullary microvasculature?

Harrison's 20th Ed. Chapter 304 Page 2102 Figure 304-4

A. PGE_2
B. Acetylcholine
C. Bradykinin
D. All of the above

1026. AKI from atheroembolic disease following percutaneous catheterization of aorta, or spontaneously, is due to?

Harrison's 20th Ed. Chapter 304 Page 2102

A. Air embolization
B. Fat embolization
C. Cholesterol crystal embolization
D. All of the above

AKI from atheroembolic disease following percutaneous catheterization of aorta, or spontaneously, is due to cholesterol crystal embolization.

1027. Intra-abdominal pressure that causes abdominal compartment syndrome is?

Harrison's 20th Ed. Chapter 304 Page 2102

A. > 20 mm Hg
B. > 30 mm Hg
C. > 40 mm Hg
D. > 50 mm Hg

Intra-abdominal pressure that causes abdominal compartment syndrome is usually >20 mm Hg.

1028. Microvascular causes of AKI include which of the following?

Harrison's 20th Ed. Chapter 304 Page 2103

A. Antiphospholipid antibody syndrome
B. Malignant nephrosclerosis
C. Scleroderma
D. All of the above

Microvascular causes of AKI include the thrombotic microangiopathies (antiphospholipid antibody syndrome, radiation nephritis, malignant nephrosclerosis and thrombotic thrombocytopenic purpura/hemolytic-uremic syndrome [TTP-HUS]), scleroderma and atheroembolic disease.

1029. Which of the following structures of the kidney are vulnerable to nephrotoxin associated injury?

Harrison's 20th Ed. Chapter 304 Page 2103

A. Tubules
B. Vasculature
C. Collecting system
D. All of the above

All structures of the kidney are vulnerable to nephrotoxin associated injury, including the tubules, interstitium, vasculature, and collecting system.

1030. Risk factor for nephrotoxin associated AKI is?

Harrison's 20th Ed. Chapter 304 Page 2103

A. Older age
B. CKD
C. Prerenal azotemia
D. All of the above

1031. Which of the following is false about the clinical course (serum creatinine) of contrast nephropathy?

Harrison's 20th Ed. Chapter 304 Page 2103

A. Begins to rise 24–48 hours after exposure
B. Peaks within 3–5 days
C. Resolves within 1 week
D. None of the above

Clinical course of contrast nephropathy is characterized by a rise in serum creatinine (SCr) beginning 24–48 hours after exposure, peaking within 3–5 days and resolving within 1 week.

1032. Which of the following diagnostic agents can cause AKI?

Harrison's 20th Ed. Chapter 304 Page 2103

A. Iodinated contrast agents
B. High-dose gadolinium
C. Oral sodium phosphate solution
D. All of the above

Iodinated contrast agents are used for cardiovascular and computed tomography (CT) imaging, high-dose gadolinium is used for magnetic resonance imaging (MRI) and oral sodium phosphate solutions is used as bowel purgative.

1033. Contrast nephropathy is due to?

Harrison's 20th Ed. Chapter 304 Page 2103

A. Hypoxia in renal outer medulla
B. Cytotoxic damage to tubules
C. Tubule obstruction with precipitated contrast material
D. All of the above

1034. Which of the following drugs binds to tubular membrane cholesterol and introduces pores?

Harrison's 20th Ed. Chapter 304 Page 2103

A. Aminoglycosides
B. Amphotericin B
C. Vancomycin
D. Acyclovir

Amphotericin B binds to tubular membrane cholesterol and introduces pores.

1035. Clinical features of amphotericin B nephrotoxicity include?

Harrison's 20th Ed. Chapter 304 Page 2103

A. Hypomagnesemia
B. Hypocalcemia
C. Nongap metabolic acidosis
D. All of the above

Clinical features of amphotericin B nephrotoxicity include polyuria, hypomagnesemia, hypocalcemia and nongap metabolic acidosis.

1036. AKI typically manifests after how many days of aminoglycoside therapy?

Harrison's 20th Ed. Chapter 304 Page 2103

A. 1–3 days
B. 3–5 days
C. 5–7 days
D. 7–10 days

AKI typically manifests after 5–7 days of aminoglycoside therapy and can present even after the drug has been discontinued. Hypomagnesemia is a common finding.

1037. Which of the following drugs precipitate in tubules and cause AKI by tubular obstruction?

Harrison's 20th Ed. Chapter 304 Page 2103

A. Aminoglycosides
B. Amphotericin B
C. Vancomycin
D. Acyclovir

Acyclovir precipitates in tubules and causes AKI by tubular obstruction, particularly when given as an intravenous bolus at high doses (500 mg/m^2) or in the setting of hypovolemia.

1038. Which of the following drugs is associated with AKI due to tubular toxicity?

Harrison's 20th Ed. Chapter 304 Page 2103

A. Foscarnet
B. Pentamidine
C. Tenofovír
D. All of the above

1039. Which of the following drugs is associated with AKI due to acute interstitial nephritis?

Harrison's 20th Ed. Chapter 304 Page 2103

A. Cephalosporins
B. Quinolones
C. Rifampin
D. All of the above

Foscarnet, pentamidine, tenofovir and cidofovir are associated with AKI due to tubular toxicity. AKI secondary to acute interstitial nephritis can occur as a consequence of exposure to many antibiotics, including penicillins, cephalosporins, quinolones, sulphonamides and rifampin.

1040. Which of the following drugs can cause injury to the glomerular microvasculature (thrombotic microangiopathy)?

Harrison's 20th Ed. Chapter 304 Page 2103

A. Cisplatin
B. Carboplatin
C. Ifosfamide
D. Bevacizumab

Antiangiogenesis agent bevacizumab can cause proteinuria and hypertension via injury to the glomerular microvasculature (thrombotic microangiopathy) as do mitomycin C and gemcitabine.

1041. Which of the following is a metabolic product of ethylene glycol?

Harrison's 20th Ed. Chapter 304 Page 2103

A. Oxalic acid
B. Glycolaldehyde
C. Glyoxylate
D. All of the above

Ethylene glycol, present in automobile antifreeze, is metabolized to oxalic acid, glycolaldehyde & glyoxylate, which may cause AKI through direct tubular injury & tubular obstruction.

1042. Which of the following is the cause of "Chinese herb nephropathy" and "Balkan nephropathy"?

Harrison's 20th Ed. Chapter 304 Page 2103

A. Aristolochic acid
B. Ethylene glycol
C. 2-hydroxyethoxyacetic acid (HEAA)
D. Melamine

Aristolochic acid was found to be the cause of "Chinese herb nephropathy" and "Balkan nephropathy" due to contamination of medicinal herbs or farming.

1043. Which of the following is an environmental toxin?

Harrison's 20th Ed. Chapter 304 Page 2103

A. Melamine
B. Diethylene glycol
C. Ethylene glycol
D. All of the above

1044. Which of the following is an endogenous nephrotoxin?

Harrison's 20th Ed. Chapter 304 Page 2103

A. Myoglobin
B. Hemoglobin
C. Myeloma light chains
D. All of the above

Endogenous nephrotoxins include calcium, myoglobin, hemoglobin, uric acid, oxalate & myeloma light chains.

1045. Endogenous nephrotoxins include all except?

Harrison's 20th Ed. Chapter 304 Page 2103

A. Calcium
B. Magnesium
C. Urate
D. Oxalate

1046. Presence of which of the following suggests a diagnosis of acute renal failure due to rhabdomyolysis?

Harrison's 20th Ed. Chapter 304 Page 2103

A. Hyperkalemia
B. Hyperphosphatemia
C. Hypocalcemia
D. All of the above

Hyperkalemia, hyperphosphatemia, hypocalcemia, hyperuricemia and raised creatine kinase (MM isoenzyme) suggest a diagnosis of rhabdomyolysis.

1047. Uromodulin is also called?

Harrison's 20th Ed. Chapter 304 Page 2103

A. Bence Jones protein
B. Tamm-Horsfall protein
C. C-reactive protein
D. Heat shock protein

Uromodulin, also known as Tamm-Horsfall protein, encoded by UMOD gene on chromosome 16, is exclusively produced in the kidney and is the most abundant protein in normal urine under physiological conditions.

1048. Tamm-Horsfall protein (uromodulin) is secreted by epithelial cells of?

Harrison's 20th Ed. Chapter 304 Page 2103

A. Proximal convoluted tubule
B. Loop of Henle
C. Distal convoluted tubule
D. All of the above

Tamm-Horsfall protein (uromodulin) is secreted by epithelial cells of the thick ascending limb of the loop of Henle.

1049. Which of the following is the pathophysiological hallmark of postrenal AKI?

Harrison's 20th Ed. Chapter 304 Page 2104

A. Abrupt increase in intratubular pressures
B. Compromised filtration barrier and blood flow
C. Damage to glomerular podocytes
D. Precipitation of proteins in renal tubules

The pathophysiology of postrenal AKI involves hemodynamic alterations triggered by an abrupt increase in intratubular pressures or increased retrograde hydrostatic pressure & interference with glomerular filtration.

1050. Which of the following point towards the presence of AKI?

Harrison's 20th Ed. Chapter 304 Page 2104

A. Rise in SCr from baseline of 0.3 mg/dL within 48 hours
B. At least 50% higher SCr than baseline within 1 week
C. Reduction in urine output to <0.5 mL/kg/hour for > 6 hours
D. All of the above

Presence of AKI is usually inferred by an elevation in SCr concentration. AKI is defined by a rise from baseline of at least 0.3 mg/dL within 48 hours or 50% higher than baseline within 1 week or a reduction in urine output to less than 0.5 mL/kg per hour for longer than 6 hours. Serial blood tests showing continued substantial rise of SCr represents clear evidence of AKI.

1051. Clue suggestive of CKD is?

Harrison's 20th Ed. Chapter 304 Page 2104

A. Small, shrunken kidneys with cortical thinning in USG
B. Evidence of renal osteodystrophy
C. Hyperphosphatemia and hypocalcemia
D. All of the above

Clues suggestive of CKD can come from radiologic studies (small, shrunken kidneys with cortical thinning on renal ultrasound or evidence of renal osteodystrophy) or laboratory tests such as normocytic anemia in the absence of blood loss or secondary hyperparathyroidism with hyperphosphatemia and hypocalcemia consistent with CKD.

1052. In AKI, presence of livedo reticularis points to the diagnosis of?

Harrison's 20th Ed. Chapter 304 Page 2104

A. Systemic vasculitis
B. Atheroembolic disease
C. Acute abdominal compartment syndrome
D. Rhabdomyolysis

Atheroembolic disease can be associated with livedo reticularis & other signs of emboli to legs.

1053. Which of the following is false about prerenal azotemia?

Harrison's 20th Ed. Chapter 304 Page 2105 Table 304-1

A. BUN/creatinine ratio > 20
B. FeNa < 1%
C. Urine osmolality > 500 mOsm/kg
D. None of the above

Response to restoration of hemodynamics is most diagnostic.

1054. Urine heme positive with few red blood cells is suggestive of?

Harrison's 20th Ed. Chapter 304 Page 2105 Table 304-1

A. Rhabdomyolysis
B. Hemolysis
C. Tumor lysis
D. Multiple myeloma

1055. Hyperphosphatemia, hypocalcemia, hyperuricemia are suggestive of?

Harrison's 20th Ed. Chapter 304 Page 2105 Table 304-1

A. Rhabdomyolysis
B. Hemolysis
C. Tumor lysis
D. Multiple myeloma

1056. Schistocytes on peripheral blood smear are suggestive of?

Harrison's 20th Ed. Chapter 304 Page 2105 Table 304-1

A. Atheroembolic disease
B. TTP/HUS
C. Glomerulonephritis/vasculitis
D. Hemolysis

"Typical HUS" refers to AKI with a diarrheal prodrome, due to Shiga toxin released from Escherichia coli. "Atypical HUS" constitutes the majority of adult cases of HUS and is due to inherited or acquired complement dysregulation. "TTP-HUS" refers to sporadic cases in adults.

1057. Eosinophilia & sterile pyuria is suggestive of?

Harrison's 20th Ed. Chapter 304 Page 2105 Table 304-1

A. Interstitial nephritis
B. Tubular injury
C. Glomerulonephritis/vasculitis
D. All of the above

1058. Hypocomplementemia & eosinophiluria is suggestive of?

Harrison's 20th Ed. Chapter 304 Page 2105 Table 304-1

A. Atheroembolic disease
B. TTP/HUS
C. Glomerulonephritis/vasculitis
D. Hemolysis

1059. Which of the following is a calcineurin inhibitor?

Harrison's 20th Ed. Chapter 304 Page 2105

A. Tacrolimus
B. Sirolimus
C. Everolimus
D. All of the above

CNI or calcineurin inhibitors include cyclosporine and tacrolimus. They have an afferent arteriolar constrictor effect on the kidney. They may cause TTP/HUS.

1060. Which of the following is a cause of complete anuria?

Harrison's 20th Ed. Chapter 304 Page 2106

A. Renal artery occlusion
B. Overwhelming septic shock
C. Severe proliferative glomerulonephritis
D. All of the above

Complete anuria early in the course of AKI is uncommon. It may however be seen in complete urinary tract obstruction, renal artery occlusion, overwhelming septic shock, severe ischemia (with cortical necrosis), or severe proliferative glomerulonephritis or vasculitis.

1061. Oliguria is defined as?

Harrison's 20th Ed. Chapter 304 Page 2106

A. Urine output < 100 mL/day
B. Urine output < 200 mL/day
C. Urine output < 300 mL/day
D. Urine output < 400 mL/day

Oliguria is defined as urine output of <400 mL/day contributing to extracellular fluid overload.

1062. Nephrogenic diabetes insipidus is characteristic of?

Harrison's 20th Ed. Chapter 304 Page 2106

A. Long-standing urinary tract obstruction
B. Tubulointerstitial disease
C. Nephrotoxicity from cisplatin or aminoglycosides
D. All of the above

Nephrogenic diabetes insipidus is characteristic of long-standing urinary tract obstruction, tubulointerstitial disease, or nephrotoxicity from cisplatin or aminoglycosides.

1063. Urine is strongly positive for heme by dipstick in?

Harrison's 20th Ed. Chapter 304 Page 2106

A. Hemoglobinuria
B. Hematuria
C. Myoglobinuria
D. All of the above

Urine is strongly positive for heme by dipstick in hemoglobinuria, hematuria & myoglobinuria. If the dipstick is positive for hemoglobin but few red blood cells are evident in the urine sediment, then rhabdomyolysis or hemolysis should be suspected.

1064. Pigmented "muddy brown" granular cast is characteristic of?

Harrison's 20th Ed. Chapter 304 Page 2106

A. Prerenal ARF
B. Ischemic or nephrotoxic ATN
C. Postrenal ARF
D. All of the above

Pigmented "muddy brown" granular cast is characteristic of ATN due to ischemic or nephrotoxic etiology. AKI from ATN due to ischemic injury, sepsis or certain nephrotoxins has characteristic urine sediment findings: pigmented "muddy brown" granular casts and tubular epithelial cell casts.

1065. Broad granular casts are characteristic of?

Harrison's 20th Ed. Chapter 304 Page 2106

A. Glomerular injury
B. Acute tubulointerstitial nephritis
C. Ischemic or nephrotoxic ATN
D. Chronic kidney disease

Broad granular casts are characteristic of chronic kidney disease.

1066. Oxalate crystal is best related with?

Harrison's 20th Ed. Chapter 304 Page 2106

A. Envelope-shaped
B. Needle-shaped
C. Round-shaped
D. Elliptical-shaped

The finding of oxalate crystals in AKI should prompt an evaluation for ethylene glycol toxicity.

1067. Hippurate crystal is best related with?

Harrison's 20th Ed. Chapter 304 Page 2106

A. Envelope-shaped
B. Needle-shaped
C. Round-shaped
D. Elliptical-shaped

Ethylene glycol toxicity causes oxalate (envelope-shaped) & hippurate (needle-shaped) crystals.

1068. Abundant uric acid crystals may be seen in?

Harrison's 20th Ed. Chapter 304 Page 2106

A. Atheroembolic disease
B. Cystitis
C. Tumor lysis syndrome
D. Ethylene glycol toxicity

Abundant uric acid crystals may be seen in the tumor lysis syndrome.

1069. In AKI, the rise in SCr is characteristically delayed in?

Harrison's 20th Ed. Chapter 304 Page 2107

A. Contrast nephropathy
B. Atheroembolic disease
C. Aminoglycoside antibiotics and cisplatin toxicity
D. All of the above

In aminoglycoside antibiotics and cisplatin toxicity, the rise in SCr is characteristically delayed for 3–5 days to 2 weeks after initial exposure.

1070. Which of the following cause kidney injury through intrarenal vasoconstriction?

Harrison's 20th Ed. Chapter 304 Page 2107

A. Radiocontrast agents
B. Cyclosporine
C. Tacrolimus
D. All of the above

Radiocontrast agents, cyclosporine & tacrolimus cause kidney injury through intrarenal vasoconstriction.

1071. In acute renal failure, systemic eosinophilia suggests?

Harrison's 20th Ed. Chapter 304 Page 2107

A. Allergic interstitial nephritis
B. Atheroembolic disease
C. Polyarteritis nodosa
D. All of the above

In acute renal failure, systemic eosinophilia suggests allergic interstitial nephritis, atheroembolic disease, polyarteritis nodosa and Churg-Strauss vasculitis. .

1072. Eosinophilia is found in which of the following causes of acute renal failure?

Harrison's 20th Ed. Chapter 304 Page 2107

A. Renal artery thrombosis
B. HUS/TTP
C. Hemolysis
D. Atheroembolic disease

Peripheral eosinophilia can accompany interstitial nephritis, atheroembolic disease, polyarteritis nodosa and Churg-Strauss vasculitis.

1073. Acute renal failure impairs which of the following?

Harrison's 20th Ed. Chapter 304 Page 2107

A. Renal excretion of sodium, potassium & water
B. Divalent cation homeostasis
C. Urinary acidification mechanisms
D. All of the above

ARF impairs renal excretion of sodium, potassium, and water and perturbs divalent cation homeostasis and urinary acidification mechanisms.

1074. In acute renal failure, severe anemia in the absence of hemorrhage suggests?

Harrison's 20th Ed. Chapter 304 Page 2107

A. Hemolysis
B. Multiple myeloma
C. Thrombotic microangiopathy
D. All of the above

In acute renal failure, severe anemia in the absence of hemorrhage suggests hemolysis, multiple myeloma, or thrombotic microangiopathy (HUS or TTP).

1075. Laboratory finding of thrombotic microangiopathy is?

Harrison's 20th Ed. Chapter 304 Page 2107

A. Schistocytes on peripheral blood smear
B. Elevated lactate dehydrogenase level
C. Low haptoglobin content
D. All of the above

Laboratory findings of thrombotic microangiopathy include thrombocytopenia, schistocytes on peripheral blood smear, elevated lactate dehydrogenase level and low haptoglobin content.

1076. Increased serum LDH is found in which of the following causes of acute renal failure?

Harrison's 20th Ed. Chapter 304 Page 2107

A. Renal artery thrombosis
B. HUS/TTP
C. Hemolysis
D. All of the above

Increased serum LDH is found in acute renal failure due to renal artery, HUS/TTP, thrombosis, hemolysis, acute urate nephropathy & tumor lysis syndrome.

1077. AKI leads to which of the following?

Harrison's 20th Ed. Chapter 304 Page 2107

A. Hyperkalemia
B. Hyperphosphatemia
C. Hypocalcemia
D. All of the above

AKI leads to hyperkalemia, hyperphosphatemia, and hypocalcemia.

1078. Which of the following occur in tumor lysis syndrome?

Harrison's 20th Ed. Chapter 304 Page 2107

A. Marked hyperphosphatemia
B. Normal or marginally elevated creatine kinase
C. Markedly elevated serum uric acid
D. All of the above

AKI causes hyperkalemia, hyperphosphatemia and hypocalcemia. Marked hyperphosphatemia with accompanying hypocalcemia suggests rhabdomyolysis or tumor lysis syndrome. Creatine phosphokinase levels & serum uric acid are elevated in rhabdomyolysis, while tumor lysis syndrome shows normal or marginally elevated creatine kinase and markedly elevated serum uric acid.

1079. High titers of which of the following is seen in glomerulonephritis and vasculitis?

Harrison's 20th Ed. Chapter 304 Page 2107

A. Antineutrophil cytoplasmic antibodies (ANCAs)
B. Antiglomerular basement membrane (Anti-GBM) antibodies
C. Cryoglobulins
D. All of the above

Findings in glomerulonephritis and vasculitis include depressed complement levels and high titers of antinuclear antibodies (ANAs), antineutrophil cytoplasmic antibodies (ANCAs), antiglomerular basement membrane (Anti-GBM) antibodies, and cryoglobulins.

1080. Disproportionate BUN elevation is seen in?

Harrison's 20th Ed. Chapter 304 Page 2107

A. Upper gastrointestinal bleeding
B. Hyperalimentation
C. Glucocorticoid use
D. All of the above

Disproportionate BUN elevation is seen in upper gastrointestinal bleeding, hyperalimentation, increased tissue catabolism and glucocorticoid use. This is due to low tubular flow rate and increased renal medullary recycling of urea seen in prerenal azotemia.

1081. Hypocomplementemia is found in which of the following causes of acute renal failure?

Harrison's 20th Ed. Chapter 304 Page 2107

A. Renal artery thrombosis
B. Ethylene glycol ingestion
C. Multiple myeloma
D. Atheroembolic disease

1082. Fractional excretion of sodium (FE_{Na}) is calculated as?

Lancet 2005;365:417-430

A. [(Urine sodium × Plasma sodium)÷ (Plasma creatinine × urine creatinine)] × 100
B. [(Urine creatinine × Plasma creatinine)÷ (Plasma sodium × Urine sodium)] × 100
C. [(Urine sodium × Urine creatinine)÷ (Plasma sodium × Plasma creatinine)] × 100
D. [(Urine sodium × Plasma creatinine)÷ (Plasma sodium × Urine creatinine)] × 100

The fractional excretion of sodium (FeNa) is the fraction of the filtered sodium load that is reabsorbed by the tubules and is a measure of both the kidney's ability to reabsorb sodium as well as endogenously and exogenously administered factors that affect tubular reabsorption. FE_{Na} relates sodium clearance to creatinine clearance. Patients with prerenal ARF typically have a FE_{Na} of <1.0%. FE_{Na} may be >1.0% in prerenal ARF if patients are on diuretics or with preexisting CKD, salt-wasting syndromes or adrenal insufficiency. In ischemic AKI, the FeNa is above 1% because of tubular injury and resultant inability to reabsorb sodium.

1083. FeNa depends on?

Harrison's 20th Ed. Chapter 304 Page 2107

A. Sodium intake
B. Effective intravascular volume
C. GFR
D. All of the above

FeNa depends on sodium intake, effective intravascular volume, GFR, diuretic intake and intact tubular reabsorptive mechanisms. Low FeNa is suggestive, but not synonymous, with effective intravascular volume depletion.

1084. FeNa below 1% may be present in?

Harrison's 20th Ed. Chapter 304 Page 2107

A. Early sepsis
B. Rhabdomyolysis
C. Contrast nephropathy
D. All of the above

FeNa below 1% may be present in sepsis (often early in the course), rhabdomyolysis and contrast nephropathy.

1085. Kidney size may be increased in which of the following chronic renal diseases?

Harrison's 20th Ed. Chapter 304 Page 2107

A. Diabetic nephropathy
B. Amyloidosis
C. HIV associated nephropathy
D. All of the above

Kidney size may be normal or increased in diabetic nephropathy, amyloidosis, polycystic kidney disease and HIV associated nephropathy.

1086. Enlarged kidneys in a patient with AKI suggests?

Harrison's 20th Ed. Chapter 304 Page 2107

A. Acute interstitial nephritis
B. Multiple myeloma
C. HIV -associated nephropathy
D. Rhabdomyolysis

Enlarged kidneys in a patient with AKI suggests acute interstitial nephritis.

1087. Nephrogenic system fibrosis (NSF) is best related to?

Harrison's 20th Ed. Chapter 304 Page 2107

A. Renal artery thrombosis
B. Ethylene glycol ingestion
C. Gadolinium-based contrast agent
D. Multiple myeloma

MRI with gadolinium-based contrast agents should be avoided in severe AKI due to the possibility of inducing nephrogenic system fibrosis.

1088. Kidney biopsy is avoided when the probable diagnosis is?

Harrison's 20th Ed. Chapter 304 Page 2107

A. Prerenal azotemia
B. Postrenal AKI
C. Ischemic or nephrotoxic AKI
D. All of the above

1089. In oliguric AKI, what urinary flow rate after IV furosemide identifies patients at higher risk of progression to severe AKI?

Harrison's 20th Ed. Chapter 304 Page 2107

A. < 100 mL over 1 hour
B. < 200 mL over 1 hour
C. < 100 mL over 2 hour
D. < 200 mL over 2 hour

In cases of oliguric AKI, in response to bolus intravenous furosemide (1.0 - 1.5 mg/kg), urine output of < 200 mL over 2 hour may identify patients at higher risk of progression to more severe AKI, and the need for renal replacement therapy.

1090. Which of the following observation is associated with severity and worsening of AKI?

Harrison's 20th Ed. Chapter 304 Page 2107

A. Inadequate response to bolus intravenous furosemide
B. ↑ed renal tubular epithelial cells in urine sediment
C. ↑ed granular casts in urine sediment
D. All of the above

1091. Which of the following about kidney injury molecule-1 (KIM-1) is false?

Harrison's 20th Ed. Chapter 304 Page 2108

A. Type 1 transmembrane protein with two extracellular domains
B. Expressed in injured proximal tubular cells
C. Not expressed in extrarenal tissues
D. None of the above

Kidney injury molecule-1 (KIM-1) is a type 1 transmembrane protein that is abundantly expressed in proximal tubular cells (S3 segment) injured by ischemia or nephrotoxins. KIM-1 is not expressed in the absence of tubular injury or in extrarenal tissues. Its role is to confer phagocytic properties to tubular cells, enabling them to clear debris from tubular lumen after kidney injury. KIM-1 can be detected shortly after ischemic or nephrotoxic injury in urine. Urinary KIM-1 can be used as a specific biomarker for early diagnosis of AKI.

1092. Which of the following about Neutrophil gelatinase associated lipocalin (NGAL) is false?

Harrison's 20th Ed. Chapter 304 Page 2108

A. Also known as lipocalin-2 or siderocalin
B. Binds to iron siderophore complexes & protects proximal tubule
C. Upregulated after inflammation and kidney injury
D. None of the above

Neutrophil gelatinase associated lipocalin (NGAL, also known as lipocalin-2 or siderocalin) is another novel biomarker of AKI. It was first discovered as a protein in granules of human neutrophils. NGAL can bind to iron siderophore complexes and may have tissue-protective effects in the proximal tubule. NGAL is highly upregulated after inflammation and kidney injury and can be detected in the plasma and urine within 2 hours of cardiopulmonary bypass-associated AKI.

1093. Which of the following is a biomarker of AKI?

Harrison's 20th Ed. Chapter 304 Page 2108

A. Neutrophil gelatinase associated lipocalin (NGAL)
B. Insulin-like growth factor binding protein 7 (IGFBP7)
C. Tissue inhibitor of metalloproteinase-2 (TIMP-2)
D. All of the above

1094. Which of the following is a biomarker of AKI?

Harrison's 20th Ed. Chapter 304 Page 2108

A. Neutrophil gelatinase associated lipocalin (NGAL)
B. Interleukin (IL) 18
C. Kidney injury molecule-1 (KIM-1)
D. All of the above

Other biomarkers of AKI include interleukin (IL) 18, a proinflammatory cytokine of the IL-1 superfamily that may mediate ischemic proximal tubular injury and L-type fatty acid binding protein, which is expressed in ischemic proximal tubule cells and may be renoprotective by binding free fatty acids and lipid peroxidation products.

1095. Which of the following is the hallmark of AKI?

Harrison's 20th Ed. Chapter 304 Page 2108

A. Elevated BUN concentration
B. Elevated creatine concentration
C. Oliguria
D. Impaired salt and water excretion

Buildup of nitrogenous waste products, manifested as an elevated BUN concentration, is a hallmark of AKI.

1096. BUN itself poses little direct toxicity at levels below?

Harrison's 20th Ed. Chapter 304 Page 2108

A. 10 mg/dL
B. 30 mg/dL
C. 70 mg/dL
D. 100 mg/dL

BUN itself poses little direct toxicity at levels below 100 mg/dL. At higher concentrations, mental status changes and bleeding complications arise. Other toxins normally cleared by the kidney may be responsible for the symptom complex known as uremia.

1097. Urine output is lowest in which of the following phases of ischemic ATN?

Harrison's 20th Ed. Chapter 304 Page 2109

A. Initiation
B. Extension
C. Maintenance
D. Recovery

During maintenance phase that lasts for 1–2 weeks, urine output is lowest due to reduced GFR and uremic complications may appear.

1098. Diuresis occurs in which of the following phases of ischemic ATN?

Harrison's 20th Ed. Chapter 304 Page 2109

A. Initiation
B. Extension
C. Maintenance
D. Recovery

Diuresis occurs in the recovery phase. Recovery from AKI can be accompanied by polyuria which if untreated can lead to significant volume depletion. The polyuric phase of recovery may be due to an osmotic diuresis from retained urea and other waste products as well as delayed recovery of tubular reabsorptive functions.

1099. Which of the following can occur during recovery phase of ARF?

Harrison's 20th Ed. Chapter 304 Page 2109

A. Hypernatremia
B. Hypokalemia
C. Hypophosphatemia
D. All of the above

Vigorous diuresis during recovery phase of ARF may lead to intravascular volume depletion causing hypernatremia, hypokalemia, hypomagnesemia, hypophosphatemia and hypocalcemia.

1100. Which of the following is not a feature of AKI?

Harrison's 20th Ed. Chapter 304 Page 2109

A. Hyperphosphatemia
B. Hypocalcemia
C. Hypomagnesemia
D. Metabolic acidosis

ARF is complicated by hyponatremia, hyperkalemia, hyperphosphatemia, hypocalcemia, hypermagnesemia and metabolic acidosis.

1101. Hyperkalemia in AKI is severe in?

Harrison's 20th Ed. Chapter 304 Page 2109

A. Rhabdomyolysis
B. Hemolysis
C. Tumor lysis syndrome
D. All of the above

Hyperkalemia in acute renal failure may be severe in patients with rhabdomyolysis, hemolysis, and tumor lysis syndrome due to release of intracellular potassium from damaged cells.

1102. Hyperphosphatemia in AKI is severe in?

Harrison's 20th Ed. Chapter 304 Page 2109

A. Rhabdomyolysis
B. Hemolysis
C. Tumor lysis syndrome
D. All of the above

AKI can lead to hyperphosphatemia, particularly in highly catabolic patients or those with AKI from rhabdomyolysis, hemolysis and tumor lysis syndrome. Metastatic deposition of calcium phosphate leads to hypocalcemia apart from derangements in vitamin D-parathyroid hormone-fibroblast growth factor-23 axis.

1103. Which of the following is a najor complication of AKI?

Harrison's 20th Ed. Chapter 304 Page 2109

A. Anemia and bleeding
B. Arrhythmias, pericarditis and pericardial effusion
C. Infections
D. All of the above

Direct hematologic effects from AKI-related uremia include decreased erythropoiesis and platelet dysfunction. Major cardiac complications of AKI are arrhythmias, pericarditis and pericardial effusion. Infections are a dreaded complication of AKI. Direct hematologic effects from AKI-related uremia include decreased erythropoiesis and platelet dysfunction.

1104. AKI due to scleroderma (scleroderma renal crisis) should be treated with?

Harrison's 20th Ed. Chapter 304 Page 2109

A. Terlipressin
B. Octreotide
C. Midodrine
D. ACE inhibitors

AKI due to scleroderma (scleroderma renal crisis) should be treated with ACE inhibitors.

1105. Which of the following is a phosphate binder?

Harrison's 20th Ed. Chapter 304 Page 2110

A. Lanthanum
B. Sevelamer
C. Aluminum hydroxide
D. All of the above

1106. Which of the following is an oral phosphate binder?

Harrison's 20th Ed. Chapter 304 Page 2110

A. Calcium carbonate
B. Calcium acetate
C. Aluminum hydroxide
D. All of the above

Hyperphosphatemia is common in AKI and can usually be treated by limiting intestinal absorption of phosphate using phosphate binders (calcium carbonate, calcium acetate, lanthanum, sevelamer, or aluminum hydroxide).

1107. Absolute indication for dialysis in ARF is?

Harrison's 20th Ed. Chapter 304 Page 2110

A. Uremic syndrome
B. Hyperkalemia
C. Acidosis
D. All of the above

Absolute indications for dialysis are symptoms or signs of uremic syndrome, refractory hypervolemia, hyperkalemia, or acidosis.

1108. In patients of AKI on dialysis, what is the recommended protein intake?

Harrison's 20th Ed. Chapter 304 Page 2110

A. 0.1–0.4 gram/kg per day
B. 0.4–0.8 gram/kg per day
C. 0.8–1.0 gram/kg per day
D. 1.0–1.5 gram/kg per day

According to the Kidney Disease Improving Global Outcomes (KDIGO) guidelines, patients with AKI should get a total energy intake of 20–30 kcal/kg per day. Protein intake should vary depending on the severity of AKI : 0.8–1.0 g/kg per day in noncatabolic AKI without the need for dialysis; 1.0–1.5 g/kg per day in patients on dialysis; and up to a maximum of 1.7 g/kg per day if hypercatabolic and receiving continuous renal replacement therapy.

1109. Uremic bleeding may respond to administration of?

Harrison's 20th Ed. Chapter 304 Page 2110

A. Desmopressin
B. Estrogens
C. Dialysis
D. All of the above

Uremic bleeding may respond to desmopressin, estrogens or dialysis.

1110. Severe complications of uremia include?

Harrison's 20th Ed. Chapter 304 Page 2110

A. Pericardial rub or effusion
B. Encephalopathy
C. Uremic bleeding
D. All of the above

Severe complications of uremia include asterixis, pericardial rub or effusion, encephalopathy and uremic bleeding. The initiation of dialysis should not await the development of a life-threatening complication of renal failure.

1111. Continuous renal replacement therapy (CRRT) is preferred in patients with?

Harrison's 20th Ed. Chapter 304 Page 2110

A. Severe hemodynamic instability
B. Cerebral edema
C. Significant volume overload
D. All of the above

CRRT is preferred in patients with severe hemodynamic instability, cerebral edema or significant volume overload.

1112. Which of the following prolong QT interval?

Harrison's 20th Ed. Chapter 304 Page 2110

A. Quinidine
B. Subarachnoid hemorrhage
C. Hypocalcemia
D. All of the above

1113. "Sine-wave" pattern in ECG is seen in?

Harrison's 20th Ed. Chapter 304 Page 2110

A. Hypokalemia
B. Hyperkalemia
C. Hypercalcemia
D. Hypothermia

1114. Which of the following may prevent or attenuate ARF?

Lancet 2005;365:417-430

A. Allopurinol
B. Forced alkaline diuresis
C. Rasburicase
D. All of the above

Allopurinol, forced alkaline diuresis, Rasburicase, N-acetylcysteine help in preventing development of ARF due to various causes.

1115. In acute renal failure, mortality is high when there is?

Lancet 2005;365:417-430

A. Multiorgan failure
B. High concentration of TNF-α
C. Low production of interleukin 10
D. All of the above

1116. Which of the following is a "salt-wasting nephropathy"?

Lancet 2005;365:417-430

A. Chronic pyelonephritis
B. Polycystic disease
C. Medullary cystic disease
D. All of the above

1117. To convert the values for urea nitrogen to millimoles/liter, multiply by?

A. 0.157
B. 0.257
C. 0.357
D. 0.457

1118. To convert the values for creatinine to micromoles/liter, multiply by?

A. 68.4
B. 78.4
C. 88.4
D. 98.4

1119. To convert the values for glucose to millimoles per liter, multiply by?

A. 0.4551
B. 0.5551
C. 0.6551
D. 0.7551

1120. To convert the values for calcium to millimoles per liter, multiply by?

A. 0.150
B. 0.250
C. 0.350
D. 0.450

1121. To convert the values for phosphorus to millimoles per liter, multiply by?

A. 0.1229
B. 0.2229
C. 0.3229
D. 0.4229

1122. To convert the values for magnesium to millimoles per liter, multiply by?

A. 0.200
B. 0.300
C. 0.400
D. 0.500

Chronic Kidney Disease

1123. The risk of CKD progression is closely linked to?

Harrison's 20th Ed. Chapter 305 Page 2111

A. Albuminuria
B. Urine output
C. Age
D. All of the above

The risk of CKD progression is closely linked to both - GFR and amount of albuminuria.

1124. Chronic kidney disease (CKD) is defined as?

Kidney International Supplements. 2018;8:91-165

A. Abnormalities of kidney structure or function
B. Present for >3 months
C. Implications for health
D. All of the above

1125. CKD is classified based on?

Kidney International Supplements. 2018;8:91-165

A. Cause
B. GFR
C. Albuminuria
D. All of the above

CKD is defined as abnormalities of kidney structure or function, present for >3 months, with implications for health. CKD is classified based on cause, GFR category (G1–G5), and albuminuria category (A1–A3), abbreviated as CGA.

1126. Chronic kidney disease (CKD) is divided into how many stages by Kidney Disease Improving Global Outcome (KDIGO)?

Harrison's 20th Ed. Chapter 305 Page 2111

A. 3
B. 4
C. 5
D. 6

CKD is divided into six stages by Kidney Disease Improving Global Outcome (KDIGO 2012) which CKD stratified by both estimated GFR and the degree of albuminuria, in order to predict risk of progression of CKD.

1127. Chronic renal failure typically corresponds to which of the following CKD stages?

Harrison's 20th Ed. Chapter 305 Page 2111

A. 1–3
B. 2–4
C. 3–5
D. 4–5

Term CRF applies to the process of continuing significant irreversible reduction in nephron number and typically corresponds to CKD stages 3–5.

1128. End-stage renal disease denotes which stage of CKD?

Harrison's 20th Ed. Chapter 305 Page 2111

A. 2
B. 3
C. 4
D. 5

End-stage renal disease denotes stage 5 of CKD.

1129. Factors that increase the risk for CKD include?

Harrison's 20th Ed. Chapter 305 Page 2111

A. Small for gestation birth weight
B. Childhood obesity
C. Family history of kidney disease
D. All of the above

Factors that increase the risk for CKD include small for gestation birth weight, childhood obesity, hypertension, diabetes mellitus, autoimmune disease, advanced age, African ancestry, family history of kidney disease, previous episode of acute kidney injury and the presence of proteinuria, abnormal urinary sediment or structural abnormalities of the urinary tract.

1130. Which of the following genes is associated with CKD?

Harrison's 20th Ed. Chapter 305 Page 2111

A. APOL1
B. APOE
C. ROSA26
D. MTHFR

1131. Normal annual mean decline in GFR with age is?

Harrison's 20th Ed. Chapter 305 Page 2111

A. ~1 mL/min per year per 1.73 m^2
B. ~1.5 mL/min per year per 1.73 m^2
C. ~2 mL/min per year per 1.73 m^2
D. ~2.5 mL/min per year per 1.73 m^2

1132. Mean value of GFR at the age of 70 years is?

Harrison's 20th Ed. Chapter 305 Page 2111

A. 70 mL/min per 1.73 m^2
B. 80 mL/min per 1.73 m^2
C. 90 mL/min per 1.73 m^2
D. 100 mL/min per 1.73 m^2

Normal annual mean decline in GFR with age is ~1 mL/min per year per 1.73 m^2, reaching a mean value of 70 mL/min per 1.73 m^2 at the age of 70 years.

1133. What is the GFR value (mL/min per 1.73 m^2) in stage 5 of chronic kidney disease (CKD)?

Harrison's 20th Ed. Chapter 305 Page 2112 Figure 305-1

A. < 15
B. 15–29
C. 30–59
D. 60–89

GFR in CKD (mL/min per 1.73 m^2) - Stage G1 = >90, stage G2 = 60–89, stage G3a = 45–59, stage G3b = 30–44, stage G4 = 15–29 and stage G5 = <15.

1134. Modification of Diet in Renal Disease (MDRD) formula for estimating GFR (mL/min per 1.73 m^2) is?

Harrison's 20th Ed. Chapter 305 Page 2113 Table 305-1

A. $1.56 \times (S_{Cr})^{-1.154} \times (age)^{-0.203}$
B. $1.66 \times (S_{Cr})^{-1.154} \times (age)^{-0.203}$
C. $1.76 \times (S_{Cr})^{-1.154} \times (age)^{-0.203}$
D. $1.86 \times (S_{Cr})^{-1.154} \times (age)^{-0.203}$

1135. Cockcroft-Gault equation for estimating creatinine clearance (ml/minute) is?

Harrison's 19th Ed. 1813 Table 335-1

A. (120-age × body weight in kg)/(72 × plasma creatinine)

B. (130-age × body weight in kg)/(72 × plasma creatinine)

C. (140-age × body weight in kg)/(72 × plasma creatinine)

D. (150-age × body weight in kg)/(72 × plasma creatinine)

1136. In the Chronic Kidney Disease Epidemiology Collaboration (CKD-EPI) equation, what is the value of constant K for males?

Harrison's 20th Ed. Chapter 305 Page 2113 Table 305-1

A. 0.3

B. 0.5

C. 0.7

D. 0.9

CKD-EPI Equation for GFR = $141 \times \min(S_{cr}/\kappa, 1)^{\alpha} \times \max(S_{cr}/\kappa, 1)^{-1.209} \times 0.993^{Age}$. Constant κ is 0.7 for females and 0.9 for males. α is –0.329 for females and –0.411 for males.

1137. Cockcroft - Gault equation is used for estimation of?

Harrison's 19th Ed. 1813

A. Urinary anion gap

B. Serum anion gap

C. Glomeruler filtration rate (GFR)

D. Fractional excretion of sodium

1138. Modification of Diet in Renal Disease (MDRD) equation is used for estimation of?

Harrison's 20th Ed. Chapter 305 Page 2113 Table 305-1

A. Urinary anion gap

B. Serum anion gap

C. Glomeruler filtration rate (GFR)

D. Fractional excretion of sodium

1139. Which of the following is a biomarker for prediction of first major cardiovascular events and death?

N Engl J Med. 2006; 355:2631-2639

A. C-reactive protein

B. B-type natriuretic peptide

C. Aldosterone

D. All of the above

1140. Which of the following is a biomarker for prediction of first major cardiovascular events and death?

N Engl J Med. 2006; 355:2631-2639

A. Renin

B. D-dimer

C. Urinary albumin-to-creatinine ratio

D. All of the above

Biomarkers for prediction of first major cardiovascular events and death include C-reactive protein, B-type natriuretic peptide, N-terminal pro–atrial natriuretic peptide, aldosterone, renin, fibrinogen, D-dimer, plasminogen-activator inhibitor type 1, lipoprotein-associated phospholipase A_2, homocysteine and urinary albumin-to-creatinine ratio.

1141. Which of the following is a biomarker of neurohormonal activity?

N Engl J Med. 2006; 355:2631-2639

A. B-type natriuretic peptide

B. Serum aldosterone

C. Plasma renin

D. All of the above

C-reactive protein is a marker of inflammation. B-type natriuretic peptide, N-terminal pro–atrial natriuretic peptide, serum aldosterone, and plasma renin are markers of neurohormonal activity. Fibrinogen is a marker of thrombosis & inflammation. Plasminogen-activator inhibitor type 1 is a marker of fibrinolytic potential & endothelial function. D-dimer is a marker of thrombosis. Homocysteine is a marker of endothelial function and oxidant stress. Urinary albumin-to-creatinine ratio is a marker of glomerular endothelial function.

1142. Which of the following about urinary albumin & creatinine excretion in healthy individuals is false?

N Engl J Med. 2006; 355:2631-2639

A. Average daily urinary protein excretion in adults is 80 mg/day

B. Albumin represents ~15% of daily urinary protein excretion

C. Creatinine excretion is ~ 1 gram per 1.73 m^2 BSA

D. None of the above

Average daily urinary protein excretion in adults is 80 mg/day, with normal excretion considered to be <150 mg/day. Albumin represents ~15% of daily urinary protein excretion in healthy people, with other plasma proteins (e.g., immunoglobulins, beta-2-microglobulin) and Tamm-Horsfall protein constituting the remaining 85%. Urinary excretion of abnormal quantities of protein for ≥3 months, with or without a decrease in glomerular filtration rate (GFR), is diagnostic of chronic kidney disease.

1143. Which of the following hypothesis relates diabetes and cardiovascular disease?

Diabetes. 1995 Apr;44(4):369-74

A. Knudson two-hit hypothesis

B. The "common soil" hypothesis

C. Threshold hypothesis

D. Grandmother hypothesis

Unlike classical microvascular complications, large-vessel atherosclerosis can precede development of diabetes, suggesting that rather than atherosclerosis being a complication of diabetes, both conditions have common genetic & environmental antecedents, i.e., they spring from a "common soil." (Stern, 1995).

1144. Which of the following about urinary albumin excretion (UAE) is false?

J Am Heart Assoc. 2016;5:e003245

A. Normoalbuminuria is <30 mg/day or UACR <30 mg/g

B. Microalbuminuria is 30–300 mg/day or UACR 30–300 mg/g

C. Macroalbuminuria is >300 mg/day or UACR >300 mg/g

D. None of the above

Urinary albumin excretion is classified as normoalbuminuria (<30 mg/day or UACR <30 mg/g), microalbuminuria (30–300 mg/day or UACR 30–300 mg/g), and macroalbuminuria (>300 mg/day or UACR >300 mg/g).

1145. In men, what value of urinary albumin to creatinine ratio (UACR) is indicative of primary kidney disease?

Harrison's 20th Ed. Chapter 305 Page 2111

A. > 4 mg albumin/gram creatinine

B. > 7 mg albumin/gram creatinine

C. > 12 mg albumin/gram creatinine

D. > 17 mg albumin/gram creatinine

1146. In women, what value of urinary albumin to creatinine ratio (UACR) is indicative of primary kidney disease?

Harrison's 20th Ed. Chapter 305 Page 2111

A. > 14 mg albumin/gram creatinine
B. > 20 mg albumin/gram creatinine
C. > 25 mg albumin/gram creatinine
D. > 33 mg albumin/gram creatinine

UACR above 17 mg albumin/gram creatinine in men and 25 mg albumin/gram creatinine in women serves as a marker for early detection of primary kidney disease, systemic microvascular disease & endothelial dysfunction.

1147. Out of the following, which is the most common cause of chronic kidney disease?

Harrison's 20th Ed. Chapter 305 Page 2113

A. Diabetes mellitus
B. Hypertension
C. Glomerulonephritis
D. Cystic kidney disease

Most frequent cause of CKD is diabetic nephropathy, secondary to type 2 diabetes mellitus. Hypertensive nephropathy is a common cause of CKD in the elderly.

1148. Uremic "Toxins" include?

Harrison's 20th Ed. Chapter 305 Page 2113

A. By-products of protein & amino acid metabolism
B. End products of aliphatic amine metabolism
C. End products of aromatic amino acid metabolism
D. All of the above

1149. Uremic "Toxins" include?

Harrison's 20th Ed. Chapter 305 Page 2113

A. Urea
B. Creatine
C. Urates and hippurates
D. All of the above

Apart from the above ones, PTH is also a uremic toxin.

1150. Which of the following is a nitrogenous excretory product?

Harrison's 20th Ed. Chapter 305 Page 2113

A. Polyamines
B. Myoinositol
C. Phenols
D. All of the above

1151. Which of the following is a nitrogenous excretory product?

Harrison's 20th Ed. Chapter 305 Page 2113

A. Benzoates
B. Indoles
C. Phenols
D. All of the above

Hundreds of toxins that accumulate in renal failure have been implicated in the uremic syndrome. These include water-soluble, hydrophobic, protein-bound, charged and uncharged compounds. Additional categories of nitrogenous excretory products include guanidino compounds, urates and hippurates, products of nucleic acid metabolism, polyamines, myoinositol, phenols, benzoates and indoles.

1152. Which of the following dysfunctions occur in uremic syndrome?

Harrison's 20th Ed. Chapter 305 Page 2113

A. Renal excretory failure
B. Progressive systemic inflammation
C. Loss of hormone regulation
D. All of the above

Uremic syndrome manifests as accumulation of toxins due to renal excretory failure, loss of fluid & electrolyte homeostasis & hormone regulation and progressive systemic inflammation with vascular & nutritional consequences.

1153. Plasma levels of which of the following hormones rise with renal failure?

Harrison's 20th Ed. Chapter 305 Page 2113

A. Parathyroid hormone (PTH)
B. Prolactin
C. Luteinizing hormone
D. All of the above

Plasma levels of many hormones like PTH, FGF-23, insulin, glucagon, steroid hormones including vitamin D and sex hormones and prolactin change in CKD as a result of reduced excretion, decreased degradation or abnormal regulation.

1154. Which of the following is not a negative acute-phase reactant?

Harrison's 20th Ed. Chapter 305 Page 2113

A. Transthyretin
B. Fetuin (AHSG)
C. Albumin
D. Fibrinogen

Fetuin (AHSG), a glycoprotein is synthesized by hepatocytes & is present in the circulation. It has the highest capacity of inhibiting soft tissue calcification.

1155. Which of the following is an acute-phase reactant?

Harrison's 20th Ed. Chapter 305 Page 2113

A. Thrombocytosis
B. Serum amyloid A (SAA)
C. Ferritin
D. All of the above

1156. Which of the following is a loop diuretic?

Harrison's 20th Ed. Chapter 305 Page 2114

A. Furosemide
B. Bumetanide
C. Torsemide
D. All of the above

1157. Combination with which of the following provides a synergistic effect in patients receiving long-term therapy with loop diuretic agents?

Harrison's 20th Ed. Chapter 305 Page 2114

A. Metolazone
B. Chlorthalidone
C. Spironolactone
D. Acetazolamide

Metolazone in combination provides a synergistic effect and is often required in patients receiving long-term therapy with loop diuretic agents. Resistance to loop diuretics in CKD often mandates use of higher doses than those used in patients with higher GFR. The combination of loop diuretics with metolazone may be helpful.

1158. In CKD, hyperkalemia may be precipitated by?

Harrison's 20th Ed. Chapter 305 Page 2114

A. Hemolysis
B. Transfusion of stored red blood cells
C. Metabolic acidosis
D. All of the above

1159. Which of the following is a potassium-sparing diuretic?

Harrison's 20th Ed. Chapter 305 Page 2114

A. Amiloride
B. Eplerenone
C. Triamterene
D. All of the above

1160. Which of the following inhibits sodium chloride co-transporter of the distal convoluted tubule?

Harrison's 20th Ed. Chapter 305 Page 2114

A. Amiloride
B. Eplerenone
C. Metolazone
D. All of the above

Metolazone inhibits the sodium chloride co-transporter of the distal convoluted tubule. It promotes renal salt excretion.

1161. Which of the following is involved in CKD with earlier & more severe disruption of K^+-secretory mechanisms?

Harrison's 20th Ed. Chapter 305 Page 2114

A. Glomerulus
B. Proximal tubule
C. Loop of Henle
D. Distal tubule

CKD can be associated with earlier & more severe disruption of K^+-secretory mechanisms in distal nephron, out of proportion to the decline in GFR.

1162. Which of the following preferentially affects distal nephron?

Harrison's 20th Ed. Chapter 305 Page 2114

A. Diabetic nephropathy
B. Sickle cell nephropathy
C. HIV nephropathy
D. Polycystic kidney disease

Obstructive uropathy & sickle cell nephropathy preferentially affect the distal nephron.

1163. Which of the following leads to hyporeninemic hypoaldosteronism?

Harrison's 20th Ed. Chapter 305 Page 2114

A. Diabetes mellitus
B. Obstructive uropathy
C. Sickle cell nephropathy
D. All of the above

In CKD, potassium levels may rise out of proportion to decline in GFR in conditions that lead to hyporeninemic hypoaldosteronism like diabetes, obstructive uropathy & sickle cell nephropathy.

1164. Which of the following promotes potassium loss through the GI tract?

Harrison's 20th Ed. Chapter 305 Page 2114

A. Calcium resonium
B. Sodium polystyrene
C. Patiromer
D. All of the above

Potassium-binding resins like calcium resonium, sodium polystyrene or patiromer promote potassium loss through the GI tract and may reduce the incidence of hyperkalemia in CKD.

1165. In adult males, persistence in urine of how much albumin per gram of creatinine signifies chronic renal damage?

Harrison's 20th Ed. Chapter 305 Page 2111

A. > 11 mg
B. > 13 mg
C. > 15 mg
D. > 17 mg

1166. In adult females, persistence in urine of how much albumin per gram of creatinine signifies chronic renal damage?

Harrison's 20th Ed. Chapter 305 Page 2111

A. > 18 mg
B. > 21 mg
C. > 23 mg
D. > 25 mg

Persistence in urine of >17 mg of albumin per gram of creatinine in adult males and 25 mg albumin per gram of creatinine in adult females signifies CKD.

1167. Which of the following suggests chronic kidney disease?

A. Anemia
B. Evidence of renal osteodystrophy
C. Small scarred kidneys
D. All of the above

Findings that suggest chronic kidney disease include anemia, evidence of renal osteodystrophy (radiologic or laboratory) and small scarred kidneys.

1168. A persistent reduction in GFR to less than what level per minute per 1.73 m^2 is defined as chronic kidney disease?

Lancet 2005;365:417-430

A. 60 mL
B. 70 mL
C. 80 mL
D. 90 mL

1169. In a case of CRF, oral acetylcysteine with hydration significantly lowers the risk of?

Lancet 2005;365:417-430

A. Contrast nephropathy
B. Uremic pericarditis
C. Uremic encephalopathy
D. All of the above

1170. Most rapid way to remove potassium in severe hyperkalemia is?

Lancet 2005;365:417-430

A. Intravenous calcium
B. Infusion of glucose & insulin
C. Na–K exchange resin (sodium polystyrene sulfonate)
D. Hemodialysis

1171. Decreased GFR occurs due to?
Lancet 2005;365:417-430

A. Reduced glomerular hydraulic pressure
B. Elevated Bowman's space hydraulic pressure
C. Rise in plasma colloid osmotic pressure
D. All of the above

1172. Decreased GFR occurs due to?
Lancet 2005;365:417-430

A. Reduced glomerular blood flow
B. Reduced glomerular permeability
C. Diminished filtration surface area
D. All of the above

1173. The molecular weight of inulin is about?
Lancet 2005;365:417-430

A. 4800
B. 5000
C. 5200
D. 5400

Molecular weight of inulin is ~5200. It pass freely across glomerular filtration barrier, appearing at approximately the same concentration in Bowman's space as in plasma.

1174. Which of the following is curve A-type solute?
Lancet 2005;365:417-430

A. Sodium
B. Urate
C. Urea
D. All of the above

Curve A-type solutes include urea and creatinine. These depend largely on glomerular filtration for urinary excretion. Their secretion contributes little to overall excretion. The clinical course of CRF usually also approximates curve A.

1175. Which of the following are curve B-type solutes?
Lancet 2005;365:417-430

A. Phosphate (PO_4^{3-})
B. Urate
C. Potassium & Hydrogen ions
D. All of the above

1176. Which of the following is not a curve B-type solute?
Lancet 2005;365:417-430

A. Sodium
B. Potassium
C. Hydrogen
D. None of the above

1177. Which of the following is a curve C-type solute?
Lancet 2005;365:417-430

A. Sodium
B. Potassium
C. Hydrogen
D. Urate

In contrast to solutes of the curve A type, plasma levels of phosphate, urate, and potassium and hydrogen ions usually do not rise until the GFR falls to a small percentage of normal. With progressive renal failure this pattern of response (curve B) reflects the participation of tubule transport mechanisms in the excretion of these substances.

1178. In CKD, principal complications of abnormalities of calcium and phosphate metabolism occur in?
Harrison's 20th Ed. Chapter 305 Page 2114

A. Skeleton
B. Vascular bed
C. Soft tissues
D. All of the above

Principal complications of abnormalities of calcium & phosphate metabolism in CKD occur in skeleton and the vascular bed, with occasional severe involvement of soft tissues.

1179. In CKD, which of the following bone disease is associated with high bone turnover?
Harrison's 20th Ed. Chapter 305 Page 2114

A. Adynamic bone disease
B. Osteomalacia
C. Osteitis fibrosa cystica
D. All of the above

1180. Which of the following is the classic lesion of secondary hyperparathyroidism?
Harrison's 20th Ed. Chapter 305 Page 2114

A. Adynamic bone disease
B. Osteomalacia
C. Osteitis fibrosa cystica
D. All of the above

In CKD, the major disorders of bone disease can be classified into those associated with high bone turnover with increased PTH levels (osteitis fibrosa cystica, classic lesion of secondary hyperparathyroidism), osteomalacia due to reduced action of the active forms of vitamin D, and low bone turnover with low or normal PTH levels (adynamic bone disease) or their combinations.

1181. Plasma concentration of which of the following remains normal throughout the course of CRF?
Harrison's 20th Ed. Chapter 305 Page 2114

A. Potassium
B. Sodium
C. Calcium
D. Hydrogen

For sodium chloride (NaCl), plasma concentrations remain normal throughout the course of CRF, despite unrestricted intake of these substances (curve C). Hyponatremia is not commonly seen in CKD patients but, when present, often responds to water restriction.

1182. Clinical manifestations of severe hyperparathyroidism include?
Harrison's 20th Ed. Chapter 305 Page 2115

A. Bone pain and fragility
B. Brown tumors
C. Erythropoietin (EPO) resistance
D. All of the above

Clinical manifestations of severe hyperparathyroidism include bone pain and fragility, brown tumors, compression syndromes, and erythropoietin (EPO) resistance related to bone marrow fibrosis.

1183. Which of the following about PTH is false?
Harrison's 20th Ed. Chapter 305 Page 2115

A. Uremic toxin
B. Stimulates Ca^{++} reabsorption in the distal convoluted tubule
C. Stimulates proximal tubular 1α-hydroxylation of vitamin D
D. None of the above

Most filtered phosphate ion is reabsorbed by the proximal tubule through a sodium-coupled cotransport process that is regulated by parathyroid hormone (PTH). FGF-23 stimulation of PTH also increases renal phosphate excretion.

1184. Which of the following growth patterns is seen when cell mass of parathyroid glands increases with CKD?

Harrison's 20th Ed. Chapter 305 Page 2115

A. Diffuse hyperplasia (polyclonal)
B. Nodular growth (monoclonal) within diffuse hyperplasia
C. Diffuse monoclonal hyperplasia ("adenoma" or tertiary autonomous hyperparathyroidism)
D. All of the above

Owing to increased PTH production from parathyroid cells, its cell mass increases progressively with CKD. Growth patterns may be diffuse hyperplasia (polyclonal), nodular growth (monoclonal) within diffuse hyperplasia or diffuse monoclonal hyperplasia ("adenoma" or tertiary autonomous hyperparathyroidism).

1185. Which of the following about FGF-23 is false?

Harrison's 20th Ed. Chapter 305 Page 2115

A. Secreted by osteocytes
B. Is part of a family of phosphatonins
C. Promotes renal phosphate excretion
D. None of the above

FGF-23 is a phosphaturic hormone relevant in pathophysiological scheme of secondary hyperparathyroidism.

1186. FGF-23 is a member of which of the following subfamily?

Harrison's 20th Ed. Chapter 305 Page 2115

A. FGF-19
B. FGF-21
C. FGF-23
D. All of the above

The FGF-19 subfamily is composed of three proteins - FGF-19, FGF-21, and FGF-23. FGF-23 is a central regulator of phosphate homeostasis and calcitriol blood levels. FGF-19 inhibits expression of enzyme cholesterol 7-α hydroxylase (CYP7A1), which is the first & rate-limiting step in bile acid synthesis. FGF-21 stimulates insulin independent glucose uptake in adipocytes & lowers triglycerides.

1187. Which of the following about FGF-23 is false?

Harrison's 20th Ed. Chapter 305 Page 2115

A. Increases renal phosphate excretion (phosphaturic hormone)
B. Stimulates PTH
C. Suppresses formation of $1,25(OH)_2D_3$
D. None of the above

FGF-23 increases renal phosphate excretion, stimulates PTH, which also increases renal phosphate excretion and suppresses formation of $1,25(OH)_2D_3$ leading to diminished phosphorus absorption from the GI tract. FGF23 forms a ternary complex with klotho protein and renal FGF receptors to reduce renal phosphate reabsorption.

1188. High levels of FGF-23 is an independent risk factor for?

Harrison's 20th Ed. Chapter 305 Page 2115

A. Coronary artery disease
B. Left ventricular hypertrophy
C. Acute pancreatitis
D. Cirrhosis liver

High levels of FGF-23 are also an independent risk factor for left ventricular hypertrophy and mortality in CKD, dialysis and renal transplant patients with a lower eGFR despite normal phosphate levels.. Higher FGF-23 level is associated with higher atherosclerosis score.

1189. FGF23 is associated with?

Harrison's 20th Ed. Chapter 305 Page 2115

A. Vascular dysfunction
B. Atherosclerosis
C. Left ventricular hypertrophy
D. All of the above

1190. Which of the following about FGF23 is false?

Harrison's 20th Ed. Chapter 305 Page 2115

A. Its increase occurs well before an elevation in PTH in CKD
B. Potent inhibitor of renal 1-alpha hydroxylase
C. Reduces $1,25(OH)_2$ vitamin D
D. None of the above

1191. Which of the following about FGF23 is false?

Harrison's 20th Ed. Chapter 305 Page 2115

A. Regulator of calcium-phosphate metabolism
B. Responsible for inception of secondary hyperparathyroidism
C. Responsible for cardiovascular morbidity & mortality in CKD
D. None of the above

In CKD, FGF-23 is a stronger predictor of mortality than serum phosphate level.

1192. Brown tumor relates best with?

Harrison's 20th Ed. Chapter 305 Page 2115

A. Subcuteneous tissue
B. Bone
C. Brain
D. Liver

Bone histology in hyperparathyroidism may show bone cysts, at times with hemorrhagic elements giving it brown color, hence the term brown tumor.

1193. Clinical clues indicating the imminent development of uremic complications are?

Harrison's 20th Ed. Chapter 305 Page 2115

A. Muscle twitching & cramps
B. Asterixis
C. Non-compliance of treatment
D. All of the above

1194. Adynamic bone disease best relates to?

Harrison's 20th Ed. Chapter 305 Page 2115

A. Aluminium-containing phosphate binders
B. Excessive PTH suppression
C. Low calcium exposure
D. All of the above

1195. Adynamic bone disease can result from?

Harrison's 20th Ed. Chapter 305 Page 2115

A. Use of vitamin D preparations
B. Excessive calcium-containing phosphate binders
C. High-calcium dialysis solutions
D. All of the above

Adynamic bone disease is a state of reduced bone volume & mineralization. It results from excessive PTH suppression from the use of vitamin D preparations or from excessive calcium exposure in the form of calcium-containing phosphate binders or high-calcium dialysis solutions.

1196. Complications of adynamic bone disease include?
Harrison's 20th Ed. Chapter 305 Page 2115

A. Increased incidence of fracture & bone pain
B. Increased vascular & cardiac calcification
C. Tumoral calcinosis
D. All of the above

Complications of adynamic bone disease include an increased incidence of fracture and bone pain and an association with increased vascular and cardiac calcification. Occasionally, the calcium will precipitate in the soft tissues into large concretions termed "tumoral calcinosis". Very low PTH levels are associated with adynamic bone disease and possible consequences of fracture and ectopic calcification.

1197. Metastatic calcification is seen in?
Harrison's 20th Ed. Chapter 405 Page 2966

A. Sarcoidosis
B. Vitamin D intoxication
C. Milk-alkali syndrome
D. All of the above

Metastatic calcification is seen in conditions associated with hypercalcemia, such as in sarcoidosis, vitamin D intoxication, milk-alkali syndrome, and primary hyperparathyroidism.

1198. Which of the following contributes to soft tissue calcifications in CKD?
Harrison's 20th Ed. Chapter 405 Page 2966

A. Increased production of parathyroid hormone (PTH)
B. Increased production of fibroblast growth factor-23
C. Klotho deficiency
D. All of the above

1199. Which of the following is a phosphaturic agent?
Harrison's 20th Ed. Chapter 405 Page 2966

A. Thyroxine
B. Vitamin D
C. Acetazolamide
D. All of the above

Acetazolamide is a phosphaturic agent.

1200. Osteomalacia best relates to?
Harrison's 20th Ed. Chapter 305 Page 2115

A. Calcium
B. PTH
C. 1,25(OH)$_2$D$_3$
D. FGF-23

Osteomalacia in CKD is consequent to reduced production and action of 1,25(OH)$_2$D$_3$, leading to non-mineralized osteoid.

1201. Calciphylaxis best relates to?
Harrison's 20th Ed. Chapter 305 Page 2115

A. Metastatic calcification
B. Calcific uremic arteriolopathy
C. Calcific chronic pancreatitis
D. Calcific tendinitis

1202. Which of the following about calciphylaxis is false?
Harrison's 20th Ed. Chapter 305 Page 2115

A. Seen almost exclusively in patients with advanced CKD
B. Preceded by livedo reticularis
C. Patches of ischemic necrosis
D. None of the above

Calciphylaxis or calcific uremic arteriolopathy is a devastating condition seen almost exclusively in patients with advanced CKD. It is heralded by livedo reticularis and advances to patches of ischemic necrosis, especially on the legs, thighs, abdomen and breasts.

1203. Which of the following about vascular calcification is false?
Harrison's 20th Ed. Chapter 305 Page 2115

A. Matrix GLA protein prevents vascular calcification
B. Low levels of fetuin permit more rapid vascular calcification
C. Diffuse vascular calcifications associated with Paget's disease
D. None of the above

1204. Which of the following about vascular calcification is false?
Harrison's 20th Ed. Chapter 305 Page 2115

A. Warfarin can cause arterial vascular calcification
B. Hyperphosphatemia & hypercalcemia increase vascular calcification
C. Ankle:brachial index >1.40 indicates vascular calcification
D. None of the above

1205. Which of the following is a phosphate binder?
Harrison's 20th Ed. Chapter 305 Page 2115

A. Calcium chloride
B. Calcium acetate
C. Calcium gluconate
D. Calcium hydroxide

Examples of phosphate binders are calcium acetate and calcium carbonate.

1206. Which of the following is a phosphate binder?
Harrison's 20th Ed. Chapter 305 Page 2115

A. Sevelamer
B. Lanthanum
C. Calcium carbonate
D. All of the above

Sevelamer & lanthanum are non-calcium-containing polymers that bind phosphates and do not predispose CKD patients to hypercalcemia. They also attenuate calcium deposition in the vascular bed. Low serum phosphate stimulates renal proximal tubular synthesis of 1,25(OH)$_2$D, by suppressing blood levels of FGF23.

1207. Which of the following is a phosphate binding agent?
Harrison's 20th Ed. Chapter 305 Page 2115

A. Calcium acetate
B. Sevelamer hydrochloride
C. Aluminum hydroxide
D. All of the above

Agents limiting intestinal absorption of phosphate (phosphate binders) are calcium carbonate, calcium acetate, lanthanum, sevelamer, & aluminum hydroxide.

1208. In CKD, increased cardiovascular mortality has a strong association with?
Harrison's 20th Ed. Chapter 305 Page 2115

A. Hypercalcemia
B. Hyperphosphatemia
C. Chronic inflammation
D. Soft tissue calcification

Epidemiologic evidence shows a strong association between hyperphosphatemia & increased cardiovascular mortality in patients with CKD.

1209. Which of the following drugs is a risk factor for Calciphylaxis?
Harrison's 20th Ed. Chapter 305 Page 2115

A. Aspirin
B. Statins
C. Warfarin
D. All of the above

Warfarin therapy decreases vitamin K–dependent regeneration of matrix GLA protein which prevents vascular calcification.

1210. Calcimimetic agents that enhance the sensitivity of the parathyroid cell to the suppressive effect of calcium is?
Harrison's 20th Ed. Chapter 305 Page 2116

A. Sevelamer
B. Calcitriol
C. Cinacalcet
D. Lanthanum

1211. Which of the following about cinacalcet is false?
Harrison's 20th Ed. Chapter 305 Page 2116

A. Oral calcimimetic agent
B. Directly lowers PTH levels
C. Increases calcium-sensing receptor to extracellular calcium
D. None of the above

Calcimimetic agents that enhance the sensitivity of the parathyroid cell to the suppressive effect of calcium. Cinacalcet, a calcimimetic agent that acts by allosteric activation of the calcium-sensing receptor on parathyroid tissue. Sevelamer and lanthanum are non-calcium-containing polymers that function as phosphate binders. They do not predispose CKD patients to hypercalcemia and may attenuate calcium deposition in the vascular bed.

1212. Which of the following trials is related to Cinacalcet therapy?
N Engl J Med. 2012; 367:2482-2494

A. HEMO Study
B. EVOLVE trial
C. AURORA Study
D. SHARP Study

Evaluation of Cinacalcet Hydrochloride Therapy to Lower Cardiovascular Events (EVOLVE) trial tested the hypothesis that treatment with cinacalcet reduces the risks of death & nonfatal cardiovascular events among patients with secondary hyperparathyroidism, who were undergoing dialysis.

1213. In CKD, target PTH level should be between?
Harrison's 20th Ed. Chapter 305 Page 2116

A. 25–100 pg/mL
B. 75–200 pg/mL
C. 150–300 pg/mL
D. 350–500 pg/mL

1214. Which of the following is a consequence of very low PTH level?
Harrison's 20th Ed. Chapter 305 Page 2116

A. Adynamic bone disease
B. Fracture
C. Ectopic calcification
D. All of the above

In CKD, target PTH level should be between 150 and 300 pg/mL. Very low PTH levels cause adynamic bone disease, fracture and ectopic calcification.

1215. The CKD-related risk factor of vascular disease is?
Harrison's 20th Ed. Chapter 305 Page 2116

A. Increased FGF-23
B. Sleep apnea
C. Generalized inflammation
D. All of the above

1216. The CKD-related risk factor of vascular disease is?
Harrison's 20th Ed. Chapter 305 Page 2116

A. Anemia
B. Hyperphosphatemia
C. Hyperparathyroidism
D. All of the above

The CKD-related risk factors comprise anemia, hyperphosphatemia, hyperparathyroidism, increased FGF-23, sleep apnea and generalized inflammation.

1217. Fetuin best relates to which of the following?
Harrison's 20th Ed. Chapter 305 Page 2113

A. Angiogenesis
B. Negative acute-phase reactant
C. NK cell function
D. B cell activation

"Negative acute-phase reactants" include serum albumin and fetuin. Serum fetuin-A concentrations are inversely associated with CAC severity independent of traditional CVD risk factors and kidney function in community-living individuals free of clinically apparent CVD.

1218. Which of the following statements about fetuin-A is false?
J Am Soc Nephrol. 2009;20:1264-1274

A. Calcification inhibitor (inhibits ectopic calcification)
B. Also called α_2-Heremans-Schmid glycoprotein
C. Synthesized and secreted by the liver
D. None of the above

1219. Which of the following statements is false?
Harrison's 20th Ed. Chapter 305 Page 2116

A. Cardiac troponin levels are elevated in CKD
B. LVH & dCMP are the strongest risk factors for CV morbidity & mortality in CKD
C. In dialysis patients, low blood pressure carries a worse prognosis than does high blood pressure
D. All of the above

1220. Which of the following is associated with poor prognosis in late-stage CKD patients?
Harrison's 20th Ed. Chapter 305 Page 2116

A. Low blood pressure
B. Reduced body mass index
C. Hypolipidemia
D. All of the above

In late-stage CKD, low BP, reduced BMI & hypolipidemia indicate the presence of a malnutrition-inflammation state, with poor prognosis.

1221. Which of the following should be the first line of therapy in CKD?
Harrison's 20th Ed. Chapter 305 Page 2117

A. Salt restriction
B. Volume management
C. Antihypertensive agent
D. Dialysis

Salt restriction should be the first line of therapy. When volume management alone is not sufficient, the choice of antihypertensive agent is similar to that in the general population.

1222. In CKD patients with diabetes or proteinuria > 1 gram/day, blood pressure should be reduced to?

Harrison's 20th Ed. Chapter 305 Page 2117

A. < 110/70 mm Hg
B. < 125/75 mm Hg
C. < 130/80 mm Hg
D. < 140/90 mm Hg

In CKD patients with diabetes or proteinuria > 1 gram/day, BP should be reduced to <130/80 mm Hg. Renoprotective effect of antihypertensive medications is gauged by consequent reduction of proteinuria.

1223. Which of the following about potassium is false?

The American Journal of Medicine. 2018;131(5):459-460

A. K^+ is absorbed in small intestine via paracellular pathway
B. K^+ is secreted in proximal colon
C. K^+ is absorbed in distal colon
D. None of the above

Majority of potassium is absorbed in small intestine via paracellular pathway, which is driven by the K^+ concentration & positive charge. Fine tuning of K^+ absorption occurs in colon. K^+ is secreted in proximal colon, mainly mediated by calcium-dependent, large-conductance potassium channel (BK or Big Potassium channel), and absorbed in distal colon, mediated by hydrogen potassium ATPase.

1224. Which of the following is a potassium-binding agent for treatment of patients with hyperkalemia?

Harrison's 20th Ed. Chapter 305 Page 2117

A. Sodium polystyrene sulfonate (SPS)
B. Sodium zirconium cyclosilicate
C. Patiromer
D. All of the above

Sodium polystyrene sulfonate (SPS) is a nonspecific sodium-cation exchange resin sometimes associated with colonic necrosis. Sodium zirconium cyclosilicate is a selective potassium cation trapping agent while Patiromer is a calcium-potassium cation exchange resin.

1225. Which of the following about sodium polystyrene sulfonate (SPS) is false?

Harrison's 20th Ed. Chapter 305 Page 2117

A. Oral synthetic cation-exchange resin
B. Binds potassium, calcium and magnesium
C. Not absorbed into the systemic circulation
D. None of the above

Sodium polystyrene sulfonate and calcium polystyrene sulfonate may cause ischemic colitis, related to coadministration with sorbitol.

1226. Nonabsorbed polymer of Patiromer binds potassium in exchange for?

N Engl J Med. 2015;372:211-21

A. Sodium
B. Calcium
C. Magnesium
D. All of the above

The active moiety of patiromer for oral suspension is a nonabsorbed polymer that binds potassium in exchange for calcium predominantly in the distal colon, where the concentration of free potassium is highest, thus increasing fecal potassium excretion and lowering serum potassium levels. Patiromer cannot be used as an emergency treatment for life-threatening hyperkalemia because of its delayed onset of action (7 hours).

1227. Which of the following is a potential side effect of Patiromer acetate?

N Engl J Med. 2015;372:211-21

A. Hypercalcemia
B. Hypomagnesemia
C. Hypokalemia
D. All of the above

Calcium released from patiromer in exchange for potassium can have multiple fates: it can bind to phosphorous and/or oxalate forming insoluble calcium phosphate and/or calcium oxalate salts and be excreted in the stool; it can rebind with patiromer; or it can be systematically absorbed leading to hypercalcemia, although it has not been reported in any major clinical trials. Patiromer also has the ability to bind to magnesium in the colon, which can result in hypomagnesemia.

1228. Which of the following about uremic pericarditis is false?

Harrison's 20th Ed. Chapter 305 Page 2117

A. Absolute indication for urgent initiation of dialysis
B. Propensity to hemorrhage in pericardial fluid
C. Hemodialysis should be performed without heparin
D. None of the above

1229. Pericardial effusion is a side effect of?

Harrison's 20th Ed. Chapter 305 Page 2117

A. Prazosin
B. Minoxidil
C. Eplerenone
D. Labetalol

Side effects of minoxidil include hypertrichosis and pericardial effusion.

1230. Normocytic, normochromic anemia is almost always present by which stage of CKD?

Harrison's 20th Ed. Chapter 305 Page 2117

A. Stage 1
B. Stage 2
C. Stage 3
D. Stage 4

Normocytic, normochromic anemia is almost always present by stage 4 of CKD.

1231. Primary cause of anemia in patients with CKD is?

Harrison's 20th Ed. Chapter 305 Page 2117

A. Insufficient erythropoietin (EPO)
B. Iron deficiency
C. Anemia of chronic disease
D. All of the above

Primary cause of anemia in patients with CKD is insufficient production of erythropoietin (EPO) by the diseased kidneys.

1232. Anemia resistant to erythropoietic-stimulating agents (ESA) when iron stores are adequate may be due to?

Harrison's 20th Ed. Chapter 305 Page 2118

A. Inadequate dialysis
B. Severe hyperparathyroidism
C. Chronic hemolysis
D. All of the above

Anemia resistant to recommended doses of ESA in the face of adequate iron stores may be due to some combination of the following: acute or chronic inflammation, inadequate dialysis, severe hyperparathyroidism, chronic blood loss or hemolysis, chronic infection or malignancy.

1233. Use of erythropoietic-stimulating agents (ESA) in CKD may be associated with?

Harrison's 20th Ed. Chapter 305 Page 2118

A. Increased risk of stroke in patients with type 2 diabetes
B. Increase in thromboembolic events
C. Faster progression of renal decline
D. All of the above

Use of ESA in CKD may be associated with an increased risk of stroke in those with type 2 diabetes, an increase in thromboembolic events, and a faster progression of renal decline.

1234. In CKD, blood transfusions increase the risk of?

Harrison's 20th Ed. Chapter 305 Page 2118

A. Hepatitis
B. Iron overload
C. Transplant sensitization
D. All of the above

Blood transfusions increase the risk of hepatitis, iron overload and transplant sensitization.

1235. In CKD, current practice is to target a hemoglobin concentration of?

Harrison's 20th Ed. Chapter 305 Page 2118

A. 9–10.5 gram/dL
B. 10–11.5 gram/dL
C. 11–12.5 gram/dL
D. 12–13.5 gram/dL

In CKD, current practice is to target a hemoglobin concentration of 10–11.5 gram/dL.

1236. Patients with later stages of CKD may have?

Harrison's 20th Ed. Chapter 305 Page 2118

A. Decreased activity of platelet factor III
B. Abnormal platelet aggregation & adhesiveness
C. Impaired prothrombin consumption
D. All of the above

Patients with later stages of CKD may have a prolonged bleeding time, decreased activity of platelet factor III, abnormal platelet aggregation and adhesiveness and impaired prothrombin consumption.

1237. Abnormal bleeding time and coagulopathy in renal failure may be reversed temporarily with?

Harrison's 20th Ed. Chapter 305 Page 2118

A. Desmopressin (DDAVP)
B. IV conjugated estrogens
C. Erythropoietin (EPO) therapy
D. All of the above

Abnormal BT & coagulopathy in renal failure may be reversed temporarily with desmopressin (DDAVP), cryoprecipitate, IV conjugated estrogens, blood transfusions and ESA therapy.

1238. Which of the following will usually correct a prolonged bleeding time in CKD patients?

Harrison's 20th Ed. Chapter 305 Page 2118

A. Desmopressin (DDAVP)
B. IV conjugated estrogens
C. Erythropoietin (EPO) therapy
D. Optimal dialysis

Optimal dialysis will usually correct a prolonged bleeding time. A brief run of hemodialysis (without heparin) may also be considered prior to renal biopsy to normalize the bleeding time.

1239. Peripheral neuropathy of CKD becomes clinically evident after which stage of CKD?

Harrison's 20th Ed. Chapter 305 Page 2118

A. Stage 1
B. Stage 2
C. Stage 3
D. Stage 4

Peripheral neuropathy usually becomes clinically evident after stage 4 of CKD.

1240. Which of the following is true for peripheral neuropathy of CKD?

Harrison's 20th Ed. Chapter 305 Page 2118

A. Sensory nerves involved more than motor
B. Lower extremities involved more than upper
C. Distal parts of extremities involved more than proximal
D. All of the above

1241. Uremic fetor is due to breakdown of urea to ammonia in?

Harrison's 20th Ed. Chapter 305 Page 2118

A. Saliva
B. Lung
C. Mucous membranes of mouth
D. All of the above

Uremic fetor (urine-like odor on breath) is due to breakdown of urea to ammonia in saliva.

1242. Which active variant of sodium glucose co-transporter (SGLT) is responsible for 90% of glucose reabsorption in kidneys?

Int J Appl Basic Med Res. 2015;5(3):161–163

A. SGLT-1
B. SGLT-2
C. SGLT-3
D. SGLT-4

Reabsorption of glucose in kidney is mediated by insulin independent sodium glucose co-transporter (SGLT), which has six active variants SGLT-1 to SGLT-6. SGLT-2 is responsible for 90% of renal proximal tubule glucose reabsorption, whereas SGLT-1 is responsible for remaining 10% reabsorption in kidneys.

1243. SGLT1 transporter is expressed in which of the following organs?

Am J Physiol Renal Physiol. 2015;309(11):F889-F900

A. Gut
B. Heart
C. Lungs
D. All of the above

SGLT1 transporter is expressed in gut, heart, and lungs. In gut, it transports glucose & galactose. SGLT2 is highly localized to the kidney.

1244. The maximum glucose transport capacity (Tm) of proximal tubule is?

Am J Physiol Renal Physiol. 2015;309(11):F889-F900

A. ~ 175 mg/minute
B. ~ 275 mg/minute
C. ~ 375 mg/minute
D. ~ 475 mg/minute

The maximum glucose transport capacity (Tm) of the proximal tubule, on average, is ~375 mg/minute. In normal individuals with a mean day-long plasma glucose concentration of ~100 mg/dL, the filtered glucose load (~125 mg/minute or 180 gram/day) is less than the maximal renal glucose transport capacity. In poorly controlled diabetic individuals, filtered glucose load may exceed 375 mg/minute, and all of the filtered glucose in excess of the Tm is excreted in the urine. In healthy individuals, plasma glucose threshold at which glucosuria begins is ~180 mg/dL due to nonlinear transition in the reabsorption and excretion curves (splay).

1245. Prototype compound of SGLT inhibitors is?

Int J Appl Basic Med Res. 2015;5(3):161–163

A. Arborizin
B. Phlorizin
C. Temporizin
D. Cetirizin

Prototype compound of SGLT inhibitors is a bitter white glycoside Phlorizin (O-glucoside phlorizin dihydrochalcones, a type of flavonoid). Phlorizin, isolated from the bark of apple trees, was the first renal sodium-glucose cotransport inhibitor to be identified.

1246. Which class of drugs approved for the treatment of T2DM reduces kidney function decline and cardiovascular events?

Harrison's 20th Ed. Chapter 305 Page 2119

A. Biguanides
B. Glucagon-like peptide 1 (GLP-1)
C. DPP-4 inhibitors
D. SGLT inhibitors

By inhibiting sodium, along with glucose, transport in proximal tubule and increasing sodium delivery to juxtaglomerular apparatus, SGLT2 inhibitors cause afferent renal arteriolar vasoconstriction, decreased intraglomerular pressure, and reduction in GFR hyperfiltration.

1247. Pregnancy is associated with high rate of spontaneous abortion, when GFR is?

Harrison's 20th Ed. Chapter 305 Page 2119

A. ~ 90 mL/minute
B. ~ 70 mL/minute
C. ~ 40 mL/minute
D. ~ 30 mL/minute

Pregnancy is associated with high rate of spontaneous abortion, when GFR is ~ 40 mL/minute. At this stage, only ~ 20% of pregnancies lead to live births.

1248. Skin pigmentation in advanced CKD is due to?

Harrison's 20th Ed. Chapter 305 Page 2119

A. Chromogens
B. Chromolytes
C. Urochromes
D. Renochromes

Patients become more pigmented in advanced CKD, even on dialysis due to deposition of retained pigmented metabolites called urochromes.

1249. Disorders associated with ESRD include?

Harrison's 20th Ed. Chapter 305 Page 2119

A. Calciphylaxis
B. Uremic frost
C. Nephrogenic fibrosing dermopathy
D. All of the above

Uremic frost is infrequently seen because of early dialytic intervention. When BUN level is high, concentration of urea in sweat is increased greatly. Evaporation results in the deposition of urea crystals on skin as fine white-to-yellow crystals that dissolve readily when challenged by a drop of water.

1250. Nephrogenic fibrosing dermopathy is similar to?

Harrison's 20th Ed. Chapter 305 Page 2119

A. Guttate morphea
B. Scleromyxedema
C. Linear scleroderma
D. Diffuse fasciitis with eosinophilia

Nephrogenic fibrosing dermopathy, seen in CKD, is a progressive subcutaneous induration on arms & legs similar to scleromyxedema.

1251. Which of the following can precipitate nephrogenic fibrosing dermopathy?

Harrison's 20th Ed. Chapter 305 Page 2119

A. Vitamin D
B. Metformin
C. Aluminum
D. Gadolinium

Exposure to magnetic resonance contrast agent, gadolinium may precipitate nephrogenic fibrosing dermopathy or nephrogenic systemic fibrosis (NSF) between 5 & 75 days following exposure.

1252. Rapid removal of gadolinium can be done by?

Harrison's 20th Ed. Chapter 305 Page 2119

A. Forced diuresis
B. IV calcium
C. Hemodialysis
D. All of the above

Rapid removal of gadolinium can be done by hemodialysis.

1253. Which of the following test must be done in all unexplained anemic with normal serum calcium CKD patients >35 years?

Harrison's 20th Ed. Chapter 305 Page 2119

A. Hepatitis B
B. Serum and urine protein electrophoresis
C. Serum concentrations of PTH
D. Serum vitamin B_{12} and folate

Serum and urine protein electrophoresis for multiple myeloma must be done in all patients >35 years with unexplained CKD, especially if there is associated anemia and elevated or even inappropriately normal serum calcium concentration.

1254. In which of the following conditions, kidney size may be normal in the face of CKD?

Harrison's 20th Ed. Chapter 305 Page 2119

A. Diabetic nephropathy
B. HIV nephropathy
C. Amyloidosis
D. All of the above

1255. Which of the following measures attenuate contrast-induced worsening of renal function?

Harrison's 20th Ed. Chapter 305 Page 2119

A. Sodium bicarbonate containing solutions
B. N acetylcysteine
C. Use of least nephrotoxic potential radiographic contrast agent
D. All of the above

1256. Contraindications to renal biopsy include?

Harrison's 20th Ed. Chapter 305 Page 2120

A. Bilaterally small kidneys
B. Uncontrolled hypertension
C. Active urinary tract infection
D. All of the above

1257. Contraindications to renal biopsy include?

Harrison's 20th Ed. Chapter 305 Page 2120

A. Bleeding diathesis
B. Ongoing anticoagulation
C. Severe obesity
D. All of the above

1258. If bleeding time is ↑ed at the time of renal biopsy, which of the following is administered immediately prior to the procedure?

Harrison's 20th Ed. Chapter 305 Page 2120

A. Protamine
B. Desmopressin
C. N acetylcysteine
D. IV calcium

If bleeding time is increased at the time of renal biopsy, desmopressin should be administered immediately prior to the procedure. A brief run of hemodialysis, without heparin, also helps.

1259. Which of the following can be a superimposed acute process in CKD?

Harrison's 20th Ed. Chapter 305 Page 2120

A. ECFV depletion
B. Urinary infection or obstruction
C. Nephrotoxin exposure
D. All of the above

Potentially reversible uper imposed acute or subacute processes like ECFV depletion, uncontrolled hypertension, urinary tract infection, new obstructive uropathy, exposure to nephrotoxic agents (NSAIDs or radiographic dye), and reactivation or flare of the original disease, such as lupus or vasculitis, may complicate CKD.

1260. Which of the following have an antiproteinuric and renoprotective effect?

Harrison's 20th Ed. Chapter 305 Page 2120

A. ACE inhibitors and ARBs
B. Diltiazem
C. Verapamil
D. All of the above

1261. CKD is likely if bilateral kidney size is?

Harrison's 20th Ed. Chapter 305 Page 2120

A. < 8.5 cm
B. < 9.0 cm
C. < 9.5 cm
D. < 10 cm

Finding of bilaterally reduced kidney size (<8.5 cm) favors CKD.

1262. Dose adjustment is not needed, if the medication's excretion by nonrenal route is?

Harrison's 20th Ed. Chapter 305 Page 2120

A. > 60%
B. > 70%
C. > 80%
D. > 90%

For those medication in which >70% excretion is by a nonrenal route (hepatic elimination), dose adjustment may not be needed.

1263. Which of the following drugs that should be avoided in CKD?

Harrison's 20th Ed. Chapter 305 Page 2120

A. Metformin
B. Meperidine
C. Gadolinium
D. All of the above

Drugs that should be avoided in CKD include metformin, meperidine & gadolinium.

1264. Clear indications for initiation of renal replacement therapy include?

Harrison's 20th Ed. Chapter 305 Page 2121

A. Pericarditis
B. Progressive neuropathy due to uremia
C. Encephalopathy
D. All of the above

1265. Clear indications for initiation of renal replacement therapy include?

Harrison's 20th Ed. Chapter 305 Page 2121

A. Muscle irritability
B. Anorexia & nausea not relieved by protein restriction
C. Refractory fluid & electrolyte abnormalities
D. All of the above

1266. Clear indications for initiation of renal replacement therapy include?

Harrison's 20th Ed. Chapter 305 Page 2121

A. Unresponsive volume overload
B. Unresponsive hyperkalemia
C. Progressive metabolic acidosis
D. All of the above

Clear indications for initiation of renal replacement therapy in CKD include pericarditis, encephalopathy, intractable muscle cramping, anorexia, nausea, malnutrition, & refractory fluid & electrolyte abnormalities (hyperkalemia).

1267. Clinical clues indicating the imminent development of uremic complications are?

Harrison's 20th Ed. Chapter 305 Page 2121

A. History of hiccoughing
B. Intractable pruritus
C. Morning nausea & vomiting
D. All of the above

Dialysis in the Treatment of Renal Failure

1268. Which of the following dialysis process is specific to the management of acute renal failure?

Harrison's 20th Ed. Chapter 306 Page 2121

A. Continuous renal replacement therapies (CRRT)
B. Prolonged intermittent renal replacement therapy (PIRRT)
C. Slow low-efficiency dialysis (SLED)
D. All of the above

1269. Which of the following is the leading cause of ESRD?

Harrison's 20th Ed. Chapter 306 Page 2122

A. Hypertension
B. Diabetes mellitus
C. Glomerulonephritis
D. Obstructive uropathy

The leading cause of ESRD is diabetes mellitus (~45% of newly diagnosed cases of ESRD). Other include hypertension (~30%), glomerulonephritis, polycystic kidney disease and obstructive uropathy.

1270. Mortality rates for patients with ESRD are lowest in?

Harrison's 20th Ed. Chapter 306 Page 2122

A. Japan
B. USA
C. Australia
D. UAE

Mortality rates for patients with ESRD are lowest in Europe and Japan.

1271. Which of the following is an accepted criteria for initiating patients on maintenance dialysis?

Harrison's 20th Ed. Chapter 306 Page 2122

A. Presence of uremic symptoms
B. Acidosis refractory to medical therapy
C. Bleeding diathesis
D. All of the above

Accepted criteria for initiating patients on maintenance dialysis include presence of uremic symptoms, presence of hyperkalemia unresponsive to conservative measures, persistent extracellular volume expansion despite diuretic therapy, acidosis refractory to medical therapy, bleeding diathesis and creatinine clearance or estimated glomerular filtration rate (GFR) below 10 mL/minute per 1.73 m^2. There is no benefit to initiating dialysis preemptively at a GFR of 10–14 mL/minute per 1.73 m^2 compared to initiating dialysis for symptoms of uremia.

1272. Complications of advanced chronic kidney disease (CKD) include?

Harrison's 20th Ed. Chapter 306 Page 2122

A. Anemia
B. Acidosis
C. Secondary hyperparathyroidism
D. All of the above

Complications of advanced chronic kidney disease (CKD) include hypertension, anemia, acidosis, and secondary hyperparathyroidism.

1273. Which of the following is the most common therapeutic modality for ESRD?

Harrison's 20th Ed. Chapter 306 Page 2122

A. Hemodialysis
B. Continuous ambulatory peritoneal dialysis (CAPD)
C. Continuous cyclic peritoneal dialysis (CCPD)
D. Reanl transplantation

In ESRD, treatment options include hemodialysis (institutional or domiciliary), peritoneal dialysis as either continuous ambulatory peritoneal dialysis (CAPD) or continuous cyclic peritoneal dialysis (CCPD) or transplantation. Hemodialysis remains the most common therapeutic modality for ESRD.

1274. What is the size of urea molecule?

Harrison's 20th Ed. Chapter 306 Page 2122

A. 50 Da
B. 60 Da
C. 70 Da
D. 80 Da

1275. What is the size of creatinine molecule?

Harrison's 20th Ed. Chapter 306 Page 2122

A. 100 Da
B. 113 Da
C. 123 Da
D. 132 Da

Size of urea molecule is 60 Da, while that of creatinine is 113 Da. According to laws of diffusion, the larger the molecule, the slower is its rate of transfer across the membrane.

1276. Middle molecules have a molecular mass between?

Harrison's 20th Ed. Chapter 306 Page 2122

A. 500 & 1500 Da
B. 1500 & 3000 Da
C. 3000 & 5000 Da
D. 5000 & 8000 Da

Compounds with a molecular mass between 500 & 1500 Da are middle molecules.

1277. Which of the following processes occur in hemodialysis?

Harrison's 20th Ed. Chapter 306 Page 2122

A. Diffusive clearance
B. Ultrafiltration
C. Convective clearance
D. All of the above

1278. The rate of diffusive transport across a semipermeable membrane depends on?

Harrison's 20th Ed. Chapter 306 Page 2122

A. Magnitude of the concentration gradient
B. Membrane surface area
C. Mass transfer coefficient of the membrane
D. All of the above

1279. Mass transfer coefficient of the semipermeable membrane depends on?

Harrison's 20th Ed. Chapter 306 Page 2122

A. Porosity and thickness of the membrane
B. Size of the solute molecule
C. Conditions of flow on two sides of the membrane
D. All of the above

1280. Convective clearance best relates to?
Harrison's 20th Ed. Chapter 306 Page 2122

A. Supersaturation
B. Solvent drag
C. Ultrafiltration
D. All of the above

Convective clearance occurs because of solvent drag, with solutes being swept along with water across the semipermeable dialysis membrane.

1281. Which of the following is a component to hemodialysis?
Harrison's 20th Ed. Chapter 306 Page 2122

A. Dialyzer
B. Composition and delivery of the dialysate
C. Blood delivery system
D. All of the above

The three essential components to hemodialysis are the dialyzer, the composition and delivery of the dialysate, and the blood delivery system.

1282. Which of the following is a category of dialysis membrane?
Harrison's 20th Ed. Chapter 306 Page 2122

A. Cellulose
B. Cellulosynthetic
C. Synthetic
D. All of the above

Categories of dialysis membranes are cellulose, substituted cellulose, cellulosynthetic and synthetic.

1283. Reprocessing agent used in a hemodialyzer include?
Harrison's 20th Ed. Chapter 306 Page 2122

A. Formaldehyde
B. Peracetic acid–hydrogen peroxide
C. Glutaraldehyde
D. All of the above

Formaldehyde, peracetic acid–hydrogen peroxide, glutaraldehyde and bleach are used as reprocessing agents.

1284. Surface area of modern dialysis membranes in adult patients is?
Harrison's 20th Ed. Chapter 306 Page 2122

A. 0.5–1.0 m^2
B. 1.5–2.0 m^2
C. 2.5–3.0 m^2
D. 3.5–4.0 m^2

Surface area of modern dialysis membranes in adult patients is ~1.5–2.0 m^2.

1285. Which of the following improve the 'Biocompatibility' of a dialysis membrane?
Harrison's 20th Ed. Chapter 306 Page 2122

A. More free hydroxyl groups on membrane surface
B. Less free hydroxyl groups on membrane surface
C. More free sulphydral groups on membrane surface
D. Less free sulphydral groups on membrane surface

Bioincompatibility is defined as the ability of dialysis membrane to activate complement cascade. Cellulosic membranes are bioincompatible because of the presence of free hydroxyl groups on membrane surface.

1286. Which of the following is a form of synthetic membrane?
Harrison's 20th Ed. Chapter 306 Page 2122

A. Polysulfone
B. Poly methyl methacrylate
C. Polyacrylonitrile
D. All of the above

Examples of synthetic membranes are polysulfone, poly methyl methacrylate, and polyacrylonitrile membranes. These are more biocompatible because of the absence of free hydroxyl groups.

1287. Which of the following is false about ion concentration of dialysate?
Harrison's 20th Ed. Chapter 306 Page 2122

A. K^+ concentration of dialysate varies from 0 to 4 mmol/L
B. Ca^+ is 1.25 mmol/L or 2.5 mEq/L
C. Na^+ concentration is 136–140 mmol/L
D. None of the above

1288. During each hemodialysis session, patient is exposed to approximately how much water as dialysate?
Harrison's 20th Ed. Chapter 306 Page 2122

A. 80 L
B. 120 L
C. 180 L
D. 250 L

Patients are exposed to ~120 liters of water during each dialysis treatment.

1289. Blood flow rate in the extracorporeal circuit in hemodialysis machine ranges from?
Harrison's 20th Ed. Chapter 306 Page 2122

A. 50 to 100 mL/minute
B. 100 to 200 mL/minute
C. 250 to 450 mL/minute
D. 500 to 750 mL/minute

Blood flow rate in extracorporeal circuit in hemodialysis machine ranges from 250–450 mL/minute.

1290. 'Breschia-Cimino fistula' is used for?
Harrison's 20th Ed. Chapter 306 Page 2123

A. Dialysis access
B. Ventriculo-atrial shunt
C. Peritono-caval shunt
D. Peripheral arterial bypass

In Brescia-Cimino fistula, cephalic vein is anastomosed end-to-side to radial artery for dialysis access (arterialization of the vein).

1291. Prosthetic material for arteriovenous graft is?
Harrison's 20th Ed. Chapter 306 Page 2123

A. Polytetrafluoroethylene (PTFE)
B. Polyethylene (PE)
C. Polyvinylidene fluoride (PVDF)
D. Polytrifluoroethylene

Polytetrafluoroethylene (PTFE) is one of the most stable polymers known.

1292. Most common dialysis access-related complication is?
Harrison's 20th Ed. Chapter 306 Page 2123

A. Infection
B. Thrombosis
C. Embolism
D. Perforation

Most important complication of AV grafts is thrombosis of the graft & graft failure, due to intimal hyperplasia at anastomosis between graft & recipient vein.

1293. Most tunneled catheters are placed in?
Harrison's 20th Ed. Chapter 306 Page 2123

A. Internal jugular vein
B. External jugular vein
C. Femoral vein
D. Subclavian vein

Most tunneled catheters are placed in the internal jugular veins. External jugular, femoral, and subclavian veins may also be used.

1294. In hemodialysis, dialysate flows in an opposite counter-current direction at the rate of?
Harrison's 20th Ed. Chapter 306 Page 2123

A. 100 to 300 mL/minute
B. 300 to 500 mL/minute
C. 500 to 800 mL/minute
D. 800 to 1000 mL/minute

Dialysate flows in an opposite counter-current direction at 500–800 mL/minute while heparinized blood is pumped through the dialyzer at a flow rate of 300–450 mL/minute.

1295. The dose of dialysis is governed by?
Harrison's 20th Ed. Chapter 306 Page 2123

A. Patient size
B. Residual kidney function
C. Dietary protein intake
D. All of the above

The dose of dialysis, which is defined as a derivation of fractional urea clearance during a single treatment, is governed by patient size, residual kidney function, dietary protein intake, the degree of anabolism or catabolism, and the presence of comorbid conditions.

1296. What level of urea reduction ratio (URR) per treatment, defines minimal standards for adequacy among ESRD patients?
Harrison's 20th Ed. Chapter 306 Page 2123

A. 35%
B. 45%
C. 55%
D. 65%

Current target is a urea reduction ratio (fractional reduction in BUN per hemodialysis session) of >65– 70% (dose of dialysis).

1297. What level of KT/V per treatment, defines minimal standards for adequacy among ESRD patients?
Harrison's 20th Ed. Chapter 306 Page 2123

A. 0.8
B. 1.0
C. 1.2
D. 1.4

Current target is body water–indexed clearance x time product (KT/V) above 1.2.

1298. For the majority of patients with ESRD, how many hours of dialysis is required each week?
Harrison's 20th Ed. Chapter 306 Page 2124

A. 3 to 9 hours
B. 9 to 12 hours
C. 12 to 24 hours
D. 24 to 36 hours

For the majority of patients with ESRD, between 9 and 12 hours of dialysis are required each week, usually divided into three equal sessions.

1299. Most common acute complication of hemodialysis is?
Harrison's 20th Ed. Chapter 306 Page 2124

A. Infection
B. Hypotension
C. Anemia
D. Muscle cramps

1300. Hypotension as the most common acute complication of hemodialysis is particularly seen in?
Harrison's 20th Ed. Chapter 306 Page 2124

A. Hypertensives
B. Diabetics
C. Heart failure
D. All of the above

Hypotension is the most common acute complication of hemodialysis, particularly among diabetics. Other complications of ESRD include a high incidence of infection, progressive debility and frailty, protein-energy malnutrition and impaired cognitive function.

1301. In dialysate, presence of which of the following is a common cause of hypotension?
Harrison's 20th Ed. Chapter 306 Page 2124

A. Acetate
B. Bicarbonate
C. Calcium
D. Aluminium

Because of the vasodilatory & cardiodepressive effects of acetate, its use as buffer in dialysate is a common cause of hypotension. Since the introduction of bicarbonate-containing dialysate, dialysis-associated hypotension has become less common.

1302. In the management of hypotension during dialysis, administration of which of the following is useful?
Harrison's 20th Ed. Chapter 306 Page 2124

A. 100 to 250 mL of isotonic saline
B. 10 mL of 23% saturated hypertonic saline
C. Salt-poor albumin
D. All of the above

Hypotension during dialysis is managed with discontinuing ultrafiltration, 100–250 mL of isotonic saline or 10 mL of 23% saturated hypertonic saline, and administration of salt-poor albumin.

1303. Hypotension during dialysis can be prevented by?
Harrison's 20th Ed. Chapter 306 Page 2124

A. Careful evaluation of dry weight
B. Withholding of antihypertensive medications
C. Avoiding heavy meals during dialysis
D. All of the above

1304. Hypotension during dialysis can be prevented by?
Harrison's 20th Ed. Chapter 306 Page 2124

A. Ultrafiltration modeling
B. Midodrine
C. Cooling of dialysate during dialysis treatment
D. All of the above

1305. Excessively rapid fluid removal during hemodialysis refers to?
Harrison's 20th Ed. Chapter 306 Page 2124

A. > 8 mL/kg per hour
B. > 13 mL/kg per hour
C. > 18 mL/kg per hour
D. > 23 mL/kg per hour

Hypotension during dialysis can be prevented by by ultrafiltration modeling, such that more fluid is removed at the beginning rather than the end of dialysis procedure. Excessively rapid fluid removal i.e. >13 mL/kg per hour should be avoided.

1306. Which of the following may prevent muscle cramps during hemodialysis?
Harrison's 20th Ed. Chapter 306 Page 2124

A. Reducing volume removal during dialysis
B. Use of sodium modeling
C. Ultrafiltration profiling
D. All of the above

1307. Which of the following is false about anaphylactoid reactions to the dialyzer?
Harrison's 20th Ed. Chapter 306 Page 2124

A. Occur with bioincompatible cellulosic-containing membranes
B. Type A reactions are hypersensitivity reaction to ethylene oxide
C. Type B reaction activate complement & release of cytokine
D. None of the above

Anaphylactoid reactions to dialyzer, particularly on its first use, occur mostly with bioincompatible cellulosic-containing membranes. Dialyzer reactions can be divided into two types, A and B. Type A reactions are attributed to an IgE mediated intermediate hypersensitivity reaction to ethylene oxide used in the sterilization of new dialyzers. This reaction typically occurs soon after initiation & can progress to full-blown anaphylaxis if the therapy is not promptly discontinued. Treatment with steroids or epinephrine may be needed. Type B reaction consists of a symptom complex of nonspecific chest & back pain, which results from complement activation & cytokine release occurring several minutes into the dialysis run & typically resolve with continued dialysis.

1308. In peritoneal dialysis, how much dextrose-containing solution is infused in the peritoneal cavity?
Harrison's 20th Ed. Chapter 306 Page 2124

A. 1.5 to 3 Liters
B. 4 to 6 Liters
C. 6 to 8 Liters
D. 10 to 12 Liters

1309. In peritoneal dialysis, for how many hours dextrose-containing solution is allowed to remain in the peritoneal cavity?
Harrison's 20th Ed. Chapter 306 Page 2124

A. 1 to 2 hours
B. 2 to 4 hours
C. 4 to 6 hours
D. 6 to 8 hours

In peritoneal dialysis, 1.5–3 liters of a dextrose-containing solution is infused into peritoneal cavity & allowed for 2–4 hours.

1310. Which of the following about peritoneal dialysis is false?
Harrison's 20th Ed. Chapter 306 Page 2124

A. Metabolic byproducts removed through convective clearance
B. Metabolic byproducts removed through diffusive clearance
C. Absorption of solutes & water occurs via peritoneal lymphatics into lymphatic circulation
D. None of the above

In PD, metabolic byproducts are removed through a combination of convective clearance generated through ultrafiltration and diffusive clearance down a concentration gradient. Absorption of solutes and water from the peritoneal cavity occurs across peritoneal membrane into peritoneal capillary circulation and via peritoneal lymphatics into lymphatic circulation.

1311. Which of the following can be used in place of dextrose in peritoneal dialysis solution?
Harrison's 20th Ed. Chapter 306 Page 2124

A. Maltodextrin
B. Cyclodextrin
C. Icodextrin
D. All of the above

Icodextrin is a nonabsorbable carbohydrate that can be used in place of dextrose.

1312. Additive to peritoneal dialysis solutions may be?
Harrison's 20th Ed. Chapter 306 Page 2124

A. Heparin
B. Antibiotics
C. Insulin
D. All of the above

Additives to peritoneal dialysis solutions are heparin, antibiotics and insulin.

1313. Advantage of continuous renal replacement therapy (CRRT) over intermittent hemodialysis in ARF is?
Harrison's 20th Ed. Chapter 306 Page 2125

A. Better tolerated hemodynamically
B. Gradual correction of biochemical abnormalities
C. Highly effective in removing fluid
D. All of the above

1314. Continuous renal replacement therapy (CRRT) techniques include?
Harrison's 20th Ed. Chapter 306 Page 2125

A. Continuous arteriovenous hemodiafiltration with dialysis
B. Continuous arteriovenous hemodiafiltration without dialysis
C. Continuous veno-venous hemodiafiltration with dialysis
D. All of the above

1315. Which of the following is a type of 'Peritoneal dialysis'?
Harrison's 20th Ed. Chapter 306 Page 2125

A. Continuous ambulatory peritoneal dialysis (CAPD)
B. Continuous cyclic peritoneal dialysis (CCPD)
C. Nocturnal intermittent peritoneal dialysis (NIPD)
D. All of the above

1316. Which of the following is false for CAPD?
Harrison's 20th Ed. Chapter 306 Page 2125

A. Dialysis solution is manually infused into peritoneal cavity
B. Dialysis solution remains in peritoneal cavity through night
C. Drainage of spent dialysate is performed manually
D. None of the above

1317. Which of the following statements is false?
Harrison's 20th Ed. Chapter 306 Page 2125

A. In CCPD, exchanges are performed in automated fashion
B. In CCPD, the last exchange remains in abdomen
C. In NIPD, the abdomen is left dry during the day
D. None of the above

1318. Preferred buffer in peritoneal dialysis solution is?
Harrison's 20th Ed. Chapter 306 Page 2125

A. Lactate
B. Bicarbonate
C. Acetate
D. All of the above

Lactate is the preferred buffer in peritoneal dialysis solutions.

1319. Which of the following is a complication of peritoneal dialysis?
Harrison's 20th Ed. Chapter 306 Page 2125

A. Peritonitis
B. Weight gain
C. Residual uremia
D. All of the above

Complications of PD are peritonitis, catheter-associated nonperitonitis infections, weight gain, metabolic disturbances and residual uremia.

1320. What value of peritoneal fluid leukocyte count denotes peritonitis?
Harrison's 20th Ed. Chapter 306 Page 2125

A. $10/mm^3$
B. $40/mm^3$
C. $80/mm^3$
D. $100/mm^3$

Peritonitis is defined by a raised peritoneal fluid leukocyte count ($100/mm^3$, 50% are PMN).

1321. Most common culprit organism in peritonitis as a complication of peritoneal dialysis is?
Harrison's 20th Ed. Chapter 306 Page 2125

A. Gram-positive cocci
B. Gram-positive bacilli
C. Gram-negative cocci
D. Gram-negative bacilli

Most common culprit organisms in peritonitis as a complication of peritoneal dialysis are gram-positive cocci including Staphylococcus, reflecting the origin from skin.

1322. Nonperitonitis catheter-associated infections are termed as?
Harrison's 20th Ed. Chapter 306 Page 2125

A. Funnel infections
B. Tunnel infections
C. Channel infections
D. Chamber infections

Nonperitonitis catheter-associated infections are often termed tunnel infections.

1323. Which of the following statements is false?
Harrison's 20th Ed. Chapter 306 Page 2125

A. Acetate in PD solution can accelerate peritoneal sclerosis
B. Bicarbonate in PD solution can precipitate calcium
C. Bicarbonate in PD solution can caramelize glucose
D. None of the above

1324. Which of the following study evaluated cardiovascular risk reduction in ESRD patients?
Harrison's 20th Ed. Chapter 306 Page 2125

A. 4D
B. AURORA
C. SHARP
D. All of the above

1325. Clinical abnormalities in uremia that develop only after initiation of dialysis therapy are all except?

A. Adynamic osteomalacia
B. Dialysis disequilibrium syndrome
C. Hypotension & arrhythmias
D. Hypothermia

1326. Clinical abnormalities in uremia that develop only after initiation of dialysis therapy are all except?

A. Hepatitis
B. Idiopathic ascites
C. Peritonitis
D. Muscular irritability

1327. Clinical abnormalities in uremia that develop only after initiation of dialysis therapy are all except?

A. Leukopenia
B. Hypocomplementemia
C. Muscle cramps
D. Hypernatremia & hyponatremia

1328. Clinical abnormalities in uremia that improve with dialysis and erythropoietin therapy are all except?

A. Fatigue
B. Impaired mentation
C. Lethargy
D. Sleep disorders

1329. Clinical abnormalities in uremia that improve with dialysis and erythropoietin therapy are all except?

A. Pallor
B. Anemia
C. Bleeding diathesis
D. Leukopenia

1330. Gastrointestinal disturbances in uremia that usually improve with optimal dialysis & related therapy are all except?

A. Anorexia, nausea and vomiting
B. Uremic fetor
C. Gastroenteritis
D. Idiopathic ascites

1331. Gastrointestinal disturbances in uremia that develop only after initiation of dialysis therapy are all except?

A. Hepatitis
B. Idiopathic ascites
C. Peritonitis
D. Uremic fetor

1332. Endocrine-metabolic disturbances in uremia that develop only after initiation of dialysis therapy are all except?

A. Carbohydrate intolerance
B. Adynamic osteomalacia
C. Secondary hyperparathyroidism
D. Vitamin D-deficient osteomalacia

1333. Endocrine-metabolic disturbances in uremia that improve with optimal dialysis & related therapy are all except?

A. Carbohydrate intolerance
B. Vitamin D-deficient osteomalacia
C. Hypothermia
D. All of the above

1334. Endocrine-metabolic disturbances in uremia that tends to persist or even progress, despite optimal dialysis & related therapy are all except?

A. Increased Lp(a) level
B. Decreased high-density lipoprotein level
C. Infertility and sexual dysfunction
D. None of the above

1335. Endocrine-metabolic disturbances in uremia that tends to persist or even progress, despite optimal dialysis & related therapy are all except?

A. Amenorrhea
B. Impaired growth & development
C. Infertility & sexual dysfunction
D. None of the above

1336. Neuromuscular disturbances in uremia that usually improve with optimal dialysis & related therapy are all except?

A. Asterixis
B. Muscular irritability
C. Coma
D. Sleep disorder

1337. Neuromuscular disturbances in uremia that develops only after initiation of dialysis therapy are all except?

A. Muscle cramps
B. Myoclonus
C. Dialysis disequilibrium syndrome
D. Myopathy

1338. Neuromuscular disturbances in uremia that improve with dialysis and erythropoietin therapy are all except?

A. Fatigue
B. Impaired mentation
C. Lethargy
D. Asterixis

1339. Cardiovascular & pulmonary disturbances in uremia that usually improve with optimal dialysis & related therapy are all except?

A. CHF/pulmonary edema
B. Pericarditis
C. Uremic lung
D. Hypotension & arrhythmias

1340. Dermatologic disturbances in uremia that usually improve with optimal dialysis & related therapy are all except?

A. Ecchymoses
B. Uremic frost
C. Pallor
D. Pruritus

Transplantation in the Treatment of Renal Failure

1341. 1-year survival in deceased-donor kidney transplants is?

Harrison's 20th Ed. Chapter 307 Page 2126

A. 76%
B. 84%
C. 92%
D. 97%

1342. 1-year survival in living-donor kidney transplants is?

Harrison's 20th Ed. Chapter 307 Page 2126

A. 76%
B. 84%
C. 92%
D. 97%

Deceased-donor kidney transplants have a 92% 1-year survival and living-donor kidney transplants have a 97% 1-year survival.

1343. Currently, the "average" (t½) life expectancy of a deceased-donor kidney transplants is around?

Harrison's 20th Ed. Chapter 307 Page 2126

A. 10 years
B. 15 years
C. 20 years
D. 25 years

1344. Currently, the "average" (t½) life expectancy of a living-donor kidney transplants is around?

Harrison's 20th Ed. Chapter 307 Page 2126

A. 7 years
B. 14 years
C. 21 years
D. 28 years

Currently, the "average" (t½) life expectancy of a living-donor kidney transplants is around 14 years and that of a deceased-donor kidney transplants is ~10 years.

1345. Mortality rates after kidney transplantation are highest in?

Harrison's 20th Ed. Chapter 307 Page 2126

A. First day
B. First week
C. First month
D. First year

Mortality rates after transplantation are highest in the first year.

1346. Most kidney transplantation patients succumb at varying rates to a chronic process consisting of?

Harrison's 20th Ed. Chapter 307 Page 2126

A. Interstitial fibrosis
B. Tubular atrophy
C. Glomerulopathy
D. All of the above

Most kidney transplantation patients succumb at varying rates to a chronic process consisting of interstitial fibrosis, tubular atrophy, vasculopathy, and glomerulopathy.

1347. Potential kidney recipients with the highest expected postransplant survival are provided with kidney donor profile index (KDPI) score of?

Harrison's 20th Ed. Chapter 307 Page 2126

A. < 10%
B. < 20%
C. < 30%
D. < 40%

Kidney donor profile Index (KDPI) score from 0 to 100% quantifies potential risk of graft failure after kidney transplant based on 10 donor factors. Lower KDPI values are associated with higher expected post-transplant survival. Kidneys with KDPI <20% are allocated to the 20% of the potential recipients with highest expected post-transplant survival.

1348. Kidneys from which of the following categories is least preferred for transplantation?

Harrison's 20th Ed. Chapter 307 Page 2126 Table 307-1

A. Brought in dead
B. Unsuccessful resuscitation
C. Awaiting cardiac arrest
D. Cardiac arrest after brainstem death

1349. Kidneys from which of the following categories is preferred for transplantation?

Harrison's 20th Ed. Chapter 307 Page 2126 Table 307-1

A. Brought in dead
B. Unsuccessful resuscitation
C. Awaiting cardiac arrest
D. Cardiac arrest in a hospital patient

The five categories of non-heart-beating donor (donation after cardiac death (DCD) are I: Brought in dead, II: Unsuccessful resuscitation, III: Awaiting cardiac arrest, IV: Cardiac arrest after brainstem death and V: Cardiac arrest in a hospital patient.

1350. Which of the following statements is false?

Harrison's 20th Ed. Chapter 307 Page 2126

A. High KDPI kidneys have a poorer survival
B. Graft survival is higher for living-donor recipients
C. Transplanted kidney is placed in the inguinal fossa
D. None of the above

1351. Which of the following is relevant for selection of donors for renal allografts is?

Harrison's 20th Ed. Chapter 307 Page 2127

A. HLA antigens
B. ABH(O) blood groups
C. Endothelial antigens
D. All of the above

1352. Which of the following statements is false?

Harrison's 20th Ed. Chapter 307 Page 2127

A. The Rh system is not expressed on graft tissue
B. T lymphocytes express class I antigens
C. B lymphocytes express both class I & class II antigens
D. None of the above

1353. Which of the following statements is false?

Harrison's 20th Ed. Chapter 307 Page 2127

A. CD4+ lymphocyte respond to class II (HLA-DR) incompatibility

B. CD8+ cytotoxic lymphocyte precursors respond to class I (HLA-A, -B) antigens

C. Graft rejection is initiated by CD4 helper T lymphocytes (TH)

D. None of the above

1354. Which of the following corresponds to complete HLA mismatch?

Harrison's 20th Ed. Chapter 307 Page 2127

A. 0/6

B. 2/6

C. 4/6

D. 6/6

1355. Which of the following assays is most sensitive for recipient - donor matching?

Harrison's 20th Ed. Chapter 307 Page 2127

A. Cytotoxic cross-match of recipient serum & donor T lymphocytes

B. Flow cytometric-based crossmatch assay

C. ABO compatibility

D. All of the above

1356. Anti-thymocyte globulin (ATG) comes under which of the following categories of induction therapy?

Harrison's 20th Ed. Chapter 307 Page 2128

A. Monoclonal antibody

B. Polyclonal antibody

C. Depletional agents

D. Nondepletional agents

1357. Alemtuzumab is directed to?

Harrison's 20th Ed. Chapter 307 Page 2128

A. CD28 protein

B. CD42 protein

C. CD52 protein

D. CD68 protein

Alemtuzumab is directed to the CD52 protein, widely distributed on immune cells such as B and T cells, natural killer cells, macrophages, and some granulocytes.

1358. In kidney transplantation patients, most frequently used combination for maintenance immunosuppressive therapy is?

Harrison's 20th Ed. Chapter 307 Page 2128

A. Prednisone + mTOR inhibitors

B. Prednisone + Calcineurin inhibitor

C. Prednisone + antimetabolite

D. Prednisone + calcineurin inhibitor + antimetabolite

All kidney transplant recipients should receive maintenance immunosuppressive therapies except identical twins. The most frequently used combination is triple therapy with prednisone, a calcineurin inhibitor, and an antimetabolite.

1359. Which of the following is used as prophylaxis for acute rejection in the immediate post renal transplant period?

Harrison's 20th Ed. Chapter 307 Page 2128, Biologics. 2009;3:319-336

A. Eculizumab

B. Daclizumab

C. Bevacizumab

D. Certolizumab pegol

Anti-interleukin-2 receptor antibodies, basiliximab and daclizumab are used for the prevention of acute rejection in renal transplantation.

1360. All kidney transplant recipients should receive maintenance immunosuppressive therapies except?

Harrison's 20th Ed. Chapter 307 Page 2129

A. Father–child

B. Mother–child

C. Identical twins

D. All of the above

All kidney transplant recipients must receive maintenance immunosuppressive therapies except identical twins.

1361. Which of the following is FDA-approved for kidney transplant recipients?

Harrison's 20th Ed. Chapter 307 Page 2129

A. Abatacept

B. Belatacept

C. Rilonacept

D. All of the above

Belatacept is a fusion protein that binds costimulatory ligands (CD80 and CD86) present on antigen presenting cells, interrupting their binding to CD28 on T cells. This inhibition leads to T cell anergy and apoptosis.

1362. Which of the following antimetabolite is used for maintenance therapy in kidney transplant recipients?

Harrison's 20th Ed. Chapter 307 Page 2129

A. Azathioprine

B. Methotrexate

C. 5-flucytosine

D. All of the above

Azathioprine and Mycophenolate mofetil are used for maintenance therapy in kidney transplant recipients.

1363. Which of the following about steroids in kidney transplant recipients is false?

Harrison's 20th Ed. Chapter 307 Page 2129

A. Prevents release of IL-6 & IL-1 by monocytes-macrophages

B. Methylprednisolone used in treatment of acute rejection

C. Methylprednisolone not effective in chronic rejection

D. None of the above

1364. Which of the following side effect is more common with tacrolimus as compared to cyclosporine?

Harrison's 20th Ed. Chapter 307 Page 2129

A. Nephrotoxicity

B. Hepatotoxicity

C. Diabetes mellitus

D. Tremor

Tacrolimus has a similar side-effect profile as cyclosporine ((nephrotoxicity, hepatotoxicity, hirsutism, tremor, gingival hyperplasia, and diabetes). Tacrolimus does not produce hirsutism or gingival hyperplasia. De novo diabetes mellitus is more common with tacrolimus.

1365. Clinical evidence of rejection is characterized by?

Harrison's 20th Ed. Chapter 307 Page 2129

A. Fever
B. Swelling
C. Tenderness over the allograft
D. None of the above

Clinical evidence of rejection is rarely characterized by fever, swelling, and tenderness over the allograft. Rejection may present only with a rise in serum creatinine, with or without a reduction in urine volume. A rise in the serum creatinine level is a late marker of rejection, but it may be the only sign.

1366. Which of the following is suggestive of cyclosporine side effect on renal biopsy?

Harrison's 20th Ed. Chapter 307 Page 2129

A. Interstitial fibrosis
B. Isometric tubular vacuolization
C. Thickening of arteriolar walls
D. All of the above

In renal biopsy, interstitial fibrosis, isometric tubular vacuolization, and thickening of arteriolar walls are suggestive of cyclosporine side effect, but not diagnostic.

1367. Which of the following is relevant to acute kidney graft rejection?

Harrison's 20th Ed. Chapter 307 Page 2130

A. Component c3
B. Component c4d
C. Component c5
D. Component c5b-9

Evidence of antibody-mediated injury is present when endothelial injury and deposition of complement component c4d is detected by fluorescence labeling.

1368. Which of the following is not an infection during early (1–6 months) period in kidney transplant recipients?

Harrison's 20th Ed. Chapter 307 Page 2130 Table 307-4

A. Herpes zoster
B. Pneumocystis carinii
C. Cytomegalovirus
D. Legionella

1369. Which of the following is an infection during late (> 6 months) period in kidney transplant recipients?

Harrison's 20th Ed. Chapter 307 Page 2130 Table 307-4

A. BK virus (polyoma)
B. Aspergillus
C. Nocardia
D. All of the above

1370. Use of which of the following drugs increase catabolism of calcineurin inhibitors resulting in low blood levels?

Harrison's 20th Ed. Chapter 307 Page 2130

A. Erythromycin
B. Phenytoin
C. Ketoconazole
D. Diltiazem

Ketoconazole, erythromycin, diltiazem & verapamil compete with calcineurin inhibitors for P450 catabolism and cause their elevated levels. Phenytoin & carbamazepine increase their catabolism to result in low levels.

1371. Which of the following about OKT3 is false?

Immunotherapy 2016;8(8):889-906

A. Stands for ortho kung T3
B. Monoclonal antibody for CD3 surface antigen on human T cells
C. Potent mitogen
D. None of the above

1372. Which of the following viruses does not belong to polyoma group?

Harrison's 20th Ed. Chapter 307 Page 2131

A. BK
B. JC
C. CMV
D. SV40

The polyoma group (BK, JC, SV40) is a class of DNA viruses that become dormant in kidneys and can be activated by immunosuppression.

1373. Which of the following tumor occurs in patients on immuno-suppressive therapy?

Harrison's 20th Ed. Chapter 307 Page 2131

A. Cancer of skin and lips
B. Carcinoma in situ of cervix
C. Non-Hodgkin's lymphoma
D. All of the above

The incidence of tumors in patients on immunosuppressive therapy is 5–6%, or ~100 times greater than that in the general population in the same age range. The most common cancers are cancer of the skin and lips and carcinoma in situ of the cervix, and non-Hodgkin's lymphoma.

1374. Many renal transplant patients have creatinine clearances of?

Harrison's 20th Ed. Chapter 307 Page 2131

A. 15–30 mL/minute
B. 30–50 mL/minute
C. 50–70 mL/minute
D. 70–90 mL/minute

Many transplant patients have creatinine clearances of 30–50 mL/minute.

Glomerular Diseases

1375. Number of glomerular capillary tufts in the two human kidneys is about?
Harrison's 20th Ed. Chapter 308 Page 2132

A. 0.6 million
B. 1.2 million
C. 1.8 million
D. 2.4 million

About 1.8 million glomerular capillary tufts are found in the two human kidneys.

1376. Each kidney contains how many glomeruli in the renal cortex?
N Engl J Med. 2006;354:1387-401

A. About 1 million
B. About 2 million
C. About 3 million
D. About 4 million

1377. Which of the following about glomerulus is false?
Harrison's 20th Ed. Chapter 308 Page 2132

A. Arteriolar portal system
B. Glomerular capillaries have fenestrated endothelial cells
C. Podocytes line the outer surface of the glomerular capillaries
D. None of the above

1378. Which of the following about glomerulus is false?
Harrison's 20th Ed. Chapter 308 Page 2132

A. Parietal epithelial cells of Bowman's capsule transition into tubular epithelia of proximal nephron
B. Parietal epithelial cells of Bowman's capsule migrate into glomerular tuft to replenish podocytes
C. Adjacent podocytes interconnect by slit-pore membranes
D. None of the above

1379. Which of the following about glomerular filtration is false?
Harrison's 20th Ed. Chapter 308 Page 2132

A. Slit-pore membrane forming a selective filtration barrier
B. Physicochemical barrier
C. Positive electrostatic charge
D. Pores in GBM & slit-pore membranes have a radius of 4 nm

Glomerular filtration takes place across a physicochemical barrier governed by pore size and negative electrostatic charge.

1380. Which of the following about albumin filtration is false?
Harrison's 20th Ed. Chapter 308 Page 2132

A. Albumin has a negative charge
B. Albumin has a physical radius of 3.6 nm
C. Albumin is reclaimed by megalin & cubilin receptors of PCT
D. None of the above

1381. Pores in the glomerular basement membrane (GBM) and slit-pore membranes have a radius of?
Harrison's 20th Ed. Chapter 308 Page 2132

A. 2 nm
B. 4 nm
C. 6 nm
D. 8 nm

Pores in GBM & slit-pore membranes have a radius of 4 nm. Albumin has a physical radius of 3.6 nm.

1382. Filtration barrier of capillary wall in glomerulus contains?
N Engl J Med. 2006;354:1387-401

A. Fenestrated endothelium
B. Glomerular basement membrane
C. Interdigitating podocyte foot processes
D. All of the above

1383. Glomerular basement membrane has a thickness of?
N Engl J Med. 2006;354:1387-401

A. 200 to 250 nm
B. 300 to 350 nm
C. 400 to 450 nm
D. 500 to 550 nm

1384. Humans with normal nephrons excrete how much albumin in daily voided urine?
Harrison's 20th Ed. Chapter 308 Page 2132

A. 1–5 mg
B. 8–10 mg
C. 15–30 mg
D. 40–60 mg

1385. Main components of glomerular basement membrane are?
N Engl J Med. 2003;348:2543-56

A. Type IV collagen
B. Laminin
C. Nidogen
D. All of the above

1386. Which of the following is instrumental in reclaiming filtered albumin along the proximal tubule?
Harrison's 20th Ed. Chapter 308 Page 2132

A. Crucin
B. Optimin
C. Megalin
D. Reglin

4000 to 9000 mg/day of albumin is filtered and is reclaimed by megalin and cubilin receptors along the proximal tubule. Humans with normal nephrons excretion average 8–10 mg of albumin in daily voided urine, approximately 20–60% of total excreted protein.

1387. Founder effect best relates to?

Harrison's 20th Ed. Chapter 308 Page 2132

A. Laplace's law
B. Hardy-Weinberg law
C. Hy's Law
D. Inverse-care law

The Hardy-Weinberg law, which is the basis of population genetics, states, in part, that in a large randommating population at equilibrium (i.e. no selection, migration or genetic drift), genotype frequencies are functions of allele frequencies and the former can be predicted from the latter.

1388. What proportion of glomerular ultrafiltrate is reabsorbed in the proximal tubules?

Lancet 2005;365:417-430

A. One-third
B. One-half
C. Two-third
D. Three-fourth

~ Two-thirds of glomerular ultrafiltrate is reabsorbed isosmotically in proximal tubule with little change in osmolality or sodium concentration of unreabsorbed fraction. With water absorption, sodium along with chloride & bicarbonate are absorbed actively to keep ultrafiltrate iso-osmotic.

1389. In earliest portion of proximal tubule, which of the following is the principal ion that accompanies reabsorption of sodium?

Lancet 2005;365:417-430

A. Chloride
B. Bicarbonate
C. Hydrogen
D. Phosphate

In the earliest portion of PCT, bicarbonate is the principal anion that accompanies reabsorption of sodium. This process occurs via a Na/H exchanger at the luminal brush border and is dependent on the activity of carbonic anhydrase.

1390. Early proximal convoluted tubule is the major site of reabsorption of?

Lancet 2005;365:417-430

A. Lactate
B. Amino acids
C. Glucose
D. All of the above

Glucose, amino acids, and organic solutes like lactate are extensively reabsorbed in the proximal tubule by cotransport mechanisms.

1391. Normally, in glomerulus, which of the following is true?

Lancet 2005;365:417-430

A. Hydraulic pressure exceeds oncotic pressure
B. Oncotic pressure exceeds hydraulic pressure
C. Oncotic pressure equals hydraulic pressure
D. All of the above

At glomerulus, hydraulic pressure exceeds oncotic pressure favoring filtration.

1392. Congenital nephrotic syndrome occurs due to mutations in?

Harrison's 20th Ed. Chapter 308 Page 2132

A. PROP-1
B. NPHS1
C. PAX-8
D. PIT-1

Congenital nephrotic syndrome occurs due to mutations in NPHS1 (nephrin) and NPHS2 (podocin).

1393. Pierson's syndrome is a form of?

N Engl J Med. 2006;354:1387-401

A. Congenital nephrotic syndrome
B. Congenital heart disease
C. Congenital bone disease
D. Congenital eye disease

1394. Focal segmental glomerulosclerosis (FSGS) occurs due to mutations in?

Harrison's 20th Ed. Chapter 308 Page 2132

A. NPHS2
B. TRPC6
C. APOL1
D. SGK1

TRPC6 cation channel mutations produce focal segmental glomerulosclerosis (FSGS) in adulthood.

1395. Polymorphisms in which of the following gene is a major risk for nondiabetic ESRD, particularly FSGS?

Harrison's 20th Ed. Chapter 308 Page 2132

A. APOL1
B. COL4A5
C. ACTN4
D. All of the above

Polymorphisms in the gene encoding apolipoprotein L1, APOL1, are a major risk for African Americans with nondiabetic end stage renal disease, particularly FSGS.

1396. Which of the following statements is false?

Harrison's 20th Ed. Chapter 308 Page 2132

A. Mutations in complement factor H cause membranoproliferative glomerulonephritis (MPGN)
B. Mutations in genes encoding for α3, α4, or α5 chains of type IV collagen cause Alport's syndrome
C. α-galactosidase A deficiency causes Fabry's disease
D. None of the above

1397. Nephrosialidosis is cause by?

Harrison's 20th Ed. Chapter 308 Page 2132

A. S-Adenosylhomocysteine hydrolase deficiency
B. N acetylneuraminic acid hydrolase deficiency
C. Glycine N-methyltransferase deficiency
D. Adenosine kinase deficiency

Nephrosialidosis is an ultra-rare disorder and lacks comprehensive information about the clinical course (<20 cases in the literature). It presents as childhood-onset, steroid resistant nephrotic syndrome and is due to a mutation in NEU1 causing N acetylneuraminic acid hydrolase deficiency.

1398. Chronic glomerulosclerosis in systemic hypertension & atherosclerosis is due to?

Harrison's 20th Ed. Chapter 308 Page 2133

A. Pressure stress
B. Ischemia
C. Lipid oxidants
D. All of the above

1399. Thickening of GBM in diabetic nephropathy is secondary to the long-standing effects of?

Harrison's 20th Ed. Chapter 308 Page 2133

A. Hyperglycemia
B. Advanced glycosylation end products
C. Reactive oxygen species
D. All of the above

Diabetic nephropathy is an acquired sclerotic injury associated with thickening of GBM secondary to long-standing effects of hyperglycemia, advanced glycosylation end products and reactive oxygen species.

1400. Glomerulonephritis refers to inflammation of?

Harrison's 20th Ed. Chapter 308 Page 2133

A. Glomerular capillaries
B. Glomerular arterioles
C. Glomerular basement membrane (GBM)
D. All of the above

Inflammation of the glomerular capillaries is called glomerulonephritis.

1401. In glomerulonephritis, cytokines & proteases damage which of the following?

Harrison's 20th Ed. Chapter 308 Page 2133

A. Mesangium
B. Capillaries
C. GBM
D. All of the above

Chemokines attract neutrophils, macrophages & T cells into glomerular tuft. These react with antigens & epitopes producing more cytokines & proteases that damage mesangium, capillaries, and/or GBM.

1402. Which of the following is an antiglomerular basement membrane disease?

Harrison's 20th Ed. Chapter 308 Page 2133

A. Membranous glomerulonephritis (MGN)
B. Goodpasture's syndrome
C. Lupus nephritis
D. Granulomatosis with polyangiitis (Wegener's)

Antiglomerular basement membrane disease producing Goodpasture's syndrome. It primarily injures both lung & kidney because of the narrow distribution of the a3 NC1 domain of type IV collagen that is the target antigen.

1403. Which of the following plays an important role in the mechanism of glomerulonephritis?

Harrison's 20th Ed. Chapter 308 Page 2133

A. Deposition of immune complexes
B. Early T cell activation
C. Complement injury
D. Systemic inflammation

While the adaptive immune response is similar to that of other tissues, early T cell activation plays an important role in the mechanism of glomerulonephritis.

1404. Which of the following is associated with immune deposits along the GBM?

Harrison's 20th Ed. Chapter 308 Page 2134

A. Poststreptococcal glomerulonephritis
B. Lupus nephritis
C. Idiopathic membranous nephritis
D. All of the above

Poststreptococcal glomerulonephritis, lupus nephritis, and idiopathic membranous nephritis typically are associated with immune deposits along the GBM.

1405. Preformed circulating immune complexes precipitate along which side of the GBM?

Harrison's 20th Ed. Chapter 308 Page 2134

A. Subendothelial side
B. Subepithelial side
C. In lumen
D. All of the above

Preformed circulating immune complexes precipitate along the subendothelial side of the GBM, while immune deposits formed in situ precipitate on the subepithelial side.

1406. Complement membrane attack complex (MAC) best relates to?

Harrison's 20th Ed. Chapter 308 Page 2134

A. C3a
B. C3b
C. C5a
D. C5b-9

The five glycoproteins C5b to C9 form a complex which is responsible for the final lytic action on cells. This membrane attack complex (MAC) is formed by successive assembly of its components. The complex C5bC6C7C8$(C9)_n$ is included as an integral membrane protein complex (membrane attack complex). The free flow of small molecules and ions through the formed pores causes osmotic cell lysis. The C5 convertase (C4b2a3b of classical pathway & C3bBbC3b of alternative pathway) cleaves C5 into C5a and C5b fragments. C5a is the most potent anaphylatoxin in the complement cascade. The C5b binds to the cell surface and serves as a platform for the membrane attack complex (MAC), which consists of C5bC6789.

1407. Which of the following is the "pore-forming molecule" of complement?

Harrison's 20th Ed. Chapter 308 Page 2134

A. C3
B. C5
C. C6
D. C9

C9, a pore-forming molecule with homology to perforin, a protein used by cytotoxic T cells and natural killer cells for killing virus-infected targets. The complex of C5b678 forms a nidus for C9 binding and polymerization.

1408. Persistent glomerulonephritis that worsens renal function is always accompanied by?

Harrison's 20th Ed. Chapter 308 Page 2134

A. Interstitial nephritis
B. Renal fibrosis
C. Tubular atrophy
D. All of the above

Persistent glomerulonephritis that worsens renal function is always accompanied by interstitial nephritis, renal fibrosis, and tubular atrophy.

1409. Renal failure in glomerulonephritis best correlates histologically with the appearance of?

Harrison's 20th Ed. Chapter 308 Page 2134

A. Tubulointerstitial nephritis
B. Papillary necrosis
C. Cystic kidney disease
D. All of the above

Renal failure in glomerulonephritis best correlates histologically with the appearance of tubulointerstitial nephritis. Early acute tubulointerstitial nephritis suggests potentially recoverable renal function whereas the development of chronic interstitial fibrosis prognosticates permanent loss.

1410. Renal fibroblasts increase through which of the following mechanisms?

Harrison's 20th Ed. Chapter 308 Page 2134

A. Epithelial or endothelial mesenchymal transitions
B. Bone marrow-derived fibrocytes
C. Proliferation of resident fibroblasts
D. All of the above

At the site of injury, interstitial fibroblasts increase in number & fibrosis occurs. Renal fibroblasts increase by epithelial or endothelial mesenchymal transitions (15%), bone marrow-derived fibrocytes (35%), and the proliferation of resident fibroblasts (50%).

1411. Which of the following is active in fibrotic damage to kidneys?

Harrison's 20th Ed. Chapter 308 Page 2134

A. Transforming growth factor-β (TGF-β)
B. Fibroblast growth factor 2 (FGF-2)
C. Hypoxemia-inducible factor 1α (HIF-1α)
D. All of the above

Transforming growth factor-β (TGF-β), fibroblast growth factor 2 (FGF-2), hypoxemia-inducible factor 1α (HIF-1α), and platelet-derived growth factor (PDGF) are active in fibrosis at the site of kidney injury.

1412. Which of the following can reverse early fibrogenesis and preserve tubular architecture?

Harrison's 20th Ed. Chapter 308 Page 2134

A. Bone morphogenetic protein 2
B. Bone morphogenetic protein 7
C. Transforming growth factor β (TGF-β)
D. All of the above

In experimental studies, bone morphogenetic protein 7 and hepatocyte growth factor can reverse early fibrogenesis and preserve tubular architecture.

1413. Cause of microscopic hematuria is?

Harrison's 20th Ed. Chapter 308 Page 2134

A. Interstitial nephritis
B. Papillary necrosis
C. Cystic kidney diseases
D. All of the above

Microscopic hematuria may appear with the onset of benign prostatic hypertrophy, interstitial nephritis, papillary necrosis, hypercalciuria, renal stones, cystic kidney diseases, or renal vascular injury.

1414. Which of the following are indicative of a glomerular disease?

Harrison's 20th Ed. Chapter 308 Page 2134

A. Microscopic hematuria
B. Urinary red blood cell casts
C. Urinary dysmorphic red blood cells
D. All of the above

Sustained proteinuria >1–2 g/24 hours is also commonly associated with glomerular disease.

1415. Normal 24-hour urine protein is?

Harrison's 20th Ed. Chapter 308 Page 2134 Table 308-1

A. < 30 mg/day
B. < 100 mg/day
C. < 150 mg/day
D. < 300 mg/day

Normal 24-hour urine protein is < 150 mg/day.

1416. Albumin comprises what percentage of total proteins excreted in the urine?

Harrison's 20th Ed. Chapter 308 Page 2134 Table 308-1

A. 10–30%
B. 20–60%
C. 30–70%
D. 40–90%

Albumin represents 20–60% of the total protein excreted in the urine.

1417. Sustained isolated proteinuria is found in?

Harrison's 20th Ed. Chapter 308 Page 2135

A. Diabetic nephropathy
B. Mesangioproliferative glomerulonephritis
C. FSGS
D. All of the above

Sustained isolated proteinuria is found in diabetic nephropathy, nil lesion, mesangioproliferative glomerulonephritis, and FSGS.

1418. Orthostatic proteinuria is evident only in?

Harrison's 20th Ed. Chapter 308 Page 2135

A. Upright position
B. Recumbent position
C. Sitting position
D. Lateral position

Proteinuria only seen with upright posture is called orthostatic proteinuria.

1419. Functional proteinuria refers to?

Harrison's 20th Ed. Chapter 308 Page 2135

A. Proteinuria in females
B. Proteinuria during fever, emotional stress
C. Proteinuria in UTI
D. Proteinuria in upright posture

Benign, functional or transient proteinuria occurs in normal population. It is nonsustained and proteinuria is <1 gram/day. Fever, exercise, obesity, sleep apnea, emotional stress & congestive heart failure cause transient proteinuria.

1420. In which of the following conditions, proteinuria is selective & composed largely of albumin?

Harrison's 20th Ed. Chapter 308 Page 2135

A. Henoch-Schönlein purpura
B. Minimal change disease
C. Churg-Strauss syndrome
D. Goodpasture's syndrome

In children with minimal change disease, proteinuria is selective & composed largely of albumin.

1421. Which of the following glomerular disease can present with gross hematuria?

Harrison's 20th Ed. Chapter 308 Page 2135

A. Focal segmental glomerulosclerosis
B. Mesangioproliferative glomerulonephritis
C. IgA nephropathy
D. Subacute bacterial endocarditis

1422. Which of the following glomerular disease can present with gross hematuria?

Harrison's 20th Ed. Chapter 308 Page 2135

A. Henoch-Schönlein purpura
B. Antiphospholipid syndrome
C. Sickle cell disease
D. Nail-patella syndrome

In IgA nephropathy & sickle cell disease, gross hematuria is present.

1423. Asymptomatic hematuria is due to?

Harrison's 20th Ed. Chapter 308 Page 2135

A. IgA nephropathy (Berger's disease)
B. Thin basement membrane (TBM) disease
C. Alport's syndrome
D. All of the above

1424. Which of the following clinical syndromes is most important according to global perspective?

Harrison's 20th Ed. Chapter 308 Page 2135

A. Acute nephritic syndrome
B. Nephrotic syndrome
C. Basement membrane syndrome
D. Infectious disease–associated syndrome

Infectious disease-associated syndrome is most important if one has a global perspective. Malaria, and schistosomiasis may be the most common causes of glomerulonephritis throughout the world, closely followed by HIV and chronic hepatitis B & C. Other syndromes include acute nephritic syndromes, pulmonary-renal syndromes, nephrotic syndromes, basement membrane syndromes, glomerular vascular syndromes.

1425. Which of the following is false about a 'crescent'?

Lancet 1999;353:1509

A. Half-moon-shaped collection of cells in Bowman's space
B. Composed of proliferating parietal epithelial cells and infiltrating macrophages
C. Crescentic glomerulonephritis is also called rapidly progressive glomerulonephritis
D. None of the above

1426. Which of the following does not present as rapidly progressive glomerulonephritis (RPGN)?

Harrison's 20th Ed. Chapter 308 Page 2135 Table 308-2

A. Poststreptococcal glomerulonephritis
B. Subacute bacterial endocarditis
C. Wegener's granulomatosis
D. Henoch-Schönlein purpura

1427. Which of the following does not present as rapidly progressive glomerulonephritis (RPGN)?

Harrison's 20th Ed. Chapter 308 Page 2135 Table 308-2

A. Poststreptococcal glomerulonephritis
B. Mesangioproliferative glomerulonephritis
C. Membranoproliferative glomerulonephritis
D. Lupus nephritis

1428. Henoch-Schönlein purpura has which of the following patterns of clinical glomerulonephritis?

Harrison's 20th Ed. Chapter 308 Page 2135 Table 308-2

A. Acute nephritic syndrome
B. Pulmonary-renal syndrome
C. Glomerular vascular syndrome
D. All of the above

1429. Wegener's granulomatosis has which of the following patterns of clinical glomerulonephritis?

Harrison's 20th Ed. Chapter 308 Page 2135 Table 308-2

A. Acute nephritic syndrome
B. Pulmonary-renal syndrome
C. Glomerular vascular syndrome
D. All of the above

1430. Cryoglobulinemia has which of the following patterns of clinical glomerulonephritis?

Harrison's 20th Ed. Chapter 308 Page 2135 Table 308-2

A. Acute Nephritic syndrome
B. Pulmonary-renal syndrome
C. Glomerular vascular syndrome
D. All of the above

1431. Churg-Strauss syndrome has which of the following patterns of clinical glomerulonephritis?

Harrison's 20th Ed. Chapter 308 Page 2135 Table 308-2

A. Acute nephritic syndrome
B. Pulmonary-renal syndrome
C. Glomerular vascular syndrome
D. All of the above

1432. Which of the following can cause pulmonary-renal syndrome?

Harrison's 20th Ed. Chapter 308 Page 2135 Table 308-2

A. Henoch-Schönlein purpura
B. Microscopic polyangiitis
C. Cryoglobulinemia
D. All of the above

1433. Which of the following can cause basement membrane syndrome?

Harrison's 20th Ed. Chapter 308 Page 2135 Table 308-2

A. Alport's syndrome
B. Nail-patella syndrome
C. Thin basement membrane disease
D. All of the above

Patients with a basement membrane syndrome either have genetically abnormal basement membranes (Alport's syndrome) or an autoimmune response to basement membrane collagen IV (Goodpasture's syndrome) associated with microscopic hematuria, mild to heavy proteinuria & hypertension with variable elevations in serum creatinine.

1434. Which of the following is the most common cause of glomerulonephritis throughout the world?

Harrison's 20th Ed. Chapter 308 Page 2135

A. HIV
B. Chronic hepatitis B
C. Chronic hepatitis C
D. Malaria

Malaria and schistosomiasis may be the most common causes of glomerulonephritis throughout the world, closely followed by HIV and chronic hepatitis B and C.

1435. Which of the following stains is used to enhance basement membrane structure in renal biopsy?

Harrison's 20th Ed. Chapter 308 Page 2136

A. Hematoxylin and eosin
B. Periodic acid-Schiff (PAS)
C. Jones-methenamine silver
D. Masson's trichrome

1436. Which of the following stains is used to stain carbohydrate moieties in the membranes of the glomerular tuft & tubules?

Harrison's 20th Ed. Chapter 308 Page 2136

A. Hematoxylin and eosin
B. Periodic acid-Schiff (PAS)
C. Jones-methenamine silver
D. Masson's trichrome

1437. Which of the following stains is used to stain amyloid deposits?

Harrison's 20th Ed. Chapter 308 Page 2136

A. Congo red
B. Periodic acid-Schiff (PAS)
C. Jones-methenamine silver
D. Masson's trichrome

1438. Which of the following stains is used to stain collagen deposition and assess the degree of glomerulosclerosis & interstitial fibrosis?

Harrison's 20th Ed. Chapter 308 Page 2136

A. Congo red
B. Periodic acid-Schiff (PAS)
C. Jones-methenamine silver
D. Masson's trichrome

Renal biopsy specimen are stained with H&E for cellularity & architecture, PAS for carbohydrate moieties in glomerular tuft & tubule membranes, Jones-methenamine silver to enhance basement membrane structure, Congo red for amyloid deposits, & Masson's trichrome to identify collagen deposition to assess degree of glomerulosclerosis & interstitial fibrosis.

1439. By light microscopy, ideally how many glomeruli should be reviewed individually for discrete lesions?

Harrison's 20th Ed. Chapter 308 Page 2137

A. 1
B. 5
C. 10
D. 20

By light microscopy, ideally 20 glomeruli should be reviewed individually for discrete lesions.

1440. When cellular proliferation extends into Bowman's space, it is called?

Harrison's 20th Ed. Chapter 308 Page 2137

A. Endocapillary proliferation
B. Extracapillary proliferation
C. Synechiae
D. Crescents

Glomeruli with increased cellularity are termed as proliferative. When cells in capillary tuft proliferate, it is called endocapillary and when cellular proliferation extends into Bowman's space, it is called extracapillary.

1441. When epithelial podocytes attach to Bowman's capsule in the setting of glomerular injury, it is called?

Harrison's 20th Ed. Chapter 308 Page 2137

A. Endocapillary proliferation
B. Extracapillary proliferation
C. Synechiae
D. Crescents

When epithelial podocytes attach to Bowman's capsule in glomerular injury, it is termed synechiae.

1442. Crescents best relate to?

Harrison's 20th Ed. Chapter 308 Page 2137

A. Endocapillary proliferation
B. Extracapillary proliferation
C. Synechiae
D. All of the above

Crescents may be extension of synechiae, develop when fibrocellular/fibrin collections fill all or part of Bowman's space.

1443. Which of the following about sclerotic glomeruli is false?

Harrison's 20th Ed. Chapter 308 Page 2137

A. Acellular
B. Amorphous accumulations of proteinaceous material
C. Loss of functional capillaries & normal mesangium
D. None of the above

1444. How can background percentage of sclerosis in age-related glomerulosclerosis be estimated?

Harrison's 20th Ed. Chapter 308 Page 2137

A. (Patient's age/10) × 2
B. (Patient's age/2) – 10
C. (Patient's age/10) + 2
D. (Patient's age/2) + 10

Background percentage of sclerosis in age-related glomerulosclerosis can be estimated by dividing the patient's age in half and subtracting 10.

1445. Which of the following occurs in interstitial fibrosis?

Harrison's 20th Ed. Chapter 308 Page 2137

A. Loss of adjacency
B. Tubular dropout
C. Collagen deposition
D. All of the above

1446. 'Focal glomeulonephritis' is said to occur when lesion involves what proportion of glomeruli?

Harrison's 20th Ed. Chapter 308 Page 2137

A. < 50%
B. < 60%
C. < 70%
D. < 80%

If <50% glomeruli are involved, lesion is considered focal, else diffuse.

1447. In renal biopsy, which of the following is an ominous sign of irreversibility and progression to renal failure?

Harrison's 20th Ed. Chapter 308 Page 2137

A. Synechiae
B. Interstitial fibrosis
C. Crescents
D. All of the above

Interstitial fibrosis is an ominous sign of irreversibility & progression to renal failure.

1448. Acute nephritic syndromes classically present with?

Harrison's 20th Ed. Chapter 308 Page 2137

A. Hypertension
B. Hematuria
C. Pyuria
D. All of the above

Acute nephritic syndromes classically present with hypertension, hematuria, red blood cell casts, pyuria, and mild to moderate proteinuria.

1449. Which of the following is prototypical for acute endocapillary proliferative glomerulonephritis?

Harrison's 20th Ed. Chapter 308 Page 2137

A. Poststreptococcal glomerulonephritis
B. Endocarditis-associated glomerulonephritis
C. Lupus nephritis
D. All of the above

1450. Circulating immune-complex formation and deposition within the glomerulus is seen in?

Harrison's 20th Ed. Chapter 308 Page 2137+

A. Subacute bacterial endocarditis (SABE)
B. Lupus nephritis
C. Hepatitis-C-related cryoglobulinemia
D. All of the above

Circulating immune-complex formation and deposition within the glomerulus is seen with SABE, lupus nephritis, & hepatitis-C-related cryoglobulinemia.

1451. Poststreptococcal glomerulonephritis is prototypical for?

Harrison's 20th Ed. Chapter 308 Page 2137

A. Acute endocapillary proliferative glomerulonephritis
B. Mesangiocapillary glomerulonephritis
C. Lobar glomerulonephritis
D. Segmental necrotizing glomerulonephritis

Poststreptococcal glomerulonephritis is prototypical for acute endocapillary proliferative glomerulonephritis.

1452. Poststreptococcal glomerulonephritis develops how many weeks after streptococcal pharyngitis?

Harrison's 20th Ed. Chapter 308 Page 2137

A. 1–3 weeks
B. 2–6 weeks
C. 3–6 weeks
D. 4–8 weeks

Acute poststreptococcal glomerulonephritis (APSGN) develops after streptococcal infection with a latent period of around 1 - 3 weeks (10 days).

1453. Poststreptococcal glomerulonephritis due to impetigo develops how many weeks after the skin infection?

Harrison's 20th Ed. Chapter 308 Page 2137

A. 1–3 weeks
B. 2–6 weeks
C. 3–6 weeks
D. 4–8 weeks

Poststreptococcal glomerulonephritis due to impetigo develops 2–6 weeks after skin infection and 1–3 weeks after streptococcal pharyngitis.

1454. Which strain of streptococci is nephritogenic?

Harrison's 20th Ed. Chapter 308 Page 2137

A. H
B. O
C. M
C. N

Skin & throat infections with particular M types strains of streptococci are nephritogenic and antedate glomerular disease.

1455. Which of the following M type strain of streptococci are seen following impetigo?

Harrison's 20th Ed. Chapter 308 Page 2137

A. 47
B. 49
C. 55
D. All of the above

1456. Which of the following M type strain of streptococci are seen with pharyngitis?

Harrison's 20th Ed. Chapter 308 Page 2137

A. 1
B. 2
C. 4
D. All of the above

1457. Which of the following M type strain of streptococci are common with both impetigo & pharyngitis?

Harrison's 20th Ed. Chapter 308 Page 2137

A. 2
B. 47
C. 55
D. 60

M types 47, 49, 55, 2, 60 & 57 are seen following impetigo and M types 1, 2, 4, 3, 25, 49 & 12 with pharyngitis.

1458. The 'humps' seen in renal biopsy in poststreptococcal glomerulonephritis best relate to?

Harrison's 20th Ed. Chapter 308 Page 2137

A. Mesangium
B. Subendothelium
C. Subepithelium
D. All of the above

In APSGN, accumulation of immune complexes, complements, and plasma proteins, forming 'humps' on the outer side of glomerular tufts (subepithelium).

1459. Which of the following is an antigen from nephritogenic streptococci?

Harrison's 20th Ed. Chapter 308 Page 2137

A. Streptococcal pyrogenic exotoxin B (SPEB)
B. Streptococcal pyrogenic endotoxin B (SPEB)
C. Streptococcal plasmin exotoxin B (SPEB)
D. Streptococcal plasmin endotoxin B (SPEB)

1460. Deposition of which of the following antigens is seen in essentially all patients with early-phase APSGN?

Harrison's 20th Ed. Chapter 308 Page 2137

A. PLA2R
B. NAPlr
C. Thomsen-Friedenreich antigen
D. All of the above

Immunofluorescence staining of the renal biopsy tissues with anti-NAPlr antibody shows glomerular NAPlr deposition in essentially all patients with early-phase acute poststreptococcal glomerulonephritis (APSGN).

1461. Which of the following about NAPlr is false?

Harrison's 20th Ed. Chapter 308 Page 2137

A. Have an affinity to plasmin and glomerular proteins
B. Activates the alternative complement pathway
C. Does not co-localize with C3 in glomerular deposits
D. None of the above

A cationic cysteine proteinase known as streptococcal pyrogenic exotoxin B (SPEB) is an antigen from nephritogenic streptococci. It is generated by proteolysis of a zymogen precursor (zSPEB) and NAPlr, the nephritis-associated plasmin receptor. These two antigens have biochemical affinity for plasmin, bind as complexes and activate the alternate complement pathway. The nephritogenic antigen, SPEB, has been demonstrated inside the subepithelial 'humps' on biopsy.

1462. Deposits of IgG, IgM, C3, C4, and C5-9 in APSGN are found in?

Harrison's 20th Ed. Chapter 308 Page 2137

A. Mesangium
B. Subendothelium
C. Subepithelium
D. All of the above

1463. Deposits of nephritogenic antigen SPEB in APSGN are found in?

Harrison's 20th Ed. Chapter 308 Page 2137

A. Mesangium
B. Subendothelium
C. Subepithelium
D. All of the above

Nephritogenic antigen, SPEB, is demonstrated inside the subepithelial 'humps' on biopsy. NAPlr is localized on the inner side of glomerular tufts (endocapillary) is consistent with the predominantly endocapillary glomerular inflammation in APSGN.

1464. Nephritogenic antigens on streptococci SPEB and NAPlr have biochemical affinity for?

Harrison's 20th Ed. Chapter 308 Page 2137

A. Platelets
B. Plasmin
C. Collagen
D. Elastin

Nephritogenic antigens on streptococci SPEB and NAPlr have biochemical affinity for plasmin. NAPlr and SPEB, both bind plasmin. They protect plasmin from physiological inhibitors (Aprotinin) and thus might cause chemotaxis of inflammatory cells and degradation of glomerular basement membranes, due to the activity of plasmin. Plasmin activity may be a common final pathway in APSGN.

1465. NAPlr deposition and plasmin activity is found in which of the following glomerular disease?

Clinical Nephrology. 2006;65(2):124 -128,

A. Dense deposit disease (DDD)
B. Henoch-Schönlein Purpura nephritis (HSPN)
C. Membranoproliferative glomerulonephritis (MPGN)
D. All of the above

1466. Which of the following is a plamin inhibitor?

Harrison's 20th Ed. Chapter 308 Page 2137

A. Renin
B. Aprotinin
C. Kallikrein
D. All of the above

Aprotinin, also known as bovine pancreatic trypsin inhibitor or BPTI, is a polypeptide extracted from bovine lung that inhibits the action of serine proteases, including plasmin and kallikrein. Aprotinin slows down fibrinolysis. It is associated with AKI and this drug was withdrawn from the market.

1467. In the immune complex theory of APSGN, which of the following is false?

Harrison's 20th Ed. Chapter 308 Page 2137

A. Glomerular deposition of nephritogenic streptococcal antigen and subsequent formation of immune complexes in situ
B. Deposition of circulating antigen-antibody complexes
C. Immune complex is localized to outer side of glomerular tufts (subepithelial site)
D. None of the above

1468. In the first week of poststreptococcal glomerulonephritis, which of the following lab. findings is false?

Harrison's 20th Ed. Chapter 308 Page 2137

A. Depressed total hemolytic complement (CH50)
B. Decreased levels of C3
C. Normal levels of C4
D. None of the above

90% patients of poststreptococcal glomerulonephritis will have depressed CH50 & decreased levels of C3 with normal levels of C4 in first week of symptoms. Positive rheumatoid factor (30–40%), cryoglobulins and circulating immune complexes (60–70%), ANCA against myeloperoxidase (10%), increased titers of ASO (30%), anti-DNAse (70%) or anti-hyaluronidase antibodies (40%) can help confirm the diagnosis.

1469. Which of the following has no role in treatment of poststreptococcal glomerulonephritis?

Harrison's 20th Ed. Chapter 308 Page 2137

A. Antibiotics
B. Antihypertensives
C. Immunosuppressive therapy
D. Dialysis

There is no role for immunosuppressive therapy in poststreptococcal glomerulonephritis even in the setting of crescents.

1470. In APSGN, complete resolution of hematuria & proteinuria occurs within what time after the onset of nephritis?

Harrison's 20th Ed. Chapter 308 Page 2137

A. 1–3 weeks
B. 3–6 weeks
C. 6–9 weeks
D. 9–12 weeks

Complete resolution of the hematuria and proteinuria in the majority of children occurs within 3–6 weeks of the onset of nephritis.

1471. 'Starry sky' appearance on immunofluorescence microscopy of renal biopsy is seen in?

Am J Kidney Dis. 2015;66(4):e31-e32

A. Acute poststreptococcal glomerulonephritis
B. Lupus nephritis
C. Glomerulonephritis in SLE
D. Goodpasture's syndrome

Post-streptococcal GN has prominent PMN infiltrate in glomerular tuft, with 'garland' or 'starry sky' appearance of IgG+C3 deposits by (immunofluorescence microscopy), & hump-shaped subepithelial deposits by EM.

1472. Which of the following is a common comorbidity of endocarditis-associated glomerulonephritis?

Harrison's 20th Ed. Chapter 308 Page 2137

A. Intravenous drug use
B. Hepatitis C
C. Diabetes mellitus
D. All of the above

Common comorbidities of endocarditis-associated glomerulonephritis are valvular heart disease, intravenous drug use, hepatitis C, and diabetes mellitus.

1473. 'Flea-bitten' kidney refers to?

Harrison's 20th Ed. Chapter 308 Page 2137

A. Subcapsular necrosis
B. Subcapsular hemorrhages
C. Subcapsular oedema
D. Subcapsular fibrosis

1474. In endocarditis-associated glomerulonephritis, immune deposits of which of the following are found in kidney?

Harrison's 20th Ed. Chapter 308 Page 2137

A. IgG
B. IgM
C. C3
D. All of the above

C3 deposition is prominent in most cases.

1475. In endocarditis-associated glomerulonephritis, immune deposits of IgG, IgM and C3 are found in?

Harrison's 20th Ed. Chapter 308 Page 2137

A. Mesangium
B. Subendothelium
C. Subepithelium
D. All of the above

Kidneys in subacute bacterial endocarditis have subcapsular hemorrhages with a 'flea-bitten' appearance. Renal biopsy reveals focal proliferation around foci of necrosis associated with abundant mesangial, subendothelial and subepithelial immune deposits of IgG, IgM and C3.

1476. Which of the following is false about endocarditis-associated glomerulonephritis?

Harrison's 20th Ed. Chapter 308 Page 2138

A. Renal deposition of circulating immune complexes in kidney
B. Complement activation
C. Circulating immune complexes
D. None of the above

1477. Which of the following may be present in endocarditis-associated glomerulonephritis?

Harrison's 20th Ed. Chapter 308 Page 2138

A. Hypocomplementemia
B. High titers of rheumatoid factor
C. High titers of type III cryoglobulins
D. All of the above

The pathogenesis of endocarditis-associated glomerulonephritis is renal deposition of circulating immune complexes in kidney with complement activation. Normocytic anemia, ↑ ESR, hypocomplementemia, high titers of rheumatoid factor, type III cryoglobulins, circulating immune complexes and ANCAs may be present.

1478. Which of the following is false about endocarditis-associated glomerulonephritis?

Harrison's 20th Ed. Chapter 308 Page 2138

A. Most commonly presents with AKI
B. Complicates staphylococcal tricuspid valve infection
C. Necrotizing and crescentic glomerulonephritis
D. None of the above

Glomerulonephritis is unusual in acute bacterial endocarditis. The most common organism in IE-associated GN is S. aureus. Streptococcus species are the next most common. Less common organisms include Bartonella henselae, Coxiella burnetii, Cardiobacterium hominis, and Gemella. The most common cardiac valve infected is tricuspid followed by mitral, aortic, pulmonic and chordae tendinae. Acute kidney injury is the most common clinical presentation and almost all patients have hematuria. Crescentic GN is the most common pattern seen on kidney biopsy specimens by light microscopy, followed by diffuse proliferative GN. Subepithelial "humps" which are classically seen in infection-related GN are infrequent.

1479. In endocarditis-associated glomerulonephritis, antibiotics are given for a period of?

Harrison's 20th Ed. Chapter 308 Page 2138

A. 1–2 weeks
B. 2–4 weeks
C. 4–6 weeks
D. 6–8 weeks

1480. Which of the following sometimes accompanies or is confused with SBE?

Harrison's 20th Ed. Chapter 308 Page 2138

A. Hepatitis B virus–associated vasculitis
B. ANCA-associated vasculitis
C. Cancer-associated vasculitis
D. Drug-induced vasculitis

ANCA-associated vasculitis sometimes accompanies or is confused with SBE and should be ruled out, as the treatment is different.

1481. Postinfectious glomerulonephritis can occur in?

Harrison's 20th Ed. Chapter 308 Page 2138

A. Ventriculoatrial shunt
B. Ventriculoperitoneal shunt
C. Infected vascular prostheses
D. All of the above

Postinfectious glomerulonephritis can occur in patients with ventriculoatrial & ventriculoperitoneal shunts, pulmonary, intraabdominal, pelvic or cutaneous infections and infected vascular prostheses.

1482. Lupus nephritis is most severe in?

Harrison's 20th Ed. Chapter 308 Page 2138

A. African-American female adolescents
B. White elderly
C. Australian aboriginals
D. Chinese young male

Lupus nephritis is most severe in African-American female adolescents as a complication of SLE.

1483. Which of the following glomerulonephritis is more common in female than in male population?

Harrison's 20th Ed. Chapter 308 Page 2138

A. Alport's syndrome
B. Goodpasture's syndrome
C. Lupus nephritis
D. Nail-patella syndrome

Lupus nephritis is two + times more in female than among male population.

1484. In lupus nephritis, the most common clinical sign of renal disease is?

Harrison's 20th Ed. Chapter 308 Page 2138

A. Hypertension
B. Active urine sediment with red blood cell casts
C. Varying degrees of renal failure
D. Proteinuria

In lupus nephritis, the most common clinical sign of renal disease is proteinuria, but hematuria, hypertension, varying degrees of renal failure and active urine sediment with red blood cell casts can be present.

1485. Remission achieved with treatment is defined as a return to near-normal renal function and proteinuria ≤?

Harrison's 20th Ed. Chapter 308 Page 2138

A. 300 mg/dL per day
B. 310 mg/dL per day
C. 320 mg/dL per day
D. 330 mg/dL per day

Remission achieved with treatment is defined as a return to near-normal renal function and proteinuria ≤ 330 mg/dL per day.

1486. Which of the following about lupus nephritis is false?

Harrison's 20th Ed. Chapter 308 Page 2138

A. Lesions limited to renal mesangium have excellent prognosis
B. Systemic lupus becomes quiescent once there is renal failure
C. Lupus nephritis class V patients are predisposed to renal-vein thrombosis
D. None of the above

1487. In lupus nephritis, which of the following antibodies correlate best with the presence of renal disease?

Harrison's 20th Ed. Chapter 308 Page 2138

A. Antiendomysial antibody
B. Anti-dsDNA antibodies
C. Anticentromere antibody
D. Anti-U3-RNP

In lupus nephritis, anti-dsDNA antibodies that fix complement correlate best with the presence of renal disease.

1488. In lupus nephritis, which of the following serves as a urinary biomarker?

J. Proteome Res. 2019; 18: 1264–1277

A. α-2-macroglobulin
B. Haptoglobin
C. α-1-antitrypsin
D. All of the above

1489. In lupus nephritis, which of the following serves as a urinary biomarker?

J. Proteome Res. 2019; 18: 1264–1277

A. Ceruloplasmin
B. Transferrin
C. Afamin
D. All of the above

Seven proteins - transferrin, α-2-macroglobulin, haptoglobin, afamin, α-1-antitrypsin, vimentin, and ceruloplasmin were confirmed to be elevated in lupus nephritis urine compared to healthy controls.

1490. Lupus nephritis is categorized in to how many classes?

Harrison's 20th Ed. Chapter 308 Page 2138 Table 308-3

A. 3
B. 4
C. 5
D. 6

1491. Which class of lupus nephritis is labeled as diffuse nephritis?

Harrison's 20th Ed. Chapter 308 Page 2138 Table 308-3

A. 3
B. 4
C. 5
D. 6

Global, diffuse proliferative lesions involving the vast majority of glomeruli are labeled as class IV. They have high anti-DNA antibody titers, low serum complement, hematuria, red blood cell casts, proteinuria, hypertension, and decreased renal function. 50% of patients have nephrotic-range proteinuria. Without treatment, this aggressive lesion has the worst renal prognosis.

1492. Which class of lupus nephritis is labeled as membranous nephritis?

Harrison's 20th Ed. Chapter 308 Page 2138 Table 308-3

A. 3
B. 4
C. 5
D. 6

1493. In lupus nephritis, lesions of which class have the most varied course?

Harrison's 20th Ed. Chapter 308 Page 2138

A. 3
B. 4
C. 5
D. 6

Class III lesions have the most varied course.

1494. Which of the following drugs is not used in the treatment of lupus nephritis?

Harrison's 20th Ed. Chapter 308 Page 2138

A. Cyclophosphamide
B. Mycophenolate mofetil
C. Ipilimumab
D. Prednisone

For lupus nephritis class 3 or 4, induction phase of treatment (high-dose corticosteroids and cyclophosphamide or MMF) generally lasts 2–6 months and is followed by a prolonged, but less intense maintenance phase (steroids and mycophenolate mofetil or azathioprine), often lasting years. It is not clear when maintenance therapy can be withdrawn.

1495. Which of the following monoclonal antibody is used in the treatment of lupus nephritis?

Harrison's 20th Ed. Chapter 308 Page 2138

A. Adalimumab
B. Belimumab
C. Certolizumab
D. Golimumab

Belimumab, a monoclonal antibody directed against the B cell survival factor BLyS, trials in nonrenal lupus showed a dose-dependent trend toward a decreased rate of renal flares in patients who had received belimumab.

1496. First name of Goodpasture was?

N Engl J Med. 2003;348:2543-56

A. Albert
B. Ellis
C. Ernest
D. Eric

Ernest Goodpasture published his observation as 'The pathology of pneumonia accompanying influenza. US Naval Med Bull 1919;13:177-97'. Stanton and Tange described the pulmonary-renal syndrome almost 40 years later, and it was they who suggested that Goodpasture's name be linked to the condition.

1497. Which of the following is not a basement membrane syndrome?

Harrison's 20th Ed. Chapter 308 Page 2139

A. Alport's syndrome
B. Goodpasture's syndrome
C. Churg-Strauss syndrome
D. Nail-patella syndrome

1498. Which of the following is true for 'anti-GBM disease'?

Harrison's 20th Ed. Chapter 308 Page 2139

A. Detectable circulating anti-GBM autoantibodies
B. Normal serum complement levels
C. Absent ANCA
D. All of the above

1499. The triad in Goodpasture's syndrome consists of all except?

Harrison's 20th Ed. Chapter 308 Page 2139

A. Lung hemorrhage
B. Renal failure
C. Proteinuria
D. Anti-GBM antibodies

Term 'Goodpasture's syndrome' is used for the triad of lung hemorrhage, renal failure and anti-GBM antibodies. 'Goodpasture's disease' or anti-GBM disease refers to glomerulonephritis caused by antibodies directed against the α3-chain of type IV collagen, with or without lung hemorrhage. Etiology is unknown.

1500. Which of the following is true for Goodpasture's syndrome?

Harrison's 20th Ed. Chapter 308 Page 2139

A. Anti-GBM nephritis
B. Lung hemorrhage
C. Autoimmune disease
D. All of the above

1501. Which of the following is a protomer of collagen IV?

N Engl J Med. 2003;348:2543-56

A. α1.α1.α2(IV)
B. α3.α4.α5(IV)
C. α5.α5.α6(IV)
D. All of the above

The six chains of collagen IV form only three sets of triple helical molecules called protomers designated as α1.α1.α2(IV), α3.α4.α5(IV), and α5.α5.α6(IV).

1502. Which chain of type IV collagen is the target antigen in Goodpasture's syndrome?

Harrison's 20th Ed. Chapter 308 Page 2139

A. α1
B. α2
C. α3
D. α4

1503. Which chain of type IV collagen is called 'Goodpasture antigen'?

Harrison's 20th Ed. Chapter 308 Page 2139

A. α3
B. α4
C. α5
D. α6

1504. Which of the following is known as 'Goodpasture protomer'?

N Engl J Med. 2003;348:2543-56

A. α3(IV) NC1
B. α5.a5.α6(IV)
C. α3.a4.α5(IV)
D. α1.a1.α2(IV)

a3.a4.a5(IV) protomer is a basement-membrane molecule of family of type IV collagens in epithelial tissues and is called the "Goodpasture protomer".

1505. α3 (IV) NC1 peptides are produced by?

N Engl J Med. 2003;348:2543-56

A. Lymph node
B. Bone marrow
C. Spleen
D. Thymus

Thymus expresses α3 (IV) NC1 peptides that can cause elimination of autoreactive CD4+ helper T cells. A few such T cells escape deletion and can engage in the production of anti–glomerular basement membrane antibodies. Linear deposits of IgG antibody along the glomerular basement membrane are seen. Autoantibodies directed against glomerular basement membrane cross-react with basement membrane of alveolar walls.

1506. Which of the following is false about Goodpasture's syndrome?

Harrison's 20th Ed. Chapter 308 Page 2139

A. Occurs in young men in late 20s
B. Occurs in men & women in 60–70s
C. Hemoptysis is largely confined to smokers
D. None of the above

1507. Exposure to which of the following can cause Goodpasture's syndrome?

Harrison's 20th Ed. Chapter 308 Page 2139

A. Infection
B. Cocaine
C. Hydrocarbon
D. All of the above

1508. Antibodies against the α1(IV) NC1 domain is seen in patients with?

Harrison's 20th Ed. Chapter 308 Page 2139

A. Leukemia
B. Paraneoplastic syndrome
C. SLE
D. All of the above

Antibodies against the α1(IV) NC1 domain is seen in patients with paraneoplastic syndrome.

1509. In Goodpasture's syndrome, which of the following indicate worse prognosis at presentation?

Harrison's 20th Ed. Chapter 308 Page 2139

A. Oliguria
B. >50% crescents on renal biopsy
C. Serum creatinine >5–6 mg/dL
D. All of the above

In Goodpasture's syndrome, prognosis at presentation is worse if there is oliguria, advanced fibrosis or >50% crescents on renal biopsy, serum creatinine >5–7 mg/dL or a need for dialysis.

1510. Patients of Goodpasture's syndrome respond to which of the following treatments?

Harrison's 20th Ed. Chapter 308 Page 2139

A. Plasmapheresis
B. Oral prednisone
C. Cyclophosphamide
D. All of the above

Patients of Goodpasture's syndrome respond to plasmapheresis, accompanied by oral prednisone and cyclophosphamide therapy.

1511. Which of the following about Goodpasture's syndrome is false?

Harrison's 20th Ed. Chapter 308 Page 2139

A. Hemoptysis is largely confined to smokers
B. Presentation with oliguria has bad outcome
C. Disease in young is usually explosive
D. None of the above

1512. Out of the following, which is the most common form of glomerulonephritis?

Harrison's 20th Ed. Chapter 308 Page 2139

A. IgA nephropathy
B. Focal sclerosing glomerulonephritis
C. Rapidly progressive/crescentic glomerulonephritis
D. Membranous glomerulonephritis

IgA nephropathy is the most common form of glomerulonephritis worldwide.

1513. IgA nephropathy is also called?

Harrison's 20th Ed. Chapter 308 Page 2139

A. Barratt disease
B. Berger disease
C. Tomino disease
D. Glassock disease

IgA nephropathy (Berger disease) is a primary glomerular disease. Berger first described it in 1968.

1514. Which of the following is false about IgA nephropathy?

Harrison's 20th Ed. Chapter 308 Page 2139

A. Female preponderance
B. Peak incidence in II & III decades of life
C. Recurrent episodes of macroscopic hematuria
D. Between episodes, urinalysis is normal

In IgA nephropathy, there is a male preponderance.

1515. IgA nephropathy resembles which of the following diseases?

Harrison's 20th Ed. Chapter 308 Page 2139

A. Wegener's granulomatosis
B. Goodpasture's syndrome
C. Henoch-Schönlein purpura
D. All of the above

Clinical and laboratory evidence suggests close similarities between Henoch-Schönlein purpura and IgA nephropathy.

1516. IgA nephropathy is differentiated from Henoch-Schönlein purpura by?

Harrison's 20th Ed. Chapter 308 Page 2139

A. Prominent systemic symptoms at a younger age (<20 years)
B. Preceding infection
C. Abdominal complaints
D. All of the above

HSP is distinguished clinically from IgA nephropathy by prominent systemic symptoms, a younger age (<20 years), preceding infection & abdominal complaints.

1517. Essentials of IgA nephropathy include?

Harrison's 20th Ed. Chapter 308 Page 2139

A. Diffuse mesangial IgA deposits
B. Clinically significant glomerular inflammation
C. Renal dysfunction
D. All of the above

1518. Deposits of IgA in glomerular mesangium are found in?

Harrison's 20th Ed. Chapter 308 Page 2139

A. Chronic liver disease
B. Crohn's disease
C. Gastrointestinal adenocarcinoma
D. All of the above

1519. Deposits of IgA in glomerular mesangium are found in?

Harrison's 20th Ed. Chapter 308 Page 2139

A. Chronic bronchiectasis
B. Idiopathic interstitial pneumonia
C. Dermatitis herpetiformis
D. All of the above

1520. Deposits of IgA in glomerular mesangium are found in?

Harrison's 20th Ed. Chapter 308 Page 2139

A. Leprosy
B. Ankylosing spondylitis
C. Sjögren's syndrome
D. All of the above

Deposits of IgA in glomerular mesangium are found in chronic liver disease, Crohn's disease, gastrointestinal adenocarcinoma, chronic obstructive bronchiectasis, idiopathic interstitial pneumonia, dermatitis herpetiformis, mycosis fungoides, leprosy, ankylosing spondylitis, relapsing polychondritis, and Sjögren's syndrome. However, IgA deposition does not produce clinically significant glomerular inflammation or renal dysfunction and therefore not called IgA nephropathy.

1521. Most IgA deposited in the kidney are derived from?

Harrison's 20th Ed. Chapter 308 Page 2139

A. Lymph node
B. Bone marrow
C. Spleen
D. Liver

IgA, particularly secretory IgA, production is done by plasma cells in bone marrow.

1522. Most IgA is cleared by?

Harrison's 20th Ed. Chapter 308 Page 2139

A. Kidney
B. Bone marrow
C. Intestines
D. Liver

IgA clearance occurs predominately in the liver.

1523. In IgA nephropathy, deposition of IgA occurs in?

Harrison's 20th Ed. Chapter 308 Page 2139

A. Glomerular capillaries
B. Glomerular mesangium
C. Glomerular basement membrane
D. All of the above

Morphologically, IgA nephropathy is characterized by diffuse deposition of IgA in glomerular mesangium. IgA deposited in the mesangium is typically polymeric and of the IgA1 subclass.

1524. Which of the following is false about IgA nephropathy?

Harrison's 20th Ed. Chapter 308 Page 2139

A. Mesangial hypercellularity
B. IgA1 subclass IgA deposits in the mesangium
C. IgM, IgG, C3 codistributed with IgA deposits
D. None of the above

1525. Which of the following is abnormal in IgA nephropathy?

Harrison's 20th Ed. Chapter 308 Page 2139

A. IgA production by plasma cells
B. IgA clearance by liver
C. Receptors for IgA
D. All of the above

1526. Which of the following is key to the pathogenesis of IgA nephropathy?

Harrison's 20th Ed. Chapter 308 Page 2139

A. Glucose-deficient IgA1
B. Galactose-deficient IgA1
C. Glucose-deficient IgA2
D. Galactose-deficient IgA2

The IgA1 produced in patients with IgA nephropathy is underglycosylated (Gd-IgA1). The galactose-deficient IgA1 may evade liver catabolism and preferentially deposit in mesangium. Susceptible individuals (second hit, such as a viral or other antigen exposure) will also produce anti–Gd-IgA1 autoantibodies (auto-Ab). The Gd-IgA1 - auto-Ab immune complexes activate the alternative pathway of complement. The immune complexes are nephritogenic, contributing to local inflammation, cellular proliferation, and ultimately fibrosis.

1527. Which of the following is a finding in patients with IgA nephropathy?

Clinical Journal of the American Society of Nephrology. 2017;12:1-10

A. Galactose-deficient IgA1
B. IgG autoantibody directed against the hinge region O-glycans
C. C3
D. All of the above

A central finding in patients with IgAN A central finding in patients with IgAN is the presence of circulating and glomerular immune complexes comprised of galactose-deficient IgA1, an IgG autoantibody directed against the hinge region O-glycans, and C3.

1528. A polymorphism which of the following gene confers susceptibility to IgA nephropathy?

Clinical Journal of the American Society of Nephrology. 2017;12:1-10

A. APOL1 gene
B. APRIL gene
C. Complement factor H regulatory proteins (CFHR's) gene
D. PKD1 gene

A polymorphism in the APRIL gene confers susceptibility to IgA nephropathy.

1529. In IgA nephropathy, histologic lesion seen on light microscopy is?

Harrison's 20th Ed. Chapter 308 Page 2139

A. DPGN
B. Segmental sclerosis
C. Segmental necrosis with cellular crescent formation
D. All of the above

Immunofluorescent pattern of IgA on renal biopsy defines IgA nephropathy, but other patterns may be seen.

1530. Which of the following about IgA nephropathy is false?

Harrison's 20th Ed. Chapter 308 Page 2140

A. Recurrent episodes of macroscopic hematuria during or immediately following an upper respiratory infection
B. Accompanied by proteinuria
C. Persistent asymptomatic microscopic hematuria
D. Nephrotic syndrome is common

Nephrotic syndrome is uncommon in IgA nephropathy.

1531. Which of the following about IgA nephropathy is false?

Harrison's 20th Ed. Chapter 308 Page 2140

A. Benign disease for the majority of patients
B. Renal function well preserved
C. Slow progression
D. Use of angiotensin-converting enzyme (ACE) inhibitors harmful

Use of angiotensin-converting enzyme (ACE) inhibitors in patients of IgA nephropathy with proteinuria or declining renal function is helpful.

1532. Which of the following is a risk factor for the loss of renal function in IgA nephropathy?

Harrison's 20th Ed. Chapter 308 Page 2140

A. Presence of hypertension
B. Presence of proteinuria
C. Absence of episodes of macroscopic hematuria
D. All of the above

In IgA nephropathy, risk factors for loss of renal function include presence of hypertension or proteinuria, absence of episodes of macroscopic hematuria, male sex, older age of onset, and extensive glomerulosclerosis or interstitial fibrosis on renal biopsy.

1533. Which out of the following has the greatest predictive power for adverse renal outcomes in IgA nephropathy?

Harrison's 20th Ed. Chapter 308 Page 2140

A. Persistent proteinuria for 6 months
B. Persistent hypertension for 6 months
C. Persistent macroscopic hematuria for 6 months
D. All of the above

Analyses of IgA nephropathy patients found persistent proteinuria for 6 months or longer to have the greatest predictive power for adverse renal outcomes.

1534. Which of the following procedures benefit select patients of IgA nephropathy?

Harrison's 20th Ed. Chapter 308 Page 2140

A. Tonsillectomy
B. Appendicectomy
C. Orchidectomy
D. None of the above

Tonsillectomy & fish oil have been suggested in small studies to benefit select patients of IgA nephropathy.

1535. When IgA nephropathy presents as RPGN, which of the following is helpful?

Harrison's 20th Ed. Chapter 308 Page 2140, N Engl J Med. 2015;373:2225-36

A. Steroids
B. Cytotoxic agents
C. Plasmapheresis
D. All of the above

Addition of immunosuppression to comprehensive supportive care was not beneficial in patients with IgA nephropathy that was characterized by moderate proteinuria & chronic kidney disease stages 1 through 3.

1536. In IgA nephropathy, which of the following is helpful?

Clinical Journal of the American Society of Nephrology. 2017;12:1-10

A. Salmeterol
B. Budesonide
C. Nifedipine
D. Tadalafil

A novel potential therapy for IgAN is a modified formulation of oral budesonide (Nefecon). This agent is proposed to act locally at the mucosal lymphoid tissue in the distal ileum and proximal large intestine to modulate IgA production.

1537. Small-vessel vasculitis rarely involves which of the following?

Harrison's 20th Ed. Chapter 308 Page 2140

A. Arterioles
B. Capillaries
C. Venules
D. Small arteries

Small-vessel vasculitis involves arterioles, capillaries, venules and rarely small arteries.

1538. ANCA stands for?

Harrison's 20th Ed. Chapter 308 Page 2140

A. Anti-neutrophilic cytoplasmic antibody
B. Anti-neutrophilic cytoplasmic autoantibody
C. Anti-neutrophilic centromeric antibody
D. Anti-neutrophilic centromeric autoantibody

1539. ANCA activates which of the following?

Harrison's 20th Ed. Chapter 308 Page 2140

A. Eosinophil
B. Basophil
C. Monocyte
D. Macrophage

ANCA, in the the pathogenesis of these small-vessel vasculitides, activates cytokine (TNFα) primed neutrophils and monocytes, which express ANCA antigens, proteinase 3 and myeloperoxidase, on their surface. B cells produce ANCAs.

1540. Which of the following is a type of ANCA?

Harrison's 20th Ed. Chapter 308 Page 2140

A. Cytoplasmic (cANCA)
B. Perinuclear (pANCA)
C. Atypical (aANCA)
D. All of the above

Cytoplasmic ANCA (C-ANCA) with specificity for PR3 are usually found in patients with GPA (Wegener granulomatosis) whereas perinuclear ANCA (P-ANCA) in patients with MPA and EGPA (Churg-Strauss syndrome). aANCA is associated with levamisole-contaminated cocaine exposure in abusers. Proteinase-3 (PR3-ANCA) is also called cANCA. Myeloperoxidase (MPO-ANCA) is also called pANCA.

1541. Which of the following about ANCA is false?

Harrison's 20th Ed. Chapter 308 Page 2140

A. P-ANCA targets & attaches to myeloperoxidase in neutrophils
B. C-ANCA targets & attaches to proteinase 3 in neutrophils
C. C-ANCA is associated with GPA, P-ANCA with MPA
D. None of the above

cANCA pattern is mostly due to the presence of anti-PR3 autoantibodies while pANCA pattern is usually due to the presence of anti-myeloperoxidase (anti-MPO) antibodies. The target proteins PR3 and MPO are both localised in the azurophile (primary) granules of polymorphonuclear cells and monocytes, from where they can be exposed on the cellular surface as a result of various inflammatory stimuli.

1542. Which of the following is false about proteinase 3 (PR3)?

Harrison's 20th Ed. Chapter 308 Page 2140

A. PR3 is GPA's main autoantigen
B. The main inhibitor of PR3 is alpha-1-antitrypsin (α1-AT)
C. PR3 allows destruction of phagocytosed bacteria in activated neutrophils favours diapedesis
D. None of the above

1543. Which of the following is a ANCA associated vasculitis?

Harrison's 20th Ed. Chapter 308 Page 2140

A. Microscopic polyangiitis (MPA)
B. Granulomatosis with polyangiitis (GPA)
C. Eosinophilic granulomatosis with polyangiitis (EGPA)
D. All of the above

Anti-neutrophil cytoplasmic antibody (ANCA)-associated vasculitis (AAV) includes microscopic polyangiitis (MPA), granulomatosis with polyangiitis (GPA, also known as Wegener's granulomatosis), eosinophilic granulomatosis with polyangiitis (EGPA, also known as Churg-Strauss syndrome) and drug-induced AAV. ANCAs have a central role in the pathogenesis of AAV because they induce excessive activation of neutrophils, which results in injury to small vessels.

1544. Which of the following antibodies play a role in the pathogenesis of AAV?

Harrison's 20th Ed. Chapter 308 Page 2140

A. Anti-GBM antibodies
B. Lysosomal-associated membrane protein 2 (LAMP-2)
C. Antibodies to ADAMTS13
D. Anti-La (SS-B) antibodies

Anti-LAMP-2 antibodies play important role in the pathogenesis of AAV. These antibodies are only found in patients with active vasculitis even those who were lacking PR3 or MPO.

1545. Which of the following is an ANCA-positive, pauci-immune glomerulonephritis?

Harrison's 20th Ed. Chapter 308 Page 2140

A. Granulomatosis with polyangiitis
B. Microscopic polyangiitis
C. Churg-Strauss syndrome
D. All of the above

1546. Anti-PR3 antibodies are more common in?

Harrison's 20th Ed. Chapter 308 Page 2140

A. Granulomatosis with polyangiitis
B. Microscopic polyangiitis
C. Churg-Strauss syndrome
D. All of the above

Anti-PR3 antibodies are more common in Wegener's granulomatosis & anti-MPO antibodies are more common in microscopic polyangiitis or Churg-Strauss syndrome.

1547. Which of the following is a classical presentation in patients with granulomatosis with polyangiitis?

Harrison's 20th Ed. Chapter 308 Page 2140

A. Significant lung disease
B. Destructive sinusitis
C. Microscopic hematuria
D. All of the above

Patients with granulomatosis with polyangiitis classically present with fever, purulent rhinorrhea, nasal ulcers, sinus pain, polyarthralgias/arthritis, cough, hemoptysis, shortness of breath, microscopic hematuria, and 0.5–1 gram/day of proteinuria. Occasionally there may be cutaneous purpura and mononeuritis multiplex.

1548. Granulomatosis with polyangiitis presenting without renal involvement is termed?

Harrison's 20th Ed. Chapter 308 Page 2140

A. Wegener's disease
B. Wegener's syndrome
C. Isolated Wegener's granulomatosis
D. Limited granulomatosis with polyangiitis

Presentation without renal involvement is termed limited granulomatosis with polyangiitis.

1549. Granulomatosis with polyangiitis is more common in?

Harrison's 20th Ed. Chapter 308 Page 2140

A. Patients exposed to epoxy resins
B. Patients exposed to silica dust
C. Patients exposed to welding fumes
D. Patients exposed to aromatic hydrocarbons

1550. Granulomatosis with polyangiitis is more common in?

Harrison's 20th Ed. Chapter 308 Page 2140

A. Folate and vitamin B12 deficiency
B. α1-antitrypsin deficiency
C. Glucose-6-phosphate dehydrogenase (G6PD) deficiency
D. Vitamin D deficiency

Granulomatosis with polyangiitis is more common in patients exposed to silica dust and those with α1-antitrypsin deficiency, which is an inhibitor of PR3.

1551. Relapse after achieving remission is more common in patients with?

Harrison's 20th Ed. Chapter 308 Page 2140

A. Microscopic polyangiitis
B. Granulomatosis with polyangiitis
C. Churg-Strauss syndrome
D. C3 Glomerulopathies

1552. In microscopic polyangiitis, which of the following is uncommon?

Harrison's 20th Ed. Chapter 308 Page 2140

A. Hematuria
B. Proteinuria
C. Significant lung disease or destructive sinusitis
D. Renal involvement

Patients of microscopic polyangiitis are similar to those with Wegener's granulomatosis, except that they rarely have significant lung disease or destructive sinusitis.

1553. Which of the following distinguishes Churg-Strauss syndrome from other small-vessel vasculitis?

Harrison's 20th Ed. Chapter 308 Page 2140

A. Pulmonary infiltrates
B. Peripheral eosinophilia
C. Glomerulonephritis
D. All of the above

Churg-Strauss syndrome is a small-vessel vasculitis associated with peripheral eosinophilia, cutaneous purpura, mononeuritis, asthma, allergic rhinitis, hypergammaglobulinemia, elevated serum IgE, and rheumatoid factor.

1554. Which of the following is a type of C3 glomerulopathy?

Harrison's 20th Ed. Chapter 308 Page 2141

A. Membranous glomerulonephritis
B. Minimal change disease
C. Dense deposit disease
D. Focal segmental glomerular sclerosis

1555. Which of the following about dense deposit disease is false?

Harrison's 20th Ed. Chapter 308 Page 2141

A. Occurs in young
B. More likely to have low serum C3 levels
C. More likely to have crescentic GN
D. None of the above

Patients with C3GN are older & have more severe arteriolar sclerosis, glomerular sclerosis & interstitial scarring on renal biopsy than patients with DDD. Older age, crescentic GN & DDD subtype were independent predictors of ESRD. Both DDD and C3GN recur after renal transplantation, often resulting in allograft loss.

1556. Mutations in which of the following complement factor regulatory protein gene causes C3 glomerulopathy?

Harrison's 20th Ed. Chapter 308 Page 2141

A. G
B. H
C. J
D. P

Factor H cleaves the active form of C3, C3b, to the inactive iC3b. Mutations in the complement factor H regulatory proteins (CFHR's) genes causes C3 glomerulopathy. The major inhibitor of the alternative pathway in the circulation is factor H which acts to block the formation of alternative pathway convertases, promotes their spontaneous dissociation and also acts as a co-factor for the cleavage of C3b to its inactive form iC3b by factor I. Properdin is the only positive regulator of the alternative pathway and acts to stabilise the alternative pathway C3 convertase.

1557. Which of the following is a principal regulator of the complement system?

Harrison's 20th Ed. Chapter 308 Page 2141

A. Complement C3
B. Membrane cofactor protein (MCP)
C. Complement factor B (CFB)
D. Complement factor H (CFH)

CFH, CFHR1–5, CFI, MCP and Thrombomodulin (THBD) inhibit or regulate the complement pathway in the fluid-phase or on the surface of host cells. C3b, CFB, CFD and properdin stabilize and activate the C3 convertase.

1558. Deficiency of complement factor H (CFH) is associated with?

Harrison's 20th Ed. Chapter 308 Page 2141

A. Focal segmental glomerular sclerosis (FSGS)
B. Atypical hemolytic uremic syndrome (aHUS)
C. Minimal change disease (MCD)
D. All of the above

Deficiency of CFH is commonly associated with aHUS.

1559. Atypical hemolytic uremic syndrome is characterized by?

Harrison's 20th Ed. Chapter 308 Page 2141

A. Microangiopathic hemolysis
B. Thrombocytopenia
C. Renal failure
D. All of the above

1560. 'Ribbons in the GBM' best relates to?

Harrison's 20th Ed. Chapter 308 Page 2141

A. Microscopic polyangiitis
B. Granulomatosis with polyangiitis
C. Dense deposit disease
D. Churg-Strauss syndrome

Dense deposit disease (DDD), formerly MPGN type II, is defined morphologically with dense deposits forming ribbons in the GBM. In its absence, the entity is categorized as C3 glomerulonephritis.

1561. Which of the following about C3 nephritic factors (C3nefs) is false?

Harrison's 20th Ed. Chapter 308 Page 2141

A. Autoantibodies
B. Stabilize the alternative pathway C3 convertase
C. Prevents C3 convertase inactivation by factor H
D. None of the above

C3 nephritic factors (C3nefs), which are autoantibodies that bind to and stabilise the alternative pathway C3 convertase by preventing its inactivation by factor H.

1562. Which of the following about C3 glomerulopathy is false?

Harrison's 20th Ed. Chapter 308 Page 2141

A. Presence of glomerular deposits composed of C3
B. Absence of significant amounts of Ig in glomerular deposits
C. Low serum C3 levels with preserved serum C4 levels
D. None of the above

1563. Histopathological & laboratory features of which of the following are indistinguishable from C3 glomerulopathy?

Harrison's 20th Ed. Chapter 308 Page 2141

A. Membranous glomerulonephritis
B. Minimal change disease
C. Post-infectious glomerulonephritis
D. Focal segmental glomerular sclerosis

Post infectious glomerulonephritis may be considered a self-limiting form of C3 glomerulopathy. Renal biopsy in post infectious GN typically shows a diffuse endocapillary glomerulonephritis with subepithelial hump-like deposits on EM. On immunofluorescence, there may be glomerular staining for IgG & C3 but some cases may show C3 deposition only. Patients usually have low levels of circulating C3.

1564. Which of the following monoclonal antibody is of use in C3 glomerulopathy?

Harrison's 20th Ed. Chapter 308 Page 2141

A. Bevacizumab
B. Eculizumab
C. Certolizumab
D. Natalizumab

Eculizumab is a monoclonal antibody directed at C5 which is activated by C3. Rational treatment of C3 glomerulopathy would involve inhibition of C3 activation.

1565. Mesangiocapillary glomerulonephritis or lobar glomerulonephritis is also called?

Harrison's 20th Ed. Chapter 308 Page 2141

A. Focal segmental glomerulosclerosis
B. Membranous glomerulonephritis
C. Membranoproliferative glomerulonephritis (MPGN)
D. Mesangioproliferative glomerulonephritis

Membranoproliferative glomerulonephritis (MPGN) is also called mesangiocapillary glomerulonephritis or lobar glomerulonephritis.

1566. Which of the following about membranoproliferative glomerulonephritis (MPGN) is false?

Harrison's 20th Ed. Chapter 308 Page 2141

A. Immune-mediated glomerulonephritis
B. Thickening of the GBM
C. Mesangioproliferative changes
D. None of the above

1567. Which of the following about membranoproliferative glomerulonephritis (MPGN) is false?

Harrison's 20th Ed. Chapter 308 Page 2141

A. Most patients have hypocomplementemia
B. Rare in African Americans
C. Usually presents in childhood or young adulthood
D. None of the above

1568. Type I membranoproliferative glomerulonephritis (MPGN) is associated with?

Harrison's 20th Ed. Chapter 308 Page 2141

A. Persistent hepatitis C infections
B. Lupus
C. Neoplastic diseases
D. All of the above

Type I MPGN is commonly associated with persistent hepatitis C infections, autoimmune diseases like lupus or cryoglobulinemia, or neoplastic diseases.

1569. Which of the following is the most proliferative type of MPGN?

Harrison's 20th Ed. Chapter 308 Page 2141

A. Type I
B. Type II
C. Type III
D. All of the above

MPGN is subdivided 'pathologically' into type I, type II, and type III disease. Type I MPGN is the most proliferative type. MPGN type I has subendothelial electron-dense deposits, type II [also called dense deposit disease DDD], with intramembranous highly electron-dense deposits and type III, with both subendothelial and subepithelial deposits.

1570. Which of the following is called 'dense deposit disease'?

Harrison's 20th Ed. Chapter 308 Page 2141

A. Type I membranoproliferative glomerulonephritis
B. Type II membranoproliferative glomerulonephritis
C. Type III membranoproliferative glomerulonephritis
D. None of the above

Low serum C3 & dense thickening of GBM containing ribbons of dense deposits and C3 characterize Type II MPGN, also called dense deposit disease.

1571. Which of the following best relates to Type I membranoproliferative glomerulonephritis?

Harrison's 20th Ed. Chapter 308 Page 2141

A. Split basement membrane
B. Tram-tracking
C. Sentinel clot
D. B ring

Renal biopsy finding in Type I MPGN shows mesangial proliferation with lobular segmentation. Mesangial interposition between the capillary basement membrane and endothelial cells, produces a double contour sometimes called 'tram-tracking'.

1572. Which of the following is false about dense deposit disease or Type II membranoproliferative glomerulonephritis?

Harrison's 20th Ed. Chapter 308 Page 2141

A. Low serum C3
B. Dense thickening of the GBM
C. Ribbons of dense deposits and C3 in GBM
D. None of the above

1573. Mesangioproliferative glomerulonephritis is seen in?

Harrison's 20th Ed. Chapter 308 Page 2142

A. IgA nephropathy
B. P. falciparum malaria
C. Resolving postinfectious glomerulonephritis
D. All of the above

Mesangioproliferative glomerulonephritis is seen in IgA nephropathy, P. falciparum malaria, resolving postinfectious glomerulonephritis, and class II lupus nephritis.

1574. Minimal change disease (MCD) is also called?

Harrison's 20th Ed. Chapter 308 Page 2142

A. Nil disease
B. Lipoid nephrosis
C. Foot process disease
D. All of the above

Minimal change disease is also called lipoid nephrosis, visceral epithelial cell disease, foot process disease, nil disease or minimal change glomerulopathy.

1575. Minimal change Disease (MCD) is associated with?

Harrison's 20th Ed. Chapter 308 Page 2142

A. Hodgkin's disease
B. Allergies
C. Use of nonsteroidal anti-inflammatory agents
D. All of the above

MCD usually presents as a primary renal disease but can be associated with Hodgkin's disease, allergies, or use of NSAID agents (secondary form). Because of the association of MCD with atopy, alimentary allergies and hypersensitivity reactions, Kark (1958), referred MCD as 'asthma of the nephron'.

1576. Minimal change disease (MCD) on electron microscopy of renal biopsy consistently shows?

Harrison's 20th Ed. Chapter 308 Page 2142

A. Mesangial proliferation
B. Mesangial interposition
C. Effacement of the foot process
D. All of the above

MCD on electron microscopy of renal biopsy consistently shows an effacement of the foot process supporting epithelial podocytes, weakening of slit-pore membranes with formation of villi on the external surface of the epithelial cells (villous transformation). There are no electron-dense deposits. This is noted along virtually the entire distribution of every capillary loop.

1577. Which of the following is false about minimal change disease?

Harrison's 20th Ed. Chapter 308 Page 2142

A. Abrupt onset of edema
B. Nephrotic syndrome (average urine protein excretion 10 g/day)
C. Severe hypoalbuminemia
D. None of the above

1578. Which of the following is false about minimal change disease?

Harrison's 20th Ed. Chapter 308 Page 2142

A. Known as nil lesion
B. Commonest cause of nephrotic syndrome in adults
C. Acellular urinary sediment
D. Selective proteinuria

80% of the MCD children are < 6 years of age. MCD is more frequent in boys than in girls.

1579. Selective proteinuria in minimal change disease is for?

Harrison's 20th Ed. Chapter 308 Page 2142

A. Albumin
B. Light chain
C. Globulin
D. All of the above

MCD causes 70–90% of nephrotic syndrome in childhood but only 10–15% of nephrotic syndrome in adults. In MCD, proteinuria is selective and largely composed of albumin. The presence of high molecular weight proteins suggests another diagnosis.

1580. Which of the following is uncommon in minimal change disease?

Harrison's 20th Ed. Chapter 308 Page 2142

A. Hematuria
B. Hypertension
C. Renal failure
D. All of the above

Hematuria, hypertension, and renal failure are uncommon.

1581. Which of the following is false about minimal change disease?

Harrison's 20th Ed. Chapter 308 Page 2142

A. No glomerular histologic changes
B. No tubulointerstitial alterations
C. No immunoglobulin or complement deposition in renal tissue
D. None of the above

1582. MCD patients with steroid resistance can develop?

Harrison's 20th Ed. Chapter 308 Page 2142

A. Focal segmental glomerulosclerosis (FSGS)
B. Mesangioproliferative glomerulonephritis
C. Microscopic polyangiitis
D. All of the above

MCD patients with steroid resistance can develop FSGS on repeat biopsy.

1583. Adults are considered steroid-resistant when there is no response after how many of therapy?

Harrison's 20th Ed. Chapter 308 Page 2142

A. 1 months
B. 2 months
C. 3 months
D. 4 months

Adults are not considered steroid-resistant until after 4 months of therapy. 80–85% of adults will achieve complete remission, but only after a longer course of 20–24 weeks.

1584. 90 to 95% of children will develop a complete remission after how many weeks of steroid therapy?

Harrison's 20th Ed. Chapter 308 Page 2142

A. 1 week
B. 4 weeks
C. 6 weeks
D. 8 weeks

90 to 95% of children will develop a complete remission after 8 weeks of steroid therapy. Primary responders are patients who have a complete remission (<0.2 mg/day of proteinuria) after a single course of prednisone.

1585. In MCD, relapses occur in what proportion of children after the first remission?

Harrison's 20th Ed. Chapter 308 Page 2142

A. 10–20%
B. 30–40%
C. 50–60%
D. 70–75%

Relapses occur in 70–75% of children after first remission. Early relapse predicts multiple subsequent relapses.

1586. Which of the following is false about minimal change disease?

Harrison's 20th Ed. Chapter 308 Page 2142

A. High levels of basal proteinuria predicts relapse
B. Frequency of relapses decreases after puberty
C. Increased risk of relapse following rapid tapering of steroids
D. None of the above

1587. Which of the following immunosuppressive drugs is used for frequent relapsers, steroid-dependent, or steroid-resistant patients?

Harrison's 20th Ed. Chapter 308 Page 2142

A. Cyclophosphamide
B. Chlorambucil
C. Mycophenolate mofetil
D. All of the above

1588. Nephrosarca best relates to?

Harrison's 20th Ed. Chapter 308 Page 2142

A. Perirenal collection of fluid
B. Intrarenal edema
C. Polyuria
D. All of the above

Nephrosarca best relates to intrarenal edema.

1589. Which of the following is common between MCD and FSGS?

Harrison's 20th Ed. Chapter 308 Page 2142

A. Proteinuria
B. Podocyte injury
C. Minimal immune deposits
D. All of the above

Distinction between MCD and FSGS is critical, because both present with proteinuria, podocyte injury, and minimal immune deposits. Light microscopy, electron microscopy, and staining for Ig and complement are critical in making the distinction between MCD and FSGS. Extensive podocyte injury with adequate numbers of normal-appearing glomeruli and nonscarred tubulointerstitium by light microscopy suggests MCD.

1590. Pathologic changes of focal segmental glomerulosclerosis (FSGS) are most prominent in glomeruli located at?

Harrison's 20th Ed. Chapter 308 Page 2142

A. Corticomedullary junction
B. Outer cortex
C. Middle cortex
D. All of the above

Pathologic changes of FSGS are most prominent in glomeruli located at corticomedullary junction.

1591. Which of the following about FSGS is false?

Harrison's 20th Ed. Chapter 308 Page 2142

A. Sclerotic lesions in glomeruli that are focal (<50%)
B. Segmental (<50% of the glomerular tuft affected)
C. Podocyte injury
D. None of the above

Podocyte injury is the earliest feature of FSGS. It is exemplified by cell body attenuation, foot process effacement, pseudocyst formation and microvillous transformation. If podocytes do not recover from initial injury, there occurs a reduction in podocyte number & a mismatch between podocyte coverage & the underlying glomerular basement membrane (GBM) surface area, leading to 'uncovered' bare areas of GBM. The glomerular parietal epithelial cells (PECs) forming the cell bridge can deposit matrix between these bridging cells to form a fibrous attachment (tuft adhesion) between the glomerular tuft and Bowman's capsule.

1592. Which of the following is considered the earliest feature of FSGS seen on light microscopy?

Harrison's 20th Ed. Chapter 308 Page 2143

A. Tubular atrophy
B. Tuft adhesion
C. Hyalinosis
D. Lipid-laden macrophages

The tuft adhesion is considered the earliest feature of FSGS seen on light microscopy in human biopsies.

1593. Which of the following gene is essential for the integrity of slit diaphragm?

Adv Chronic Kidney Dis. 2014 ;21(5):408-416

A. Nephrin
B. Podocin
C. CD2AP
D. All of the above

Nephrin, podocin, CD2AP, TRPC6, GLEPP1, MYO1E are essential for the integrity of slit diaphragm.

1594. Which of the following gene is essential for foot process-GBM interaction?

Adv Chronic Kidney Dis. 2014 ;21(5):408-416

A. α-actinin 4
B. LAMB2
C. Formin
D. TRPC6

LAMB2 and ITGA3 are essential for foot process-GBM interaction.

1595. Human conditions associated with glomerulomegaly include?

Adv Chronic Kidney Dis. 2014 ;21(5):408-416

A. Obesity
B. Hypertension
C. Oligonephronia seen in low birth weight subjects
D. All of the above

Human conditions typically associated with glomerulomegaly include obesity, hypertension and the reduced nephron number (oligonephronia) seen in low birth weight subjects.

1596. In the adult human kidney, how many podocytes are present per glomerular tuft?

Adv Chronic Kidney Dis. 2014 ;21(5):408-416

A. ~ 50–60
B. ~ 100–200
C. ~ 300–500
D. ~ 500–600

In the adult human kidney, there are ~500–600 podocytes per glomerular tuft, and turnover of adult podocytes has never been demonstrated under physiological conditions. As adult podocytes are terminally differentiated epithelial cells with a very limited ability to proliferate, podocyte loss following injury can result in a reduction in podocyte number. With the loss of <20% of podocytes, glomerulus could recover, however, > 20% podocyte loss results in FSGS.

1597. The podocyte foot processes wrap around and attach to the GBM predominantly through?

Adv Chronic Kidney Dis. 2014 ;21(5):408-416

A. α3β1 integrin
B. αvβ3 integrin
C. α-dystroglycan/β-dystroglycan
D. All of the above

The podocyte foot processes wrap around and attach to the GBM predominantly through α3β1 and αvβ3 integrins, and α-dystroglycan/β-dystroglycan.

1598. Podocytes adhere tightly to the glomerular basement membrane (GBM) via interactions between?

Adv Chronic Kidney Dis. 2014 ;21(5):408-416

A. Actin cytoskeleton
B. Integrins α3β1 and αvβ3
C. GBM components laminin 521 and type IV collagen
D. All of the above

Podocytes adhere tightly to the glomerular basement membrane (GBM) via interactions between the actin cytoskeleton, integrins α3β1 and αvβ3, and the GBM components laminin 521 and type IV collagen.

1599. Which of the following is relevant in the pathogenesis of FSGS?

Harrison's 20th Ed. Chapter 308 Page 2142

A. T cell–mediated circulating permeability factor
B. Increased soluble urokinase receptor levels
C. TGF-β–mediated cellular proliferation & matrix synthesis
D. All of the above

Possible mechanisms in FSGS include a T cell–mediated circulating permeability factor, increased soluble urokinase receptor levels, TGF-β–mediated cellular proliferation and matrix synthesis, and podocyte abnormalities associated with genetic mutations. Risk polymorphisms at the APOL1 locus encoding apolipoprotein L1 expressed in podocytes substantially explain the increased burden of FSGS among African-Americans with or without HIV-associated disease.

1600. Which of the following about APOL1 FSGS is false?

Harrison's 20th Ed. Chapter 308 Page 2143

A. Most common form in African descent populations
B. More rapid progression to ESRD
C. Strongly associated with collapsing glomerulopathy
D. None of the above

1601. Histologically, FSGS may manifest as?

Harrison's 20th Ed. Chapter 308 Page 2143, Clin J Am Soc Nephrol. 2018;13(12):1889

A. Tip variant
B. Collapsing variant
C. NOS variant
D. All of the above

1602. Which of the following variant of FSGS has better prognosis?

Harrison's 20th Ed. Chapter 308 Page 2143

A. Collapsing glomerulopathy
B. Hilar stalk lesion
C. Glomerular tip lesion
D. Endocapillary hypercellularity

1603. The clinical findings of FSGS largely manifest as?

Harrison's 20th Ed. Chapter 308 Page 2143

A. Hematuria
B. Proteinuria
C. Renal failure
D. All of the above

The clinical findings of FSGS largely manifest as proteinuria.

1604. Which of the following agents is useful in primary FSGS?
Harrison's 20th Ed. Chapter 308 Page 2143

A. Steroids over 6–9 months
B. Cyclosporine
C. Plasmapheresis
D. All of the above

Calcineurin inhibitors, including cyclosporin and tacrolimus, are mainstays of FSGS therapy for both steroid-sensitive individuals who cannot tolerate continued steroid therapy and steroid-resistant FSGS.

1605. Which of the following agents is useful in secondary FSGS?
Harrison's 20th Ed. Chapter 308 Page 2144

A. Steroids
B. Cyclosporine
C. Rituximab
D. None of the above

The treatment of secondary FSGS rests on treating the underlying cause and controlling proteinuria. There is no role for steroids or other immunosuppressive agents in secondary FSGS.

1606. What value of protein:creatinine ratio indicates nephrotic range proteinuria?
Clin J Am Soc Nephrol. 2018;13(12):1889

A. > 100–150 mg/mmol
B. > 200–250 mg/mmol
C. > 250–300 mg/mmol
D. > 300–350 mg/mmol

A protein:creatinine ratio value > 300–350 mg/mmol indicates nephrotic range proteinuria.

1607. What value of urine protein-to-creatinine ratio (uPCR) is considered as nephrotic range?
Clin J Am Soc Nephrol. 2018;13(12):1889

A. ≥ 0.8 gram/gram
B. ≥ 1.2 gram/gram
C. ≥ 1.6 gram/gram
D. ≥ 2 gram/gram

Nephrotic range proteinuria is urine protein-to-creatinine ratio (uPCR) ≥2 gram/gram.

1608. Complete remission (CR) is defined as uPCR of?
Clin J Am Soc Nephrol. 2018;13(12):1889

A. < 0.8 gram/gram
B. < 1.2 gram/gram
C. < 1.6 gram/gram
D. < 2 gram/gram

Complete remission (CR) is defined as uPCR < 0.2 g/g, and partial remission (PR) is defined as having 50% reduction from baseline proteinuria and uPCR < 2 g/g.

1609. Majority of children with nephrotic syndrome are due to?
Harrison's 20th Ed. Chapter 308 Page 2144

A. Minimal change disease (MCD)
B. Focal and segmental glomerulosclerosis (FSGS)
C. Membranous glomerulopathy
D. Membranoproliferative glomerulonephritis (MPGN)

1610. Most common cause of nephrotic syndrome in the elderly is?
Harrison's 20th Ed. Chapter 308 Page 2144

A. Minimal change disease (MCD)
B. Focal segmental glomerulosclerosis (FSGS)
C. Membranous glomerulonephritis (MGN)
D. Mesangioproliferative glomerulonephritis

Membranous glomerulonephritis (MGN) is the most common cause of nephrotic syndrome in the elderly. Idiopathic membranous nephropathy (IMN) is rare in childhood.

1611. Most common cause of nephrotic syndrome in black patients is?
Am J Kidney Dis 1996;27:647-51

A. Minimal change disease (MCD)
B. Focal segmental glomerulosclerosis (FSGS)
C. Membranous glomerulonephritis (MGN)
D. Mesangioproliferative glomerulonephritis

Membranous nephropathy is the most common cause of nephrotic syndrome in white, while FSGS is the most common cause in black patients.

1612. Experimental model of membranous glomerulonephritis (MGN) in rat is called?
Clin J Am Soc Nephrol. 2017;12:983-997

A. Lewis nephritis
B. Kupin nephritis
C. Heymann nephritis
D. Pickering nephritis

1613. Which of the following podocyte antigen is involved in neonatal membranous glomerulonephritis?
Clin J Am Soc Nephrol. 2017;12:983-997

A. Neutral endopeptidase (NEP)
B. Aryl sulfatase
C. M-type phospholipase A2 receptor type 1 (PLA2R1)
D. Thrombospondin type 1 domain containing 7A (THSD7A)

Antigens expressed by podocytes are neutral endopeptidase NEP, also called CD10 or common acute lymphoblastic leukemia antigen (CALLA) in newborns, cationic bovine serum albumin (BSA) and aryl sulfatase in childhood, the M-type phospholipase A2 receptor type 1 (PLA2R1) and thrombospondin type 1 domain containing 7A (THSD7A) in adults.

1614. Membranous glomerulonephritis (MGN) can be secondary to?
Harrison's 20th Ed. Chapter 308 Page 2144

A. Solid tumors of breast, lung, colon
B. Hepatitis B
C. Malaria
D. All of the above

MGN can be secondary to solid tumors of breast, lung, colon, hepatitis B, syphilis, malaria, schistosomiasis, & lupus, rheumatoid arthritis, IgG4 diseases or drug exposure. Worldwide, malaria and schistosomiasis are the most common causes of secondary MGN. In US, the most important causes of secondary MGN are systemic lupus erythematosus (SLE), neoplasia, hepatitis B infection, and drugs.

1615. Which of the following is false about idiopathic membranous nephropathy (IMN)?
Harrison's 20th Ed. Chapter 308 Page 2144

A. Uniform thickening of BM along peripheral capillary loops
B. Diffuse granular subepithelial deposits of IgG and C3
C. Autoantibodies against M-type phospholipase A2 receptor
D. None of the above

Membranous glomerulonephritis (MGN) is the most common primary cause of the nephrotic syndrome, accounting for ~ 20% of cases. It is characterized by basement membrane thickening and subepithelial immune deposits without cellular proliferation or infiltration. Idiopathic disease has a male and adult predominance. The peak incidence is between 30 and 50 year, and MGN is particularly likely in patients over 50 years of age who present with nephrotic syndrome.

1616. Most cases of idiopathic membranous nephropathy (IMN) have circulating IgG4 autoantibody against?

Harrison's 20th Ed. Chapter 308 Page 2144

A. IL28B
B. PLA2R
C. RIG-1
D. PNPLA3

The detection of anti-PLA2R1 antibodies in patients with nephrotic syndrome is considered as a biomarker for the diagnosis of primary/idiopathic membranous nephropathy (IMN). signifcant sensitivity, Specifcity of anti-PLA2R1 antibodies for IMN has been proposed close to 100%.

1617. Patients of idiopathic membranous nephropathy (IMN) have circulating IgG4 autoantibody against?

Harrison's 20th Ed. Chapter 308 Page 2144

A. α3 NC1 domain of collagen IV
B. Thrombospondin type-1 domain containing 7A (THSD7A)
C. LIM domain region of LMX1B
D. X linked inhibitor of apoptosis protein (XIAP)

Most cases of idiopathic membranous nephropathy (IMN) have circulating IgG4 autoantibody to the podocyte membrane antigen PLA2R. In 70% of cases of IMN, autoantibodies against M-type phospholipase A2 receptor (PLA2R) circulate and bind to a conformational epitope present in PLA2R on human podocytes, producing characteristic in situ deposits. 5–10% of IMN patients have autoantibodies to thrombospondin type-1 domain containing 7A (anti-THSD7A). Both antigens co-localize within glomerular subepithelial deposits with IgG4. Low or absent levels of autoantibodies to PLA2R assist in predicting both spontaneous and treatment associated remissions.

1618. Anti-PLA2R & anti-THSD7A autoantibodies are absent in membranous glomerulopathy due to?

Harrison's 20th Ed. Chapter 308 Page 2144

A. Hepatitis A
B. Hepatitis B
C. Hepatitis C
D. All of the above

Anti-PLA2R & anti-THSD7A autoantibodies are absent in membranous glomerulopathy due to Hepatitis B and sarcoidosis.

1619. In idiopathic membranous nephropathy (IMN), presence of anti-THSD7A antibodies is associated with increased risk of?

Harrison's 20th Ed. Chapter 308 Page 2144

A. Connective tissue disorders
B. Malignancy
C. Alzheimer's disease
D. All of the above

Anti-PLAR1 antibodies are very rare or absent in patients with malignancy.

1620. Which of the following associated with worse prognosis in membranous glomerulonephritis?

Harrison's 20th Ed. Chapter 308 Page 2144

A. Male gender
B. Older age
C. Hypertension
D. All of the above

Male gender, older age, hypertension, and the persistence of proteinuria are associated with worse prognosis in membranous glomerulonephritis.

1621. Which of the following is predictive of progression of membranous glomerulonephritis?

Harrison's 20th Ed. Chapter 308 Page 2144

A. Degree of tubular atrophy
B. Interstitial fibrosis
C. Levels of autoantibodies to PLA2R
D. All of the above

Degree of tubular atrophy or interstitial fibrosis is more predictive of progression of MGN than is the stage of glomerular disease. Increasing or persistently elevated anti-PLA2R levels suggest that development of spontaneous remission is unlikely and support early initiation of immunosuppressive treatment.

1622. Which of the following causes of nephrotic syndrome has the highest incidences of renal vein thrombosis, pulmonary embolism, and deep vein thrombosis?

Harrison's 20th Ed. Chapter 308 Page 2144

A. Minimal change disease (MCD)
B. Focal segmental glomerulosclerosis (FSGS)
C. Membranous glomerulonephritis (MGN)
D. Diabetic nephropathy

Thrombotic complications occur in nephrotic syndrome. MGN has the highest incidence of renal vein thrombosis, pulmonary embolism & deep vein thrombosis. Risk of venous thrombosis is higher when serum albumin is <2–2.5 gram/dL.

1623. Immunosuppressive therapy is indicated in membranous glomerulonephritis in?

Clin J Am Soc Nephrol. 2017;12:983-997

A. Those with elevated anti-PLA2R/THSD7A levels
B. Those with proteinuria >3.5 g/d at diagnosis
C. Those who fail to reduce proteinuria to <3.5 g after 6 months of supportive care or have complications of nephrotic syndrome
D. All of the above

1624. In primary MGN, immunosuppressive drugs recommended include all except?

Harrison's 20th Ed. Chapter 308 Page 2144

A. Methotrexate
B. Chlorambucil
C. Mycophenolate mofetil
D. Cyclosporine

1625. Which of the following is useful in the treatment of primary MGN?

Am J Nephrol 2018;47(suppl 1):30-42

A. Adrenocorticotropic hormone (corticotropin)
B. Bortezomib
C. Belimumab
D. All of the above

1626. Which of the following is an anti-CD20 antibody?

Am J Nephrol 2018;47(suppl 1):30-42

A. Rituximab
B. Obinutuzumab
C. Ofatumumab
D. All of the above

1627. Which of the following is a proteasome inhibitor?
Am J Nephrol 2018;47(suppl 1):30-42

A. Bortezomib
B. Delanzomib
C. Carfilzomib
D. All of the above

1628. Risk factors for the development of diabetic nephropathy include?
Harrison's 20th Ed. Chapter 308 Page 2144

A. Smoking
B. Family history of diabetic nephropathy
C. Gene polymorphisms affecting activity of RAAS axis
D. All of the above

Risk factors for the development of diabetic nephropathy include hyperglycemia, hypertension, dyslipidemia, smoking, family history of diabetic nephropathy, and gene polymorphisms affecting activity of renin angiotensin-aldosterone axis.

1629. How many years after the onset of clinical diabetes, morphologic changes appear in kidneys?
Harrison's 20th Ed. Chapter 308 Page 2144

A. 1–2 years
B. 3–4 years
C. 5–7 years
D. 7–9 years

Within 1–2 years after the onset of clinical diabetes, morphologic changes appear in the kidney.

1630. In Types 1 or 2 diabetes, microalbuminuria appears how many years after the onset of diabetes?
Harrison's 20th Ed. Chapter 308 Page 2145

A. 2–5
B. 5–10
C. 10–15
D. 15–20

In types 1 or 2 diabetes, microalbuminuria appears 5–10 years after its onset.

1631. The glomerular filtration barrier is composed of?
Harrison's 20th Ed. Chapter 308 Page 2145

A. Fenestrated endothelium
B. GBM
C. Podocyte foot processes and slit diaphragms
D. All of the above

Glomerular filtration barrier is composed of fenestrated endothelium, GBM, podocyte foot processes and slit diaphragms.

1632. Podocytes are injured in?
Harrison's 20th Ed. Chapter 308 Page 2145

A. Minimal-change disease
B. FSGS
C. Collapsing glomerulopathy
D. All of the above

Podocytes are injured in minimal-change disease, FSGS, collapsing glomerulopathy, lupus nephritis & DN.

1633. Morphologic changes in diabetic nephropathy affect which of the following renal compartments?
Arch Pathol Lab Med. 2013;137:351-359

A. Glomeruli
B. Tubules
C. Interstitium
D. All of the above

Morphologic changes in diabetic nephropathy affect all 4 renal compartments: glomeruli, tubules, interstitium, and vessels.

1634. The morphologic renal lesions in type 1 diabetes (T1DM) predominantly affect which of the following?
Semin Nephrol. 2007 ;27(2):195-207

A. Glomeruli
B. Renal tubules
C. Interstitium
D. Arterioles

The morphologic lesions in type 1 diabetes (T1DM), predominantly affect the glomeruli, with thickening of glomerular basement membrane (GBM) and mesangial expansion, although also the podocytes, renal tubules, interstitium and arterioles undergo substantial changes, especially at later stages of disease.

1635. Which of the following is first to appear in type 1 diabetes (T1DM)?
Semin Nephrol. 2007 ;27(2):195-207

A. Thickening of glomerular basement membrane (GBM)
B. Thickening of tubular basement membrane (TBM)
C. Mesangial expansion due to increase in mesangial matrix
D. Afferent and efferent arteriolar hyalinosis

GBM thickening, the first measurable change, has been detected as early as 1.5 to 2.5 years after the onset of T1DM.

1636. Which of the following is a late manifestation in type 1 diabetes (T1DM)?
Semin Nephrol. 2007 ;27(2):195-207

A. Mesangial expansion due to increase in mesangial matrix
B. Afferent and efferent arteriolar hyalinosis
C. Abnormalities of the glomerular-tubular junction (GTJA)
D. Thickening of tubular basement membrane (TBM)

Abnormalities of the glomerular-tubular junction (GTJA) as late manifestations of the disease predominantly in patients with proteinuria. GTJA were almost entirely restricted to proteinuric patients, being rare in normoalbuminuric (NA) or microalbuminuric patients (MA).

1637. In diabetes, there is loss of which of the following in the GBM?
Harrison's 20th Ed. Chapter 308 Page 2144

A. Leucine-rich proteins
B. Heparan sulfate moieties
C. Collagenases
D. All of the above

The composition of the GBM is altered in diabetes, particularly the loss of heparan sulfate moieties that form the negatively charged filtration barrier. This results in increased filtration of serum proteins into the urine, predominately negatively charged albumin.

1638. Which of the following histopathological findings occur in diabetic kidneys?
Harrison's 20th Ed. Chapter 308 Page 2144

A. Thickening of GBM
B. Expansion of mesangial matrix
C. Nodular glomerulosclerosis
D. All of the above

Diffuse thickening of GBMs is usually the earliest structural change in diabetes. Tubular basement membranes of nonatrophic tubules are also thickened. Mesangial regions are expanded, predominantly due to accumulation of mesangial matrix. There are no immune complexes. Podocytes show variable foot process effacement, especially in advanced stages.

1639. Key diagnostic feature of diabetic nephropathy is?

Am J Kidney Dis. 2015;66(5):e37-e38

A. Increased mesangial matrix
B. Nodular glomerulosclerosis with diffuse GBM thickening
C. Concomitant hyalinosis of afferent & efferent arterioles
D. All of the above

The pathologic hallmark of diabetic nephropathy is diabetic glomerulosclerosis that results from a progressive increase in extracellular matrix in the glomerular mesangium and glomerular basement membranes.

1640. Diabetic nephropathy is most commonly complicated by which of the following kidney disease?

Arch Pathol Lab Med. 2013;137:351-359

A. Membranous nephropathy
B. Acute postinfectious glomerulonephritis
C. IgA nephropathy
D. Lupus nephritis

Hyperglycaemia may cause different patterns of renal injury in T1DM compared to T2DM patients. T2DM diabetic nephropathy is probably the most common renal disease to be complicated by another distinct identifiable kidney disease, membranous nephropathy is by far the most common. Other non-diabetic renal diseases with DN include acute post-infectious glomerulonephritis, IgA nephropathy, crescentic glomerulonephritis, membranoproliferative glomerulonephritis (types I and II), lupus nephritis, nonspecific immune complex disease, and amyloid.

1641. Light microscopy characteristic features of diabetic nephropathy include?

Arch Pathol Lab Med. 2013;137:351-359

A. Glomerular hypertrophy
B. Uniform thickening of glomerular basement membrane (GBM)
C. Increase of mesangial matrix – diffuse
D. All of the above

1642. Light microscopy characteristic features of diabetic nephropathy include?

Arch Pathol Lab Med. 2013;137:351-359

A. Kimmelstiel–Wilson nodules
B. Podocyte hypertrophy & foot process broadening & effacement
C. Hyalinosis of glomerular peripheral capillaries (plasmatic insudation)
D. All of the above

1643. Light microscopy characteristic features of diabetic nephropathy include?

Arch Pathol Lab Med. 2013;137:351-359

A. Aneurysmal peripheral glomerular capillaries
B. Capsular drops
C. Extracapillary proliferation (fibro-cellular crescents)
D. All of the above

1644. Light microscopy characteristic features of diabetic nephropathy include?

Arch Pathol Lab Med. 2013;137:351-359

A. Hyalinosis of afferent and efferent arterioles
B. Thickening of the tubular basement membrane (TBM)
C. Chronic interstitial inflammation and fibrosis
D. All of the above

1645. Ultrastructural characteristic features of diabetic nephropathy include?

Arch Pathol Lab Med. 2013;137:351-359

A. Typical uniform thickening of GBM & TBM
B. Capsular drops
C. Plasmatic insudation of glomerular capillaries
D. All of the above

Glomerular insudative lesions are one of the characteristic histological features of diabetic nephropathy (DN). They are commonly known as capsular drops and fibrin caps, which are located between the parietal epithelium and Bowman's capsule or within the glomerular capillary lumen, respectively.

1646. Which of the following is pathognomic of diabetic nephropathy?

Arch Pathol Lab Med. 2013;137:351-359

A. Well-formed, intercapillary, nodular mesangial lesions
B. Thickened glomerular and tubular basement membranes
C. Hyaline arteriolosclerosis
D. All of the above

The well-formed, intercapillary, nodular mesangial lesions, along with thickened glomerular basement membranes and tubular basement membranes, and hyaline arteriolosclerosis are virtually pathognomic of diabetic nephropathy.

1647. Kimmelstiel-Wilson lesion relates best with which of the following histopathological findings in diabetic kidney?

Harrison's 20th Ed. Chapter 308 Page 2144

A. Thickening of GBM
B. Expansion of mesangial matrix
C. Nodular glomerulosclerosis
D. Hyaline arteriosclerosis

Kimmelstiel-Wilson (1936) nodules or nodular glomerulosclerosis are eosinophilic, PAS⁺ & Jones silver stain⁺ nodules. Nodular lesions are the pathological hallmark of human diabetic nephropathy (DN). The classic Kimmelstiel Wilson nodules are postulated to be the consequence of repeated mesangiolysis, with an exuberant repair response.

1648. Which of the following about Kimmelstiel-Wilson nodules is false?

Arch Pathol Lab Med. 2013;137:351-359

A. Measure 40 to 100 μm in diameter
B. Acellular
C. PAS^+ and $silver^+$
D. None of the above

The characteristic KW nodules measure 40 to 100 μm in diameter. These nodules are PAS^+ and $silver^+$ and are usually acellular, although nuclei may be present in the periphery in a circumferential manner.

1649. Which of the following lesions can be seen in diabetic nephropathy?

Arch Pathol Lab Med. 2013;137:351-359

A. Fibrin cap
B. Capsular drop
C. Tubular atrophy, tubular apoptosis, thickened tubular BM
D. All of the above

1650. Which of the following is false about hyalinotic/exudative lesion/fibrin cap in diabetic nephropathy?

Arch Pathol Lab Med. 2013;137:351-359

A. Accumulation of hyaline, eosinophilic, homogeneous material between endothelial cells & GBM of capillary loops
B. Made up of trapped plasma proteins (IgM & C1q)
C. May occlude capillary lumen
D. None of the above

Term insudative lesion is preferable over 'exudative lesion' because these lesions are localized 'inside' the lumen. The term fibrin cap is poorly chosen because these lesions actually consist of plasma proteins with a homogeneous, glassy, and hyaline appearance, as well as lipid droplets, but do not contain fibrin.

1651. Which of the following lesion is associated with the renal prognosis of DN patients?

Harrison's 20th Ed. Chapter 308 Page 2145

A. Glomerular and arteriolar insudative lesions
B. Interstitial fibrosis
C. Tubular atrophy
D. All of the above

Recent studies of biopsy-proven DN have demonstrated that glomerular and arteriolar insudative lesions are associated with the renal prognosis of DN patients, although the association is not as strong as interstitial fibrosis and tubular atrophy (IFTA) or nodular lesions.

1652. The Armanni-Ebstein lesion is associated with?

Forensic Sci Med Pathol. 2012;8(1):19-22

A. Membranous nephropathy
B. Diabetic ketoacidosis
C. Renal amyloidosis
D. Fabry's disease

The Armanni-Ebstein lesion is a histological change in the kidney consisting of sub-nuclear vacuolation of the proximal tubules. It has been most associated with diabetic ketoacidosis.

1653. Nodular glomerulosclerosis can also be seen in?

Am J Kidney Dis. 2015;66(5):e37-e38

A. Monoclonal immunoglobulin deposition disease (MIDD)
B. Amyloidosis
C. Membranoproliferative glomerulonephritides
D. All of the above

Nodular glomerulosclerosis can also be seen in monoclonal immunoglobulin deposition disease (MIDD), amyloidosis, idiopathic nodular glomerulosclerosis, membranoproliferative glomerulonephritides.

1654. Which of the following renal morphological lesion stain positive by silver stain?

Arch Pathol Lab Med. 2013;137:351-359

A. Diabetic Nephropathy
B. Monoclonal Immunoglobulin Deposition Disease
C. Amyloidosis
D. Immunotactoid Glomerulonephritis

1655. Which of the following renal morphological lesion does not stain positive by periodic acid–Schiff (PAS)?

Arch Pathol Lab Med. 2013;137:351-359

A. Diabetic Nephropathy
B. Monoclonal Immunoglobulin Deposition Disease
C. Amyloidosis
D. Immunotactoid Glomerulonephritis

1656. Which of the following renal morphological lesion does not stain positive by Congo red?

Arch Pathol Lab Med. 2013;137:351-359

A. Diabetic Nephropathy
B. Monoclonal Immunoglobulin Deposition Disease
C. Amyloidosis
D. Immunotactoid Glomerulonephritis

1657. Which of the following is different between type 1 & type 2 diabetes?

Harrison's 20th Ed. Chapter 308 Page 2145

A. Natural history of diabetic nephropathy
B. Renal biopsy findings
C. Onset of microalbuminuria
D. Presence of diabetic retinopathy

Renal biopsies from patients with Types 1 and 2 diabetes are largely indistinguishable. Natural history of diabetic nephropathy in patients with Types 1 and 2 diabetes is similar. >90% of Type 1 diabetics with nephropathy have diabetic retinopathy while only 60% of Type 2 diabetics with nephropathy have diabetic retinopathy.

1658. The pathologic changes in diabetic nephropathy are the result of?

Harrison's 20th Ed. Chapter 308 Page 2145

A. Intraglomerular hypertension
B. Direct effects of hyperglycemia on actin cytoskeleton of renal mesangial & vascular smooth-muscle cells
C. Diabetes-associated changes in circulating factors
D. All of the above

1659. Diabetes-associated changes occur in which of the following circulating factors?

Harrison's 20th Ed. Chapter 308 Page 2145

A. Atrial natriuretic factor
B. Angiotensin II
C. Insulin-like growth factor (IGF)
D. All of the above

1660. Sustained glomerular hypertension leads to?

Harrison's 20th Ed. Chapter 308 Page 2145

A. Increased mesangial matrix production
B. Alterations in GBM with disruption in filtration barrier
C. Glomerulosclerosis
D. All of the above

1661. In diabetic nephropathy, mesangial matrix production is altered by?

Harrison's 20th Ed. Chapter 308 Page 2145

A. Accumulation of advanced glycosylation end products (AGE)
B. Growth hormone
C. IGF-I
D. All of the above

1662. In diabetic nephropathy, mesangial matrix production is altered by?

Harrison's 20th Ed. Chapter 308 Page 2145

A. Angiotensin II
B. Connective tissue growth factor
C. TGF-β
D. All of the above

1663. In microalbuminuria, the range of albuminuria is?

Harrison's 20th Ed. Chapter 308 Page 2145

A. <150 mg/day
B. 20–200 mg/day
C. 30–300 mg/day
D. 40–400 mg/day

Albuminuria in the range of 30 - 300 mg/day is called microalbuminuria. Or, microalbuminuria is defined as urinary albumin excretion ≥30 and <300 mg/gCr.

1664. Dipstick positive level of albuminuria is?

Harrison's 20th Ed. Chapter 308 Page 2145

A. >30 mg
B. >150 mg
C. >300 mg
D. >500 mg

Dipstick positive level of proteinuria is >300 mg albuminuria. Macroalbuminuria is urinary albumin excretion ≥300 mg/gCr and overt proteinuria is macroalbuminuria exceeding 1 g/day.

1665. In diabetes, renal functions unrelentingly decline after what level of proteinuria?

Harrison's 20th Ed. Chapter 308 Page 2145

A. >500 mg/day
B. >1000 mg/day
C. >1500 mg/day
D. >2500 mg/day

1666. From the earliest stages of microalbuminuria, it takes how many years to reach end-stage renal disease (ESRD)?

Harrison's 20th Ed. Chapter 308 Page 2145

A. 5–10 years
B. 10–20 years
C. 20–30 years
D. >30 years

After proteinuria level of >500 mg/day, renal function decline relentlessly. From the stage of microalbuminuria, it usually takes 10–20 years to reach ESRD.

1667. Which of the following statements is false?

Harrison's 20th Ed. Chapter 308 Page 2145

A. >90% patients with type 1 diabetes & nephropathy have diabetic retinopathy
B. 60% patients with type 2 diabetes with nephropathy have diabetic retinopathy
C. Significant correlation between presence of retinopathy & presence of Kimmelstiel-Wilson nodules
D. None of the above

1668. Which of the following class of drugs may be of benefit in diabetic nephropathy?

Harrison's 20th Ed. Chapter 308 Page 2145

A. Sodium glucose transport 2 inhibitors
B. Endothelin antagonists
C. Aldosterone antagonists
D. All of the above

1669. Which of the following is a renin inhibitor?

Harrison's 20th Ed. Chapter 308 Page 2145

A. Bosentan
B. Aliskiren
C. Empagliflozin
D. Eplerenone

1670. Which of the following is an endothelin antagonist?

Harrison's 20th Ed. Chapter 308 Page 2145

A. Bosentan
B. Aliskiren
C. Empagliflozin
D. Eplerenone

1671. Which of the following is a SGLT2 inhibitor?

Harrison's 20th Ed. Chapter 308 Page 2145

A. Bosentan
B. Aliskiren
C. Empagliflozin
D. Eplerenone

1672. Which of the following is an aldosterone antagonist?

Harrison's 20th Ed. Chapter 308 Page 2145

A. Bosentan
B. Aliskiren
C. Empagliflozin
D. Eplerenone

Aliskiren is an oral, nonpeptide competitive inhibitors of the enzymatic activity of renin. Bosentan is an endothelin antagonist. Spironolactone & eplerenone are aldosterone antagonists. Empagliflozin, canagliflozin & dapagliflozin are SGLT2 inhibitors.

1673. Which of the following about Light Chain Deposition Disease (LCDD) is false?

Harrison's 20th Ed. Chapter 308 Page 2145

A. Produce kappa light chains
B. Light-chain deposits are not fibrillar
C. Light-chain deposits do not stain with Congo red
D. None of the above

Light Chain Deposition Disease (LCDD) produces nephrotic syndrome with renal failure. Congo red negative nodular deposition of nonamyloid immunoglobulin light chains is the most common pathologic finding in light chain deposition disease in light microscopy. Immunoflurescent microscopy usually demonstrates the presence of monotypic kappa light chain. Nodular glomerulosclerosis of LCDD resembles diabetic Kimmelstiel-Wilson.

1674. Which of the following about Light Chain Deposition Disease (LCDD) is false?

J Renal Inj Prev. 2013; 2(4): 127–128

A. Clinical picture is like rapidly progressive glomerulonephritis
B. Proteinuria is a combination of light chain and albumin
C. Nodular glomerulosclerosis resembles diabetic KW lesion
D. None of the above

1675. Which of the following causes renal failure but not heavy proteinuria?

Harrison's 20th Ed. Chapter 308 Page 2145

A. Amyloidosis
B. Light chain deposition disease
C. Cast nephropathy (myeloma kidney)
D. All of the above

1676. Renal vein thrombosis is common in patients with nephrotic syndrome due to?

Harrison's 20th Ed. Chapter 308 Page 2145

A. Membranous glomerulopathy
B. Membranoproliferative glomerulonephritis
C. Amyloidosis
D. All of the above

1677. Clinical features that suggest acute renal vein thrombosis include all except?

Harrison's 19th Ed. 1845

A. Sudden onset of flank or abdominal pain
B. Gross hematuria
C. Right-sided varicocele
D. Acute decline in GFR

Clinical features that suggest acute renal vein thrombosis include light-sided varicocele.

1678. Congo red stains are positive in?

Harrison's 20th Ed. Chapter 308 Page 2145

A. AA & AL amyloidosis
B. Fibrillary-Immunotactoid Glomerulopathy
C. Light chain deposition disease
D. All of the above

AA and AL amyloid fibrils are detectable with Congo red.

1679. Organs that amyloid infiltrates include?

Harrison's 20th Ed. Chapter 308 Page 2145

A. Peripheral nerves
B. Upper pharynx
C. Kidney
D. All of the above

Amyloid infiltrates the liver, heart, peripheral nerves, carpal tunnel, upper pharynx, and kidney.

1680. In systemic AL amyloidosis (primary amyloidosis), excess light chain are made into fragments by?

Harrison's 20th Ed. Chapter 308 Page 2145

A. Lymphocytes
B. Eosinophils
C. Macrophages
D. All of the above

In systemic AL amyloidosis, also called primary amyloidosis, light chains produced in excess by clonal plasma cell dyscrasias are made into fragments by macrophages leading to self-aggregation at an acid pH.

1681. Which of the following statements about primary amyloidosis is false?

Harrison's 20th Ed. Chapter 308 Page 2145

A. Excess light chains produced by clonal plasma cell dyscrasias
B. Predominant light chains are of lambda class
C. Light chain fragments self-aggregate at acid pH
D. None of the above

1682. AL amyloidosis occurs in the setting of?

Harrison's 20th Ed. Chapter 308 Page 2145

A. Multiple myeloma (MM)
B. Waldenström's macroglobulinemia
C. Lymphoma
D. All of the above

AL amyloidosis occurs in the setting of multiple myeloma (MM), Waldenström's macroglobulinemia, lymphoma, other plasmacytomas, or lymphoproliferative disorders, or without any other identifiable disease.

1683. Which of the following is true about AA amyloidosis or secondary amyloidosis?

Harrison's 20th Ed. Chapter 308 Page 2145

A. Deposition of α-pleated sheets of serum amyloid A protein
B. Deposition of β-pleated sheets of serum amyloid A protein
C. Deposition of γ-pleated sheets of serum amyloid A protein
D. Deposition of δ-pleated sheets of serum amyloid A protein

AA amyloidosis (secondary amyloidosis) is due to deposition of β-pleated sheets of serum amyloid A protein.

1684. Which of the following is true about serum amyloid A protein?

Harrison's 20th Ed. Chapter 308 Page 2145

A. Acute phase reactant
B. Membrane cofactor protein
C. Complement-regulatory protein
D. Lithogenic factor

Serum amyloid A (SAA) protein is an apolipoprotein of high-density lipoproteins that serves as a dynamic acute phase reactant. It is synthesized as a precursor by hepatocytes in response to transcriptional stimuli from various proinflammatory cytokines, such as interleukin (IL)-1, IL-6, and tumor necrosis factor (TNF) alpha.

1685. Which of the following is a positive acute-phase reactant?

Harrison's 20th Ed. Chapter 308 Page 2145

A. Ceruloplasmin
B. C-reactive protein
C. Transferrin
D. All of the above

1686. Which of the following is not a positive acute-phase reactant?

Harrison's 20th Ed. Chapter 308 Page 2145

A. Ferritin
B. Thrombocytosis
C. Serum amyloid A (SAA)
D. Albumin

Negative acute-phase reactants are albumin and fetuin. Serum amyloid A protein (SAA), a hepatic acute phase reactant.

1687. Which of the following is the function of serum amyloid A protein?

Harrison's 20th Ed. Chapter 308 Page 2146

A. Cholesterol transport
B. Immune cell attraction
C. Metalloproteases activation
D. All of the above

Serum amyloid A protein, an acute phase reactant whose physiologic functions include cholesterol transport, immune cell attraction and metalloproteases activation.

1688. Which of the following is the most common type of amyloidosis worldwide?

Clin Epidemiol. 2014;6:369-377

A. Primary AL amyloidosis
B. Secondary amyloid A (AA) amyloidosis
C. Familial amyloidosis
D. β2-microglobulin related amyloidosis

AA amyloidosis is the most common type of amyloidosis worldwide.

1689. Familial amyloidosis best relates to?

Clin Epidemiol. 2014;6:369-377

A. Serum amyloid A protein
B. Mutant transthyretin
C. β2-microglobulin
D. Light chains

1690. Amyloid A hereditary (AH) best relates to?

Clin Epidemiol. 2014;6:369-377

A. Serum amyloid A protein
B. Mutant transthyretin
C. β2-microglobulin
D. Light chains

1691. Which of the following diseases is related to serum amyloid A protein?

Harrison's 20th Ed. Chapter 308 Page 2146

A. Rheumatoid arthritis
B. Familial Mediterranean fever (FMF)
C. Muckle–Wells syndrome
D. All of the above

Autoimmune diseases such as rheumatoid arthritis, ankylosing spondylitis, chronic juvenile arthritis, and inflammatory bowel disease, or hereditary inflammatory diseases, such as FMF, TNF receptor-associated periodic syndrome, or Muckle–Wells syndrome, account for up to 90% of recent cases of AA amyloidosis.

1692. Which of the following is the most frequent clinical manifestation that should raise suspicion of AA amyloidosis?

Harrison's 20th Ed. Chapter 308 Page 2146

A. Hematuria
B. Proteinuria
C. Hepatosplenomegaly
D. Adrenal insufficiency

Proteinuria leading to nephrotic syndrome and renal insufficiency is the earliest and most frequent clinical manifestation that should raise suspicion of AA amyloidosis.

1693. Which of the following is the preferred site for biopsy for the diagnosis of amyloidosis?

Harrison's 20th Ed. Chapter 308 Page 2146

A. Rectal mucosa
B. Gingival mucosa
C. Abdominal fat pad aspirates
D. Minor salivary gland biopsy

In 1973, Westermark & Stenkvist described subcutaneous abdominal fat tissue aspiration as a new, noninvasive technique, and this has now become the preferred initial option in most centers throughout the world.

1694. Which of the following drugs is useful in the treatment for primary amyloidosis?

Harrison's 20th Ed. Chapter 308 Page 2146

A. Busulfan
B. Melphalan
C. Cyclophosphamide
D. Chlorambucil

The median survival of patients with primary amyloidosis is <2 years, with death usually from progressive congestive heart failure or renal failure. Chemotherapy with melphalan, prednisone, and colchicine, to reduce the concentration of monoclonal proteins, and autologous stem cell transplantation may prolong survival. Melphalan inhibits mitosis by cross-linking DNA strands. Colchicine decreases leukocyte motility and phagocytosis in inflammatory responses.

1695. Which of the following is false about fibrillary-immunotactoid glomerulopathy?

Harrison's 20th Ed. Chapter 308 Page 2146

A. Glomerular accumulation of nonbranching randomly arranged fibrils
B. Nonamyloid fibrillary disease not associated with a systemic illness
C. Congo red stains are negative
D. None of the above

The cause of this "nonamyloid" immunotactoid glomerulopathy is idiopathic, with an occasional association with chronic lymphocytic leukemia or B cell lymphoma.

1696. Which of the following best relates to Fabry's Disease?

Harrison's 20th Ed. Chapter 308 Page 2146

A. Glucosylceramide
B. Galactosylceramide
C. Globotriaosylceramide
D. Ceramide

Fabry disease is an X-linked inborn error of globotriaosylceramide metabolism secondary to deficient lysosomal α-galactosidase A activity (mutations in α-galactosidase gene), resulting in excessive intracellular storage of globotriaosylceramide.

1697. Organ affected in Fabry's disease is?

Harrison's 20th Ed. Chapter 308 Page 2146

A. Heart
B. Brain
C. Kidney
D. All of the above

Organs affected in Fabry's disease include the vascular endothelium, heart, brain, and kidneys.

1698. Classically, Fabry's disease presents with?

Harrison's 20th Ed. Chapter 308 Page 2146

A. Acroparesthesias
B. Angiokeratoma
C. Hypohidrosis
D. All of the above

Classically, Fabry's disease presents in childhood in males with acroparesthesias, angiokeratoma, and hypohidrosis.

1699. Clinical manifestations of Fabry's disease include all except?

Harrison's 20th Ed. Chapter 411 Page 3007, N Engl J Med. 2001;345:9-16

A. Angiokeratomas
B. Corneal and lenticular opacities
C. Small-vessel disease of the kidney
D. Macrocephaly

Fabry's disease is also known as angiokeratoma corpus diffusum or Anderson-Fabry disease. Clinically, Fabry's disease manifests as angiokeratomas (telangiectatic skin lesions), hypohidrosis, corneal and lenticular opacities (cornea verticillata), painful acroparesthesia, and small-vessel disease of kidney, heart, & brain.

1700. Which of the following is false about Fabry's disease?

Harrison's 20th Ed. Chapter 411 Page 3007

A. X-linked dominant disorder
B. Due to mutations in GALA that encodes α-galactosidase A
C. Accumulation of ceramide trihexoside in nerves, blood vessels
D. None of the above

1701. Angiokeratomas is a clinical feature of?

Br J Dermatol 1997;136594- 597

A. Fabry's disease
B. β-Mannosidosis
C. Fucosidosis
D. All of the above

Angiokeratomas are also seen in mannosidosis, fucosidosis, sialidosis, and β-galactosidase and β-hexosaminidase deficiency.

1702. In Fabry's disease, angiokeratomas are most dense?

Harrison's 20th Ed. Chapter 308 Page 2146

A. Over nape of the neck
B. Over fingertips
C. Between umbilicus and knees
D. Over forehead

In Fabry's disease, angiokeratomas (telangiectatic skin lesions) are most dense between umbilicus and knees "the bathing suit area" but may occur anywhere, including mucosal surfaces.

1703. In renal biopsy, "Zebra bodies" is a histopathological hallmark of?

Harrison's 20th Ed. Chapter 308 Page 2146

A. Fabry's disease
B. β-Mannosidosis
C. Fucosidosis
D. All of the above

In Fabry's disease, electron microscopy of renal biopsy shows enlarged glomerular visceral epithelial cells packed with vacuoles containing globotriaosylceramide in parallel arrays called zebra bodies.

1704. Nephropathy of Fabry's disease typically progresses to renal failure in which decade of life?

Harrison's 20th Ed. Chapter 308 Page 2146

A. First
B. Second
C. Third
D. Fourth

Nephropathy of Fabry's disease progresses to renal failure by the fourth or fifh decade. Nephropathy typically presents in the third decade of life as mild to moderate proteinuria, sometimes with microscopic hematuria or nephrotic syndrome.

1705. Which of the following is found in the urine of patients with Fabry's disease?

Harrison's 20th Ed. Chapter 308 Page 2146

A. Eosinophils
B. Maltese cross
C. Randall's plaque
D. Waxy casts

In Fabry's disease, urinalysis may reveal oval fat bodies and birefringent glycolipid globules under polarized light called maltese cross.

1706. In Fabry's disease, neutral glycosphingolipids accumulate in which orgenelle of glomerular cells?

Harrison's 20th Ed. Chapter 308 Page 2146

A. Mitochondria
B. Golgi apparatus
C. Lysosome
D. Nucleus

1707. The dose of recombinant α-galactosidase A in Fabry's disease is?

N Engl J Med. 2001;345:9-16

A. 1 mg/kg
B. 2 mg/kg
C. 3 mg/kg
D. 4 mg/kg

The dose of 1 mg of recombinant α-galactosidase A per kilogram every other week for about six months to one year safely and effectively reversed the accumulation of microvascular endothelial deposits of globotriaosylceramide in the kidneys, heart, and skin.

1708. Which of the following is included in pulmonary renal syndromes?

Harrison's 20th Ed. Chapter 308 Page 2146

A. Goodpasture's syndrome
B. Henoch-Schonlein purpura
C. Cryoglobulinemia
D. All of the above

Pulmonary renal syndromes present with catastrophic hemoptysis and glomerulonephritis associated with varying degrees of renal failure. The usual causes include Goodpasture's syndrome, granulomatosis with polyangiitis, microscopic polyangiitis, Churg-Strauss vasculitis and Henoch-Schonlein purpura or cryoglobulinemia.

1709. Which of the following is a component of glomerular basement membrane?

Harrison's 20th Ed. Chapter 308 Page 2146

A. Collagen IV
B. Laminins
C. Nidogen
D. All of the above

1710. Kidney basement membrane is made of?

Harrison's 20th Ed. Chapter 308 Page 2146

A. Collagen IV with laminins
B. Nidogen
C. Sulfated proteoglycans
D. All of the above

kidney epithelia, including podocytes, rest on basement membranes assembled into a planar surface through the interweaving of collagen IV with laminins, nidogen and sulfated proteoglycans.

1711. Which of the following triple-helical protomer is present in glomerular & tubular basement membrane?

Harrison's 20th Ed. Chapter 308 Page 2146

A. α1.α1.α2(IV) collagen
B. α3.α4.α5(IV) collagen
C. α5.α5.α6(IV) collagen
D. All of the above

1712. Which of the following triple-helical protomer is present along Bowman's capsule in the kidney?

Harrison's 20th Ed. Chapter 308 Page 2146

A. α1.α1.α2(IV) collagen
B. α3.α4.α5(IV) collagen
C. α5.α5.α6(IV) collagen
D. All of the above

All epithelial basement membranes early in human development are composed of interconnected triple-helical protomers rich in α1.α1.α2(IV) collagen. The α1 (IV) and α2 (IV) chains are ubiquitous in all basement membranes. Specialized tissues like kidney (glomerular and tubular basement membrane), lung, testis, cochlea, and eye undergo a developmental switch replacing α1.α1.α2(IV) protomers with an α3.α4.α5(IV) collagen network. In skin, smooth muscle, esophagus and along Bowman's capsule in the kidney, α5.α5.α6(IV) collagen network appears. This modification provides more resistance to proteases and ensures the structural longevity of critical tissues.

1713. Which of the following is false about Alport's syndrome?
Harrison's 20th Ed. Chapter 308 Page 2146

A. Hematuria
B. Thinning and splitting of GBMs
C. Mild proteinuria
D. None of the above

1714. The triad of clinical findings of Alport syndrome includes all except?
Harrison's 20th Ed. Chapter 308 Page 2147

A. Hemorrhagic nephritis
B. Proteinuria
C. Sensorineural hearing loss
D. Characteristic ocular findings

Alport syndrome is an oculo-renal syndrome characterized by a triad of clinical findings consisting of hemorrhagic nephritis, sensorineural hearing loss and characteristic ocular findings.

1715. Which of the following is false about Alport's syndrome?
Harrison's 20th Ed. Chapter 308 Page 2147

A. Inherited tubulointerstitial disease
B. Due to mutation in COL4A5 gene
C. Hematuria, glomerulosclerosis & renal failure
D. Usually X linked

Chronic glomerulosclerosis is a feature of Alport's syndrome. Mutations in COL4A5 (X-linked), COL4A3, or COL4A4 (both autosomal recessive) genes result in defective synthesis of collagen type IV with consequent dysfunction and inflammation of the glomerular basement membrane.

1716. Which of the following is related to Alport's syndrome?
Harrison's 20th Ed. Chapter 308 Page 2147

A. Ataxia
B. Sensorineural deafness
C. Alopecia
D. Jaundice

Alport's syndrome consists of hematuria, proteinuria (<1 to 2 gram/day), progressive renal failure and sensorineural deafness. In the early stages, hearing impairment is detectable only by audiometry, with bilateral hearing loss of high tones in frequencies ranging from 2000-8000 hertz (Hz).

1717. Ocular manifestations of Alport's syndrome include?
Harrison's 20th Ed. Chapter 308 Page 2147

A. Anterior lenticonus
B. Dot-and-fleck retinopathy
C. Temporal macular thinning
D. All of the above

In Alport's syndrome, central part of the lens projects anteriorly 3-4 mm in an axial projection as seen on biomicroscopic examination. The condition is usually bilateral & causes a slowly progressive axial myopia. Numerous bilateral, white and yellow perimacular dots and flecks occur in this condition. These spare the fovea but can spread to the periphery. No associated visual impairment or night blindness occurs. Typically, dot-and-fleck retinopathy does not fluoresce with angiography.

1718. Which of the following is considered pathognomonic of Alport's syndrome?
Harrison's 20th Ed. Chapter 308 Page 2147

A. Anterior lenticonus
B. Sensorineural hearing loss
C. Hematuria
D. Leiomyomatosis

Anterior lenticonus is the most specific & is pathognomonic extrarenal manifestation of Alport's syndrome (AS). It also is a valuable marker of the severity of AS, being consistently associated with both a rapid progression to renal failure and hearing loss. Lenticonus is never present at birth.

1719. Positive "oil droplet sign" in Alport's syndrome pertains to?
N Engl J Med. 2003;348:2543-56, Harrison's 20th Ed. Chapter 308 Page 2147

A. Ocular lens
B. Tongue
C. Nails
D. Nose

In Alport's syndrome, lenticonus of anterior lens capsule is termed as positive "oil droplet sign". Distinctive oil droplet appearance on the red reflex on slit lamp examination is characteristic of Alport's syndrome.

1720. Which of the following suggests a poorer prognosis in Alport's syndrome?
Harrison's 20th Ed. Chapter 308 Page 2147

A. Early severe deafness
B. Lenticonus
C. Proteinuria
D. All of the above

Early severe deafness, lenticonus, or proteinuria suggests a poorer prognosis.

1721. In Alport's syndrome, skin biopsy revealing the lack of which of the following collagen chain helps in diagnosis?
Harrison's 20th Ed. Chapter 308 Page 2147

A. $\alpha 2$(IV)
B. $\alpha 3$(IV)
C. $\alpha 4$(IV)
D. $\alpha 5$(IV)

Since α5(IV) collagen is expressed in the skin, some X-linked Alport's patients can be diagnosed with a skin biopsy revealing the lack of the α5(IV) collagen chain on immunofluorescent analysis.

1722. Hereditary disorder that may include renal involvement and hearing loss is?
Kidney International. 1999;56:760-775

A. Muckle-Wells syndrome
B. Cockayne's syndrome
C. Alström's syndrome
D. All of the above

1723. Hereditary disorder that may include renal involvement and hearing loss is?
Kidney International. 1999;56:760-775

A. Bardet-Biedl syndrome
B. Refsum's disease
C. Charcot-Marie-Tooth syndrome
D. All of the above

A specific mitochondrial DNA (mtDNA) mutation (a guanine for adenine substitution at position 3243) is responsible for a syndrome combining diabetes mellitus, sensorineural deafness, & progressive renal failure.

1724. Thin basement membrane disease (TBMD) is typically associated with?
Harrison's 20th Ed. Chapter 308 Page 2147

A. Proteinuria
B. Hypertension
C. Loss of renal function
D. None of the above

Thin basement membrane disease (TBMD) characterized by persistent or recurrent hematuria is not typically associated with proteinuria, hypertension, or loss of renal function or extrarenal disease.

1725. Which of the following is false about thin basement membrane disease (TBMD)?

Harrison's 20th Ed. Chapter 308 Page 2147

A. Also called benign familial hematuria
B. Genetic defects in type IV collagen
C. Diffuse thinning of GBM
D. None of the above

1726. Which of the following is a heritable form of CKD?

Harrison's 20th Ed. Chapter 308 Page 2147

A. Alport's syndrome
B. Fabry disease
C. Cystinosis
D. All of the above

Alport syndrome, Fabry disease and cystinosis are a heritable form of CKD.

1727. Which of the following statements about 'Nail-patella syndrome' is false?

N Engl J Med. 2006;354:1387-401, Harrison's 20th Ed. Chapter 308 Page 2147

A. It an autosomal dominant disease
B. More common in females
C. Primarily affect patella, elbows and nails
D. None of the above

Skeletal features include absent or hypoplastic patellae, patella dislocations, elbow abnormalities, talipes, and iliac horns on X-ray. NPS is caused by loss of function mutations in the transcription factor LMX1B at 9q34.

1728. Nail-patella syndrome (NPS) is also known as?

Journal of Medical Genetics 2003;40:153-162

A. Hereditary osteo-onychodysplasia (HOOD)
B. Fong disease
C. Turner-Kieser syndrome
D. All of the above

Nail-patella syndrome (NPS) (OMIM 161200), also known as hereditary osteo-onychodysplasia (HOOD), Fong disease, Turner-Kieser syndrome, and Österreicher-Turner syndrome, is a pleiotropic condition with a classical clinical tetrad involving the nails, knees, elbows, and the presence of iliac horns.

1729. Which of the following is a clinical feature of Nail-patella syndrome?

Journal of Medical Genetics. 2003;40:153-162

A. Abnormal muscle distribution in upper arms
B. Nails may be absent, hypoplastic, or dystrophic
C. Patellae may be small, irregularly shaped, or absent
D. All of the above

Lean body habitus, poorly developed biceps & triceps muscles with full development of deltoids & forearm muscles are seen in Nail-patella syndrome. The nail changes may be limited to triangular lunules. A sensitive sign of digital involvement in NPS is loss of the creases in the skin overlying the distal interphalangeal (DIP) joints of the fingers.

1730. Which of the following is a clinical feature of Nail-patella syndrome?

Journal of Medical Genetics. 2003;40:153-162

A. Iliac horns
B. High forehead and hairline
C. Irregular thickening of GBM ("moth eaten" appearance)
D. All of the above

Features of Nail-patella syndrome are iliac horns which are bilateral, conical, bony processes that project posteriorly & laterally from central part of iliac bones of the pelvis. Also, irregular thickening of GBM giving it a mottled "moth eaten" appearance is seen. Lester's sign consists of a zone of darker pigmentation around the central part of iris, which is roughly a cloverleaf or flower shaped.

1731. Which of the following is a clinical feature of Nail-patella syndrome?

Journal of Medical Genetics. 2003;40:153-162

A. Cleft lip and palate
B. Deafness
C. Mental retardation
D. None of the above

1732. Which of the following statements about Nail-patella syndrome is false?

N Engl J Med. 2006;354:1387-401, Harrison's 20th Ed. Chapter 308 Page 2147

A. Glomerular basement membrane is thickened with splitting and fibrillar collagen deposits
B. Caused by loss-of-function mutations in *LMX1B*
C. *LMX1B* is expressed in kidney primarily by podocytes
D. None of the above

1733. LMX1B regulates the expression of genes encoding?

Harrison's 20th Ed. Chapter 308 Page 2147

A. α3 and α4 chains of collagen IV
B. Interstitial type III collagen
C. Podocin
D. All of the above

LMX1B regulates the expression of genes encoding α3 and α4 chains of collagen IV, interstitial type III collagen, podocin and CD2AP that help form the slit-pore membranes connecting podocytes.

1734. Which of the following may be present in Nail-patella syndrome?

Harrison's 20th Ed. Chapter 308 Page 2148

A. Neural-sensory hearing impairment
B. Glaucoma
C. Iliac horns on the pelvis
D. All of the above

Iliac horns are bilateral, conical, bony processes that project posteriorly and laterally from the central part of the iliac bones of the pelvis and are considered "pathognomonic" of NPS.

1735. Which of the following is a finding in renal biopsy in Nail-patella syndrome?

Harrison's 20th Ed. Chapter 308 Page 2148

A. Focal sclerosing glomerulonephritis
B. Lucent damage to the lamina densa of GBM
C. Increase in collagen III fibrils along glomerular capillaries and in mesangium
D. All of the above

In Nail-patella syndrome, renal biopsy shows focal sclerosing glomerulonephritis with specific lucent damage to lamina densa of the GBM, an increase in collagen III fibrils along glomerular capillaries and in the mesangium, and damage to slit-pore membrane.

1736. What magnitude of glomeruli are normally sclerotic by the age of 60 years?

Harrison's 20th Ed. Chapter 308 Page 2148

A. 10%
B. 20%
C. 30%
D. 40%

~10% of glomeruli are normally sclerotic by age 40, rising to 20% by age 60 and 30% by age 80.

1737. Which of the following is false about apolipoprotein E (ApoE)?
Harrison's 20th Ed. Chapter 308 Page 2148

A. Plasma glycoprotein
B. Helps lipoprotein clearance from circulation
C. Structural protein of chylomicrons, VLDL, IDL, HDL
D. None of the above

Apolipoprotein E (ApoE) is a plasma glycoprotein and helps lipoprotein clearance from circulation. ApoE is a structural protein of chylomicrons, very-low-density lipoproteins, intermediate-density lipoproteins, and high-density lipoproteins, and serves as a ligand for the uptake of ApoE-containing lipoproteins by the hepatic ApoE receptor or low-density lipoprotein (LDL) receptor. ApoE gene polymorphisms are associated with atherosclerosis and play critical roles in lipid metabolism.

1738. Lipoprotein glomerulopathy best relates to?
Harrison's 20th Ed. Chapter 308 Page 2148

A. E2 allele
B. E3 allele
C. E4 allele
D. All of the above

E4 allele is accompanied by increases in serum cholesterol and is more closely associated with atherogenic profiles in patients with renal failure. Mutations in E2 alleles, particularly in Japanese patients, produces lipoprotein glomerulopathy associated with glomerular lipoprotein thrombi & capillary dilation.

1739. Systemic hypertension causes permanent damage to kidneys in what percentage of patients with elevated blood pressure?
Harrison's 20th Ed. Chapter 308 Page 2148

A. ~ 6%
B. ~ 14%
C. ~ 26%
D. ~ 46%

Systemic hypertension causes permanent damage to kidneys in ~6% of patients with elevated BP.

1740. What percentage of patients with end-stage kidney disease have hypertension as a primary cause?
Harrison's 20th Ed. Chapter 308 Page 2148

A. 27%
B. 38%
C. 52%
D. 70%

~27% of patients with end-stage kidney disease (ESRD) have hypertension as a primary cause.

1741. Risk alleles associated with APOL1, a functional gene for apolipoprotein L1, expressed in?
Harrison's 20th Ed. Chapter 308 Page 2148

A. Glomerular basement membrane
B. Tubular basement membrane
C. Podocytes
D. All of the above

Risk alleles associated with APOL1, a functional gene for apolipoprotein L1 expressed in podocytes.

1742. Systemic hypertension associated risk factor for progression to end-stage kidney disease is?
Harrison's 20th Ed. Chapter 308 Page 2148

A. Smoking
B. Low birth weight
C. Preexisting renal injury
D. All of the above

Systemic hypertension associated risk factors for progression to ESRD include increased age, male gender, race, smoking, hypercholesterolemia, duration of hypertension, low birth weight, and preexisting renal injury.

1743. Kidney biopsies in patients with hypertension, microhematuria, and moderate proteinuria show all except?
Harrison's 20th Ed. Chapter 308 Page 2148

A. Arteriolosclerosis
B. Chronic nephrosclerosis
C. Interstitial fibrosis
D. Immune deposits

Kidney biopsies in patients with hypertension, microhematuria, and moderate proteinuria demonstrate arteriolosclerosis, chronic nephrosclerosis, and interstitial fibrosis in the absence of immune deposits.

1744. Hemodynamic stress of malignant hypertension leads to?
Harrison's 20th Ed. Chapter 308 Page 2148

A. Fibrinoid necrosis of small blood vessels
B. Thrombotic microangiography
C. Acute renal failure
D. All of the above

The hemodynamic stress of malignant hypertension leads to fibrinoid necrosis of small blood vessels, thrombotic microangiopathy, a nephritic urinalysis, and acute renal failure.

1745. In atherosclerosis, cholesterol crystals are showered into the circulation due to?
Harrison's 20th Ed. Chapter 308 Page 2148

A. Spontaneously
B. Endovascular procedure with manipulation of aorta
C. With use of systemic anticoagulation
D. All of the above

1746. Release of cholesterol fragments from atherosclerotic plaques can lead to which of the following?
Harrison's 20th Ed. Chapter 308 Page 2148

A. Cerebral transient ischemic attacks
B. Livedo reticularis in lower extremities
C. Hollenhorst plaques in retina with visual field cuts
D. All of the above

Release of cholesterol fragments from atherosclerotic plaques can lead to cerebral transient ischemic attacks, livedo reticularis in lower extremities, Hollenhorst plaques in retina with visual field cuts, necrosis of toes, acute glomerular capillary injury leading to FSGS and fever, eosinophilia, or eosinophiliuria.

1747. Which out of the following is false about sickle cell disease?
Harrison's 20th Ed. Chapter 308 Page 2148

A. Hyposthenuria
B. Infarction of the renal medulla
C. Predisposition to volume depletion
D. None of the above

Individuals with SA-hemoglobin are usually asymptomatic, but most will gradually develop hyposthenuria due to subclinical infarction of renal medulla, thus predisposing them to volume depletion.

1748. In sickle cell disease, vessel occlusion in kidney produces which of the following?
Harrison's 20th Ed. Chapter 308 Page 2148

A. Glomerular hypertension
B. FSGS
C. Interstitial nephritis
D. All of the above

In sickle cell disease, vessel occlusion in kidney produces glomerular hypertension, FSGS, interstitial nephritis, and renal infarction associated with hyposthenuria, microscopic hematuria, and even gross hematuria.

1749. TTP & HUS share features of?
Harrison's 20th Ed. Chapter 308 Page 2148

A. Idiopathic thrombocytopenic purpura
B. Preeclampsia/HELLP
C. Antiphospholipid syndrome
D. All of the above

1750. TTP/HUS is seen with the use of?
Harrison's 20th Ed. Chapter 308 Page 2149

A. Quinine
B. Calcineurin inhibitors
C. Ticlopidine and clopidogrel
D. All of the above

1751. TTP/HUS is seen in?
Harrison's 20th Ed. Chapter 308 Page 2149

A. Pregnancy
B. With the use of oral contraceptives
C. HIV infection
D. All of the above

1752. Shiga toxin best relates to which of the following?
Harrison's 20th Ed. Chapter 308 Page 2149

A. Tetrodotoxin
B. Verotoxin
C. Excitotoxin
D. Crinotoxin

Shiga toxin producing Escherichia coli (STEC) HUS is caused by the Shiga toxins (Stx1 and Stx2), which are also referred to as verotoxin.

1753. Shiga toxin binds to which of the following?
Harrison's 20th Ed. Chapter 308 Page 2149

A. Heparan sulfate–like surface receptors
B. Glycolipid surface receptor globotriaosylceramide (Gb3)
C. Low-density lipoprotein receptor–related proteins (LRPs)
D. vascular endothelial growth factor (VEGF)

Shiga toxin binds to glycolipid surface receptor globotriaosylceramide (Gb3), which is richly expressed on cells of the renal microvasculature.

1754. Shiga toxin inhibits the endothelial production of?
Harrison's 20th Ed. Chapter 308 Page 2149

A. Fibroblast growth factor (FGF)
B. ADAMTS13
C. Vascular endothelial growth factor (VEGF)
D. IL-1α, β

Shiga toxin inhibits the endothelial production of ADAMTS13.

1755. ADAMTS13 best relates to?
Harrison's 20th Ed. Chapter 308 Page 2149

A. Epidermal growth factor
B. Transcription factors STAT3 and STAT6
C. von Willebrand's factor
D. Factor H

ADAMTS13 metalloprotease cleaves large multimers of von Willebrand's factor. In the absence of ADAMTS13, large multimers cause platelet clumping and intravascular hemolysis.

1756. Atypical HUS (aHUS) best relates to?
Harrison's 20th Ed. Chapter 308 Page 2149

A. Shiga toxin (verotoxin)
B. Thrombospondin receptor
C. Complement protein deficiencies
D. Plasminogen-activator inhibitor 1 (PAI-1)

Atypical HUS or complement mediated HUS is the result of complement dysregulation which may be congenital or acquired. Affected patients have low C3 and normal C4 levels, characteristic of alternative pathway activation. Factor H deficiency is the most common defect.

1757. Adult TTP/HUS with ADAMTS13 antibodies is treated with?
Harrison's 20th Ed. Chapter 308 Page 2149

A. Rituximab
B. Steroids
C. Plasmapheresis
D. Splenectomy

Treatment of adult TTP/HUS with ADAMTS13 antibodies is daily plasmapheresis with fresh frozen plasma.

1758. The lesion in HIV-associated nephropathy (HIVAN) is resembles that of?
Harrison's 20th Ed. Chapter 308 Page 2149

A. Minimal change disease
B. Focal segmental glomerulosclerosis (FSGS)
C. Membranous glomerulonephritis
D. Renal amyloidosis

The lesion in HIVAN is FSGS, with characteristic collapsing glomerulopathy. There occurs visceral epithelial cell swelling, microcystic dilatation of renal tubules, and tubuloreticular inclusion. Tubular microcysts and interstitial inflammation distinguish it from idiopathic FSGS.

1759. HIVAN develops almost exclusively in patients of black race origin who have which of the following variant?
Harrison's 20th Ed. Chapter 308 Page 2149

A. PKHD1
B. APOL1
C. UMOD
D. IL28B

1760. Which of the following about HIV-associated nephropathy (HIVAN) is false?
Harrison's 20th Ed. Chapter 308 Page 2149

A. Significant proteinuria and rapidly progressive kidney disease
B. Normal blood pressure
C. Normal to enlarged kidneys
D. None of the above

HIVAN usually presents in patients with advanced HIV disease, with low CD4 count and detectable viral load. HIVAN occurs almost exclusively in patients who are of African descent.

1761. Which of the following is not present in nephrotic syndrome associated with HIV infection?
Harrison's 20th Ed. Chapter 308 Page 2149

A. Hypertension
B. Edema
C. Hyperlipidemia
D. All of the above

1762. Which of the following about HIV immune complex kidney disease (HIVICK) is false?

Harrison's 20th Ed. Chapter 308 Page 2149

A. Complication of active HIV viremia
B. Glomerular lesions
C. ART was not associated with improved renal outcomes
D. None of the above

HIVICK, HIV immune complex kidney disease is a group of immune complex-mediated glomerular lesions seen in HIV patients, and on biopsy can look like other glomerular lesions including postinfectious glomerulonephritis, MGN, MPGN, DPGN, MCD, and IgA nephropathy. The HIVICK effect is a complication of active HIV viremia.

1763. After what duration does HIV-associated nephropathy begin?

Harrison's 20th Ed. Chapter 308 Page 2149

A. ~ 3 months
B. ~ 6 months
C. ~ 1 year
D ~ 2.5 years

HIV-associated nephropathy begins ~ 2.5 years after HIV infection.

1764. HIV infection is most commonly associated with which of the following glomerulopathies?

Harrison's 20th Ed. Chapter 308 Page 2149

A. Aggressive focal segmental glomerulosclerosis
B. Acute diffuse proliferative glomerulonephritis
C. IgA nephropathy
D. Membranous glomerulopathy

1765. Term HIV-associated nephropathy (HIVAN) is used for?

Harrison's 20th Ed. Chapter 308 Page 2149

A. Aggressive focal segmental glomerulosclerosis
B. Acute diffuse proliferative glomerulonephritis
C. IgA nephropathy
D. Membranous glomerulopathy

1766. Which of the following is false for HIV-associated nephropathy (HIVAN)?

Harrison's 20th Ed. Chapter 308 Page 2149

A. May be the first manifestation of HIV infection
B. More common in blacks
C. More frequent in intravenous drug abusers
D. Slow clinical course

1767. HIV patients with FSGS present with nephrotic-range proteinuria & hypoalbuminemia but without?

Harrison's 20th Ed. Chapter 308 Page 2149

A. Hypertension
B. Edema
C. Hyperlipidemia
D. All of the above

HIV patients with FSGS typically present with nephrotic-range proteinuria and hypoalbuminemia, but without hypertension, edema, or hyperlipidemia.

1768. There is a close association between hepatitis B infection and?

Harrison's 20th Ed. Chapter 308 Page 2149

A. Renal amyloidosis
B. Lymphoma
C. Polyarteritis nodosa with vasculitis
D. Parvovirus infection

There is a close association between hepatitis B infection and polyarteritis nodosa with vasculitis appearing generally in the first 6 months following infection.

1769. Renal manifestations of hepatitis B infection include?

Harrison's 20th Ed. Chapter 308 Page 2149

A. Renal artery aneurysms
B. Renal infarction
C. Renal ischemic scars
D. All of the above

Renal manifestations of hepatitis B infection include renal artery aneurysms, renal infarction & renal ischemic scars.

1770. Glomerular lesion associated with HBV infection include?

Harrison's 20th Ed. Chapter 308 Page 2149

A. Membranous glomerulonephritis (MGN)
B. Membrane proliferative glomerulonephritis (MPGN)
C. Cryoglobulinemic glomerulonephritis
D. All of the above

1771. Which out of the following viral antigen is most commonly found in the renal deposits in HBV infection?

Harrison's 20th Ed. Chapter 308 Page 2149

A. HBsAG
B. HBeAG
C. HBcAG
D. All of the above

HBeAG viral antigen is most commonly found in the renal deposits in HBV infection.

1772. What proportion of children with HBV infection achieve spontaneous remission within 4 years?

Harrison's 20th Ed. Chapter 308 Page 2149

A. 40–45%
B. 50–55%
C. 60–65%
D. 70–75%

60 - 65% of children with HBV infection achieve spontaneous remission within 4 years.

1773. Renal lesion most commonly seen in chronic hepatitis C infection is?

Harrison's 20th Ed. Chapter 308 Page 2149

A. Cryoglobulinemic glomerulonephritis
B. Membranous glomerulonephritis (MGN)
C. Type I Membrane proliferative glomerulonephritis (MPGN)
D. IgA nephropathy

Renal lesions most commonly seen in chronic hepatitis C infection, in order of decreasing frequency, are cryoglobulinemic glomerulonephritis, MGN, and type I MPGN.

1774. HCV-induced immune-complex disease is associated with which of the following?

Harrison's 20th Ed. Chapter 308 Page 2149

A. Cryoglobulinemic glomerulonephritis
B. MPGN
C. Membranous glomerulopathy
D. All of the above

The renal lesions most commonly seen in chronic hepatitis C infection in order of decreasing frequency are cryoglobulinemic glomerulonephritis, MGN and type I MPGN.

1775. Dengue hemorrhagic fever causes?

Harrison's 20th Ed. Chapter 308 Page 2150

A. Anti-GBM disease
B. Mesangioproliferative glomerulonephritis
C. Endocapillary proliferative glomerulonephritis
D. Focal glomerulornephritis

Like measles, dengue hemorrhagic fever causes endocapillary proliferative glomerulonephritis.

1776. Leprosy is classified by which of the following criteria?

Harrison's 20th Ed. Chapter 308 Page 2150

A. Manning criteria
B. Bethesda criteria
C. Ridley Jopling criteria
D. Rome criteria

Leprosy is classified by Ridley Jopling criteria into tuberculoid, borderline tuberculoid, mid-borderline and borderline lepromatous and lepromatous.

1777. Renal involvement is more severe in infection with?

Harrison's 20th Ed. Chapter 308 Page 2150

A. Plasmodium falciparum
B. Plasmodium malariae
C. Plasmodium vivax
D. Plasmodium ovale

In quartan malaria from infection with Plasmodium malariae, children are more commonly affected and renal involvement is more severe.

1778. Which of the following cells of kidney do not proliferate?

Harrison's 16th Ed. 1678

A. Mesangial cells
B. Endothelial cells
C. Visceral epithelial cells
D. All of the above

1779. 'Crescents' are composed of?

A. Infiltrating monocytes
B. Proliferating parietal epithelial cells
C. Fibrin
D. All of the above

1780. Intrarenal vasoconstrictors include all except?

Am Fam Physician. 2012;86(7):631-639

A. Leukotrienes
B. Nitric oxide
C. Thromboxanes
D. Platelet-activating factor

1781. Intrarenal vasoconstrictors include all except?

Am Fam Physician. 2012;86(7):631-639

A. Endothelins
B. Prostacyclin
C. Adenosine
D. Angiotensin II

Intrarenal vasoconstrictors include Angiotensin II, Endothelin, Thromboxane, Adenosine, Leukotrienes, Platelet-activating factor. Intrarenal vasodilators are endothelium derived nitric oxide (EDNO), bradykinin and prostaglandin I2 (PGI2).

1782. Which of the following is true for Henoch Schonlein purpura?

A. Normal complement levels
B. Negative anti-GBM serology
C. Negative ANCA serology
D. All of the above

1783. Which of the following glomerulopathies is most commonly associated with Hodgkin's lymphoma?

A. FSGS
B. MCD
C. MPGN
D. Membranous glomerulopathy

Polycystic Kidney Disease and Other Inherited Disorders of Tubule Growth and Development

1784. Ciliary dysfunction in ciliopathies manifest as?
Pediatr Nephrol. 2011;26:1039-1056

A. Retinal degeneration
B. Renal disease
C. Cerebral anomalies
D. All of the above

Ciliopathies comprise a group of disorders associated with genetic mutations encoding defective proteins, which result in abnormal formation or function of cilia. As cilia are a component of almost all cells, ciliary dysfunction can manifest as a constellation of features that include primarily retinal degeneration, renal disease and cerebral anomalies.

1785. Which of the following is a renal ciliopathic syndrome?
Pediatr Nephrol. 2011;26:1039-1056

A. Polycystic kidney disease (PKD)
B. Renal medullary cystic disease
C. Cystic renal dysplasia
D. All of the above

1786. Characteristic clinical features of a "Ciliopathy" includes all except?
Pediatr Nephrol. 2011;26:1039-1056

A. Renal disease
B. Retinal disease
C. Cerebral malformations
D. Ectopic thyroid

1787. Ciliopathic syndromes include all except?
Pediatr Nephrol. 2011;26:1039-1056

A. Joubert syndrome
B. Bardet–Biedl syndrome
C. Orofaciodigital syndrome
D. Atypical hemolytic uremic syndrome

1788. Retinitis pigmentosa is a feature of which of the following inherited diseases associated with a cystic phenotype?
Harrison's 20th Ed. Chapter 309 Page 2151 Table 309-1

A. Bardet-Biedl syndrome
B. Sensenbrenner syndrome
C. Leber congenital amaurosis
D. All of the above

1789. Gout is a feature of which of the following inherited diseases associated with a cystic phenotype?
Harrison's 20th Ed. Chapter 309 Page 2151 Table 309-1

A. Autosomal dominant polycystic kidney disease
B. Medullary cystic kidney
C. Nephronophthisis
D. Tuberous sclerosis

1790. Polydactyly is a feature of which of the following inherited diseases associated with a cystic phenotype?
Harrison's 20th Ed. Chapter 309 Page 2151 Table 309-1

A. Sensenbrenner syndrome
B. Bardet-Biedl syndrome
C. Meckel-Gruber syndrome
D. All of the above

1791. Pheochromocytoma is a feature of which of the following inherited diseases associated with a cystic phenotype?
Harrison's 20th Ed. Chapter 309 Page 2151 Table 309-1

A. Tuberous sclerosis
B. Nephronophthisis
C. Von Hippel-Lindau disease
D. Medullary cystic kidney

1792. Liver fibrosis is a feature of which of the following inherited diseases associated with a cystic phenotype?
Harrison's 20th Ed. Chapter 309 Page 2151 Table 309-1

A. Autosomal recessive polycystic kidney disease
B. Medullary cystic kidney
C. Nephronophthisis
D. Tuberous sclerosis

1793. Renal cell carcinoma is a feature of which of the following inherited diseases associated with a cystic phenotype?
Harrison's 20th Ed. Chapter 309 Page 2151 Table 309-1

A. Autosomal recessive polycystic kidney disease
B. Medullary cystic kidney
C. Nephronophthisis
D. Tuberous sclerosis

1794. Obesity is a feature of which of the following inherited diseases associated with a cystic phenotype?
Harrison's 20th Ed. Chapter 309 Page 2151 Table 309-1

A. Bardet-Biedl syndrome
B. Sensenbrenner syndrome
C. Senior-Loken syndrome
D. Von Hippel-Lindau disease

1795. UMOD gene is associated with which of the following inherited diseases associated with a cystic phenotype?
Harrison's 20th Ed. Chapter 309 Page 2151 Table 309-1

A. Autosomal recessive polycystic kidney disease
B. Medullary cystic kidney
C. Nephronophthisis
D. Tuberous sclerosis

1796. Which of the following gene is associated with autosomal recessive polycystic kidney disease?
Harrison's 20th Ed. Chapter 309 Page 2151 Table 309-1

A. PKD1
B. PKD2
C. PKHD1
D. NPHP1-20

1797. Which of the following gene is associated with tuberous sclerosis?

Harrison's 20th Ed. Chapter 309 Page 2151 Table 309-1

A. TCTN2
B. TSC1
C. TMEM67
D. All of the above

1798. Which of the following is a monogenic disorder?

Harrison's 20th Ed. Chapter 309 Page 2150

A. Autosomal dominant polycystic kidney disease (ADPKD)
B. Glucocorticoid-remediable primary hyperaldosteronism
C. Cystic fibrosis (CF)
D. All of the above

Monogenic disorders include primary hyperoxaluria, cystinuria, monogenic forms of DM, mutations of the amyloid precursor protein in familial Alzheimer's disease, the microtubule-associated protein tau (MAPT) in frontotemporal dementia, α-synuclein in Parkinson's disease, cerebral autosomal recessive arteriopathy with subcortical infarcts and leukoencephalopathy (CARASIL), hereditary endotheliopathy, retinopathy, nephropathy and stroke (HERNS), Glucocorticoid-remediable primary hyperaldosteronism, cystic fibrosis (CF), autosomal dominant polycystic kidney disease (ADPKD).

1799. Which of the following statements is false about polycystic kidney disease?

Harrison's 20th Ed. Chapter 309 Page 2150

A. ADPKD is seen predominantly in childhood
B. ARPKD is mainly a disease of adults
C. They infrequently cause kidney failure
D. All of the above

Autosomal dominant polycystic kidney disease (ADPKD) is seen predominantly in adults, whereas autosomal recessive polycystic kidney disease (ARPKD) is mainly a disease of childhood. They frequently causes kidney failure.

1800. What percentage of total nephrons are involved in ADPKD?

Harrison's 20th Ed. Chapter 309 Page 2150

A. < 1%
B. < 2%
C. < 3%
D. < 5%

In ADPKD, <5% of total nephrons (tubules) are involved.

1801. The cellular defect in ADPKD is?

Harrison's 20th Ed. Chapter 309 Page 2150

A. Increased cell proliferation and fluid secretion
B. Decreased cell differentiation
C. Abnormal extracellular matrix
D. All of the above

The cellular defects in ADPKD are increased cell proliferation and fluid secretion, decreased cell differentiation, and abnormal extracellular matrix.

1802. Which of the following is a PKD-1 encoded protein?

Harrison's 20th Ed. Chapter 309 Page 2150

A. Fibrocystin
B. Polycystin-1
C. Caveolin 3
D. FMR-1 protein

ADPKD results from mutations in either PKD-1 (85% of cases) or PKD-2 gene. PKD-1 encodes polycystin-1 (PC1), whereas PKD-2 gene product is polycystin-2 (PC2).

1803. Which of the following statements about 'Autosomal dominant polycystic kidney disease is false?

Harrison's 20th Ed. Chapter 309 Page 2150

A. PC1 is a large 11-transmembrane protein that functions like a G-protein coupled receptor
B. PC2 is a Ca^{++}-permeable 6 transmembrane protein that belongs to transient receptor potential (TRP) cation channel family
C. PKD1 is called 1st disease gene & PKD2 2nd disease gene
D. PKD1 is on chromosome 16 and PKD2 is on chromosome 6

The first disease gene (PKD1) is localized to the region of the alpha-globin gene on chromosome 16p13, and a second disease gene (PKD2) locus is mapped to chromosome 4q21-q23.

1804. Which of the following statements about polycystin-1 (PC1) is false?

Harrison's 20th Ed. Chapter 309 Page 2150

A. Large 11-transmembrane protein that functions like a GPCR
B. Widely expressed in almost all tissues and organs
C. Expression is high in development and low in the adult
D. None of the above

1805. Which of the following statements about polycystin-2 (PC2) is false?

Harrison's 20th Ed. Chapter 309 Page 2150

A. Ca^{++}-permeable 6 transmembrane protein of transient receptor potential (TRP) cation channel family
B. Widely expressed in almost all tissues and organs
C. Expression is relatively constant
D. None of the above

1806. Which of the following statements about PC1/2 is false?

Harrison's 20th Ed. Chapter 309 Page 2151

A. Found on the primary cilium
B. PC1 & PC2 bind together to form receptor-channel complex
C. Defect causes ciliopathies
D. None of the above

1807. Which of the following statements about primary cilia is false?

Harrison's 20th Ed. Chapter 309 Page 2152 Figure 309-1

A. "9+0" organization of microtubule doublets
B. Proteins are transported into cilium by motor protein kinesin 2
C. Proteins are transported out of the cilium by dynein
D. None of the above

Primary cilia differ from motile cilia (9+2 cilia) in their lack of central microtubule doublet, so they are described as having a "9+0" arrangement. 9+0 cilia are immotile and do not beat. Ciliary axoneme (shaft) is only 0.25 μm in diameter but its length can be up to 2 mm. The basal body is a cylindrical structure measuring 0.4 by 0.2 μm positioned perpendicular to the cell membrane, anchoring cilium in the cytoplasm. It also acts as the nucleation point from which the cilium extends out from the cell. The basal body consists of nine triplets of microtubules arranged in a ring from which extend three microtubules: A, B, and C. All three fibres project from the basal body into the proximal region of the cilium known as the transition zone. This is the region from which a nascent cilium grows. Further along the cilium is the middle zone composed of nine doublets consisting of just A and B filaments. The axoneme terminates with the distal zone, comprised primarily of microtubule singlets.

1808. Which of the following statements about PC1/2 protein complex is false?

Harrison's 20th Ed. Chapter 309 Page 2151

A. Serves as a mechanosensor or chemical sensor
B. Regulates calcium and G protein signaling
C. Regulate cellular functions & signaling pathways
D. None of the above

PC1/2 protein complex serves as a mechanosensor or chemical sensor and regulates calcium and G protein signaling.

1809. Which of the following cellular functions is regulated by PC1/2 protein complex?

Harrison's 20th Ed. Chapter 309 Page 2151

A. Cell cycle
B. Actin cytoskeleton
C. Planar cell polarity (PCP)
D. All of the above

PC1/2 protein complex also directly regulates cellular functions including the cell cycle, the actin cytoskeleton, planar cell polarity (PCP), and cell migration.

1810. Which of the following signaling pathways is regulated by PC1/2 protein complex?

Harrison's 20th Ed. Chapter 309 Page 2151

A. Wnt
B. Mammalian target of rapamycin (mTOR)
C. STAT3
D. All of the above

1811. Which of the following signaling pathways is regulated by PC1/2 protein complex?

Harrison's 20th Ed. Chapter 309 Page 2151

A. cMET
B. Phosphoinositide 3-kinase (PI3K/Akt)
C. G protein–coupled receptor (GPCR)
D. All of the above

PC1/2 protein complex has also been implicated in regulating a number of signaling pathways, including Wnt, mammalian target of rapamycin (mTOR), STAT3, cMET, phosphoinositide 3-kinase (PI3K/Akt), G protein–coupled receptor (GPCR), and epidermal growth factor receptor (EGFR), as well as in the localization and activity of cystic fibrosis transmembrane conductance regulator (CFTR).

1812. Loss of ciliary function of PC1 and PC2 in ADPKD kidneys leads to?

Harrison's 20th Ed. Chapter 309 Page 2151

A. Aberrant calcium signaling
B. Cyst growth by promoting proliferation
C. Fluid secretion of cyst-lining cells through Cl^- & AQP channels
D. All of the above

Loss of ciliary function of PC1 and PC2 in ADPKD kidneys leads to aberrant Ca^{++} signaling and consequent increase of adenylyl cyclase activity & decrease of phosphodiesterase activity, which, in turn, causes increased cellular cAMP. Increased cAMP promotes protein kinase A activity, and, in turn, leads to cyst growth by promoting proliferation and fluid secretion of cyst-lining cells through chloride & aquaporin channels.

1813. Which of the following statements about autosomal dominant polycystic kidney disease (ADPKD) is false?

Harrison's 20th Ed. Chapter 309 Page 2151

A. Inherited as an autosomal dominant trait
B. Complete penetrance
C. Variable expressivity
D. None of the above

ADPKD is inherited as an autosomal dominant trait with complete penetrance, but variable expressivity.

1814. Which of the following gene causes autosomal dominant polycystic kidney disease (ADPKD)?

Harrison's 20th Ed. Chapter 309 Page 2151

A. IFT80
B. GANAB
C. REN
D. MKS1

A third gene GANAB, encoding glucosidase IIa subunit, can cause ADPKD through mutations. All have polycystic liver disease also, and their kidney disease is milder than that in classic ADPKD.

1815. Which of the following statements about 'autosomal dominant polycystic kidney disease (ADPKD)' is false?

Harrison's 20th Ed. Chapter 309 Page 2150

A. ADPKD-1 gene is on chromosome 16p13.3
B. ADPKD-2 gene is on chromosome 4q21-23
C. Cysts are distributed throughout cortex & medulla
D. Erythropoietin production is low

1816. In ADPKD, cyst formation begins?

Harrison's 20th Ed. Chapter 309 Page 2152

A. In utero
B. In early childhood
C. In adolescence
D. In adulthood

In ADPKD, cyst formation begins in utero. It is the most common, life-threatening single-gene disease in adults.

1817. Extrarenal manifestation of ADPKD is?

Harrison's 20th Ed. Chapter 309 Page 2152

A. Intracranial aneurysm
B. Cardiac valvular abnormalities
C. Colonic diverticulae
D. All of the above

Intracranial aneurysm, cardiac valvular abnormalities (MVPS, AR), hepatic cysts, colonic diverticulae, inguinal hernias occur with a higher frequency than in the general population in ADPKD.

1818. Which of the following is the most common extrarenal complication in ADPKD?

Harrison's 20th Ed. Chapter 309 Page 2152

A. Intracranial aneurysm
B. Colonic diverticulae
C. Liver cysts
D. Abdominal wall hernias

Liver cysts derived from the biliary epithelia are the most common extrarenal complication.

1819. Autosomal dominant polycystic liver disease (ADPLD) is caused by mutations in?

Harrison's 20th Ed. Chapter 309 Page 2152

A. CRTAP
B. FKBP10
C. PRKCSH
D. IFITM5

Polycystic liver disease associated with ADPKD is different from autosomal dominant polycystic liver disease (ADPLD) which is caused by mutations in PRKCSH & SEC63 genes, and does not progress to renal failure. Massive polycystic liver disease occurs almost exclusively in women with ADPKD, particularly those with multiple pregnancies.

1820. Which of the following statements about 'Autosomal dominant polycystic kidney disease (ADPKD)' is false?

Harrison's 20th Ed. Chapter 309 Page 2153

A. Standard diagnostic criteria is at least 3 to 5 cysts in each kidney
B. Cysts may be found in brain, thyroid
C. Mitral valve prolapse found in 30% of patients
D. Intracranial aneurysms are 4–5 times more frequent

1821. In ADPKD, cysts can also develop in?

Harrison's 20th Ed. Chapter 309 Page 2153

A. Liver
B. Pancreas
C. Arachnoid membranes
D. All of the above

Cysts can also develop in liver, pancreas, spleen, arachnoid membranes & seminal vesicles in men.

1822. Vascular abnormalities in ADPKD patients include?

Harrison's 20th Ed. Chapter 309 Page 2153

A. Diffuse arterial dolichoectasias of anterior & posterior cerebral circulation
B. Left ventricular hypertrophy (LVH)
C. Stroke
D. All of the above

Vascular abnormalities in ADPKD patients include diffuse arterial dolichoectasias of the anterior & posterior cerebral circulation, which can predispose to arterial dissection and stroke.

1823. Which of the following valvular abnormalities is seen in ADPKD patients?

Harrison's 20th Ed. Chapter 309 Page 2153

A. Mitral valve prolapse
B. Tricuspid valve prolapse
C. Aortic insufficiency
D. All of the above

Mitral valve prolapse occurs in ~30% of patients with ADPKD, tricuspid valve prolapse is less common. Other valvular abnormalities include insufficiency of mitral, aortic, and tricuspid valves.

1824. Which of the following abnormalities is seen in ADPKD?

Harrison's 20th Ed. Chapter 309 Page 2153

A. Colonic diverticulae
B. Abdominal wall hernias
C. Stroke
D. All of the above

The prevalence of colonic diverticulae & abdominal wall hernias are increased in ADPKD patients.

1825. Diagnostic criteria for ADPKD in young include?

Harrison's 20th Ed. Chapter 309 Page 2153

A. ≥ 2
B. ≥ 3
C. ≥ 4
D. ≥ 5

1826. Diagnostic criteria for ADPKD in > 60 year old include?

Harrison's 20th Ed. Chapter 309 Page 2153

A. ≥ 1
B. ≥ 2
C. ≥ 3
D. ≥ 4

Diagnostic criteria for ADPKD require two or more cysts in kidney (unilateral or bilateral) in young subjects (15 and 29 years), but four or more in subjects older than 60 years. Presence of at least two cysts in each kidney is required for the diagnosis among at-risk subjects aged 30–59 years.

1827. Which of the following clinical trials is related to control of hypertension in ADPKD?

Harrison's 20th Ed. Chapter 309 Page 2153

A. STOP-PKD
B. HALT-PKD
C. CONTROL-PKD
D. SLOW-PKD

The HALT-PKD trial was a prospective randomized study to test whether dual blockade of RAAS using ACEI and ARB combination therapy delay normal progression of kidney disease compared to ACEI monotherapy. Results showed that in the early stages of ADPKD, dual inhibition of RAAS did not significantly decrease the rate of total kidney volume growth.

1828. What level of BP is recommended by JNC VIII for reducing CV complications in ADPKD & renal disease progression?

Harrison's 20th Ed. Chapter 309 Page 2153

A. 110/70 mm Hg
B. 120/80 mm Hg
C. 140/80 mm Hg
D. 140/90 mm Hg

Blood pressure control to a target of 140/90 mm Hg is recommended according to the guidelines from the eighth report of the Joint National Committee on Prevention, Detection, Evaluation, and Treatment of High Blood Pressure (JNC VIII) for reducing cardiovascular complications in ADPKD and renal disease progression. More rigorous blood pressure control does not equal greater clinical benefits.

1829. Which of the following antibiotics is not preferred for cyst infection in ADPKD?

Harrison's 20th Ed. Chapter 309 Page 2153

A. Cephalosporins
B. Trimethoprim-sulfamethoxazole
C. Quinolones
D. Chloramphenicol

Lipid-soluble antibiotics against common gram-negative enteric organisms such as trimethoprim-sulfamethoxazole, quinolones and chloramphenicol are preferred for cyst infection because most renal cysts are not connected to glomerular filtration and antibiotics that are capable of penetrating the cyst walls are likely to be more effective. Treatment often requires 4–6 weeks.

1830. Which of the following drugs are useful in ADPKD?

Harrison's 20th Ed. Chapter 309 Page 2154

A. Sirolimus
B. Tolvaptan
C. Octreotide
D. All of the above

1831. Autosomal recessive polycystic kidney disease (ARPKD) gene is called?

Harrison's 20th Ed. Chapter 309 Page 2154

A. ARPKD-1
B. ARPKD-2
C. PKHD1
D. PKHD2

ARPKD gene, on chromosome 6p21.1-6p12.2, is called PKHD1 (polycystic kidney & hepatic disease 1) gene. Mutations in PKHD1 cause all the clinical presentations of ARPKD.

1832. Protein expressed by PKHD1 is termed?

Harrison's 20th Ed. Chapter 309 Page 2154

A. Nephrocystin
B. Inversin
C. Fibrocystin/polyductin (FPC)
D. Polycystin-3

Protein expressed by PKHD1 is termed fibrocystin/polyductin (FPC).

1833. Fibrocystin/polyductin (FPC) is localized on the primary cilia of epithelia cells of?

Harrison's 20th Ed. Chapter 309 Page 2154

A. Cortical collecting ducts
B. Medullary collecting ducts
C. Cholangiocytes of bile ducts
D. All of the above

Single transmembrane FPC is localized on the primary cilia of epithelia cells of cortical & medullary collecting ducts and cholangiocytes of bile ducts. FPC is also expressed on the basal body and plasma membrane.

1834. Which of the following relate to classic ARPKD?

Harrison's 20th Ed. Chapter 309 Page 2154

A. Oligohydraminos
B. Pulmonary hypoplasia
C. Biliary dysgenesis
D. All of the above

In classic ARPKD, reduced fetal urine production contributes to oligohydraminos and pulmonary hypoplasia. Biliary dysgenesis due to a primary ductal plate malformation with associated periportal fibrosis occurs (congenital hepatic fibrosis).

1835. Which of the following statements about 'autosomal recessive polycystic kidney disease (ARPKD)' is false?

Harrison's 20th Ed. Chapter 309 Page 2154

A. Distal tubules & collecting ducts are dilated
B. Portal hypertension & esophageal varices are frequent
C. Unilateral abdominal mass is common
D. Death in neonates is due to pulmonary hypoplasia

Enlarged kidneys are detected soon after birth as bilateral abdominal masses.

1836. Caroli's disease best relates to?

Harrison's 20th Ed. Chapter 309 Page 2154

A. Dilatation of intrahepatic bile ducts
B. Biliary dysgenesis
C. Liver cysts
D. All of the above

Caroli's disease refers to dilatation of intrahepatic bile ducts & may need porto-systemic shunting.

1837. The hallmark of ARPKD liver disease is?

Harrison's 20th Ed. Chapter 309 Page 2154

A. Liver cysts
B. Biliary dysgenesis
C. Cholangiocarcinoma
D. Hepatic steatosis

The hallmarks of ARPKD liver disease are biliary dysgenesis due to a primary ductal plate malformation with associated periportal fibrosis—congenital hepatic fibrosis (CHF) and dilatation of intrahepatic bile ducts (Caroli's disease).

1838. The slow progression of renal disease in ARPKD is due to?

Harrison's 20th Ed. Chapter 309 Page 2154

A. Increasing fibrosis
B. Development of cysts
C. Systemic hypertension
D. All of the above

The slow progression of renal disease in ARPKD is due to increasing fibrosis rather than development of cysts. Systemic hypertension is common in all ARPKD patients, even those with normal renal function.

1839. Which of the following about ultrasonography in ARPKD is false?

Harrison's 20th Ed. Chapter 309 Page 2154

A. Large, echogenic kidneys
B. Poor corticomedullary differentiation
C. Diagnosis can be made in utero >24 weeks of gestation
D. None of the above

USG in ARPKD reveals large, echogenic kidneys with poor corticomedullary differentiation. The diagnosis can be made in utero after 24 weeks of gestation in severe cases.

1840. Which of the following about Tuberous sclerosis (TS) is false?

Harrison's 20th Ed. Chapter 309 Page 2154

A. Autosomal recessive
B. Caused by mutations in TSC1 encoding hamartin
C. Caused by mutations in TSC2 encoding tuberin
D. Kidney cysts are frequent

Tuberous sclerosis (TS) is a rare autosomal dominant syndrome caused by mutations in one of two genes, TSC1 encoding hamartin or TSC2 encoding tuberin.

1841. Essentially all TS patients have associated?

Harrison's 20th Ed. Chapter 309 Page 2154

A. Skin lesions
B. Neurologic lesions
C. Cardiac lesions
D. Renal lesions

TS is a syndrome affecting multiple organ systems that includes benign growths in nervous system, eyes, heart, lung, liver, and skin. Essentially all TS patients have such skin lesions, and a large proportion of patients have neurologic and cognitive manifestations.

1842. Abnormalities of kidney in tuberous sclerosis (TS) include?

Harrison's 20th Ed. Chapter 309 Page 2154

A. Renal cysts
B. Renal angiomyolipomas
C. Renal cell carcinoma
D. All of the above

Renal TS occurs as renal cysts, renal angiomyolipomas & renal cell carcinoma.

1843. The TSC2 gene is adjacent to which of the following genes in the human genome?

Harrison's 20th Ed. Chapter 309 Page 2154

A. PKD1
B. PKD2
C. PKHD1
D. All of the above

The TSC2 gene is adjacent to PKD1 in the human genome. Inactivation of these two genes may have manifestations of both ADPKD and TS.

1844. The most common kidney finding in TS is the presence of?
Harrison's 20th Ed. Chapter 309 Page 2154

A. Angiomyolipomas
B. Renal cell carcinoma
C. Renal cyst
D. Nephrolithiasis

The most common kidney finding in TS is the presence of angiomyolipomas. Multiple, bilateral and benign, surgical removal is recommended for angiomyolipomas larger than 4 cm in diameter. In contrast to ADPKD, there is a clearly increased risk of renal cell carcinoma in TS patients.

1845. Which of the following about TS is false?
Harrison's 20th Ed. Chapter 309 Page 2155

A. May lead to significant CKD & progress to ESRD
B. Unremarkable urine sediment
C. Minimal to mild proteinuria
D. None of the above

1846. Which of the following about cysts in TS is false?
Harrison's 20th Ed. Chapter 309 Page 2155

A. Radiographically similar to those seen in ADPKD
B. Pose an increased risk of renal cell carcinoma
C. Rarely become large and hemorrhagic
D. None of the above

1847. Tuberin & hamartin protein complex is localized to?
Harrison's 20th Ed. Chapter 309 Page 2155

A. Base of the cilia
B. Transition zone of cilia
C. Ciliary membrane
D. Nucleus

1848. Tuberin & hamartin protein complex is best related to?
Harrison's 20th Ed. Chapter 309 Page 2155

A. Wnt
B. Mammalian target of rapamycin (mTOR)
C. STAT3
D. G protein–coupled receptor (GPCR)

TSC1 & TSC2 gene products tuberin & hamartin interact physically. This protein complex is localized to the base of the cilia and inhibits intracellular signaling processes mediated by mTOR (mammalian target of rapamycin), leading to abnormal growth in tissues.

1849. Which of the following is false about Von Hippel-Lindau disease (VHL)?
Harrison's 20th Ed. Chapter 309 Page 2155

A. Inherited cancer syndrome
B. Autosomal dominant
C. Caused by mutations in VHL tumor-suppressor gene
D. None of the above

Von Hippel-Lindau disease (VHL) is an inherited cancer syndrome with renal manifestations. VHL is an autosomal dominant condition caused by mutations in the VHL tumor-suppressor gene. VHL is localized to the primary cilia and is necessary for the formation of primary cilia.

1850. Which of the following is a manifestation of VHL?
Harrison's 20th Ed. Chapter 309 Page 2155

A. Multiple bilateral kidney cysts
B. Renal cell carcinoma
C. Pheochromocytoma
D. All of the above

1851. Which of the following is a manifestation of VHL?
Harrison's 20th Ed. Chapter 309 Page 2155

A. Cerebellar hemangioblastomas
B. Retinal hemangiomas
C. Pheochromocytoma
D. All of the above

Kidney manifestations of VHL include multiple bilateral kidney cysts & renal cell carcinomas. Kidney cysts & carcinoma affect the majority of VHL patients. Nonrenal features of VHL include pheochromocytoma, cerebellar hemangioblastomas and retinal hemangiomas.

1852. Large renal cysts are seen in?
Harrison's 20th Ed. Chapter 309 Page 2155

A. Von Hippel-Lindau disease (VHL)
B. Tuberous sclerosis (TS)
C. Autosomal dominant polycystic kidney disease (ADPKD)
D. All of the above

1853. Medullary Cystic Kidney Disease Type I is due to mutation in?
Harrison's 20th Ed. Chapter 309 Page 2155

A. MUC1
B. UMOD
C. REN
D. KIF3A

Patients with Medullary Cystic Kidney Disease Type I (MCKD I) have mutations in the mucin 1 gene (MUC1).

1854. UMOD mutations cause which of the following diseases?
Harrison's 20th Ed. Chapter 309 Page 2155

A. Medullary Cystic Kidney Disease Type II
B. Familial juvenile hyperuricemic nephropathy (HNFJ1)
C. Glomerulocystic kidney disease (GCKD)
D. All of the above

UMOD mutations cause Medullary Cystic Kidney Disease Type II, familial juvenile hyperuricemic nephropathy (HNFJ1) and glomerulocystic kidney disease (GCKD).

1855. Uromodulin is also known as?
Harrison's 20th Ed. Chapter 309 Page 2155

A. Hop protein
B. Bence-Jones protein
C. Tamm-Horsfall protein
D. R-binder protein

UMOD gene encodes protein uromodulin which is also known as Tamm-Horsfall protein.

1856. Uromodulin is found on?
Harrison's 20th Ed. Chapter 309 Page 2155

A. Centrosome
B. Mitotic spindle
C. Primary cilia
D. All of the above

Uromodulin is found on centrosome, mitotic spindle, and the primary cilia. It colocalizes with nephrocystin-1 & KIF3A on the cilia. The products of the NPHP genes are referred to as nephrocystins.

1857. Which of the following is false about Medullary Cystic Kidney Disease Type II?

Harrison's 20th Ed. Chapter 309 Page 2155

A. Benign urine sediments
B. Absence of significant proteinuria
C. Hyperuricemia
D. None of the above

MCKD II should be suspected clinically in patients with a family history of late onset kidney disease, benign urine sediments, absence of significant proteinuria and hyperuricemia.

1858. Presence of hyperuricemia and gout point towards the diagnosis of which of the following?

Harrison's 20th Ed. Chapter 309 Page 2155

A. Autosomal recessive polycystic kidney disease
B. Medullary cystic kidney disease 2
C. Bartter's syndrome
D. Nephronophthisis (NPHP)

Most patients with medullary cystic kidney disease 2 (MCKD2) have severe hyperuricemia and precocious onset of gout.

1859. Presence of hyperuricemia and gout point towards the diagnosis of which of the following?

Harrison's 20th Ed. Chapter 309 Page 2155

A. Autosomal recessive polycystic kidney disease
B. ADKTKD-REN
C. ADTKD-MUC1
D. Nephronophthisis (NPHP)

Patients with mutations in renin gene REN (leading to ADTKD-REN) demonstrate hyporeninemia with mild hyperkalemia, hyperuricemia and gout.

1860. Which of the following is the most common genetic cause of ESRD in childhood?

Harrison's 20th Ed. Chapter 309 Page 2155

A. Autosomal recessive polycystic kidney disease
B. Medullary sponge kidney (MSK)
C. Bartter's syndrome
D. Nephronophthisis (NPHP)

Nephronophthisis (NPHP) is the most common inherited childhood form of kidney failure requiring kidney replacement therapy.

1861. Which of the following relates to nephronophthisis (NPHP)?

Harrison's 20th Ed. Chapter 309 Page 2155

A. Autosomal recessive pattern of inheritance
B. Ciliopathy
C. Most common inherited childhood form of kidney failure
D. None of the above

1862. Which of the following is a feature of nephronophthisis?

Harrison's 20th Ed. Chapter 309 Page 2155

A. Tubulointerstitial fibrosis
B. Corticomedullary cysts
C. Progressive CKD leading to renal failure
D. All of the above

NPHP share common features, including tubulointerstitial fibrosis, corticomedullary cysts and progressive CKD leading to renal failure. Proteinuria is absent or mild and the urine sediment is not active.

1863. Products of the NPHP genes are referred to as?

Harrison's 20th Ed. Chapter 309 Page 2155

A. Nephronocystins
B. Nephrocystins
C. Nephricystins
D. Nephritic cystins

Products of the NPHP genes are referred to as nephrocystins.

1864. Which of the following form of NPHP is most frequent?

Harrison's 20th Ed. Chapter 309 Page 2156

A. Infantile
B. Juvenile
C. Adolescent
D. Adult

NPHP is divided into infantile, juvenile, and adolescent forms. The juvenile form is the most frequent.

1865. Infantile form NPHP is caused by mutations in?

Harrison's 20th Ed. Chapter 309 Page 2156

A. NPHP1 gene
B. NPHP2 gene
C. NPHP3 gene
D. NPHP4 gene

1866. Juvenile form NPHP is caused by mutations in?

Harrison's 20th Ed. Chapter 309 Page 2156

A. NPHP1 gene
B. NPHP2 gene
C. NPHP3 gene
D. NPHP4 gene

1867. Senior-Loken syndrome, besides juvenile nephronophthisis, best relates to?

Harrison's 20th Ed. Chapter 309 Page 2156

A. Intracranial aneurysm
B. Retinitis pigmentosa
C. Colonic diverticulae
D. All of the above

When juvenile NPHP has retinitis pigmentosa as an extrarenal manifestation, the syndrome is called Senior-Loken syndrome.

1868. Joubert's syndrome best relates to?

Harrison's 20th Ed. Chapter 309 Page 2156

A. Retinal dystrophy
B. Cystic dilatation of renal collecting ducts
C. Hypoplasia of the cerebellar vermis
D. All of the above

1869. Which of the following is not a feature of Bardet-Biedl syndrome (BBS)?

Harrison's 20th Ed. Chapter 309 Page 2156

A. Polydactyly
B. Retinal hemangioma
C. Kidney cysts
D. Truncal obesity

The multisystem disease Bardet-Biedl syndrome (BBS) features truncal obesity, cognitive impairment, retinal dystrophy, polydactyly, developmental urogenital abnormalities and kidney cysts.

1870. Which of the following is a disease of abnormal ciliary function?

Harrison's 20th Ed. Chapter 309 Page 2156

A. Autosomal dominant polycystic kidney disease (ADPKD)
B. Nephronophthisis (NPHP)
C. Bardet-Biedl syndrome (BBS)
D. All of the above

Tubulointerstitial Diseases of the Kidney

1871. Which of the following about tubulointerstitial nephritis (TIN) is false?

Harrison's 20th Ed. Chapter 310 Page 2157

A. Tubules & interstitium primarily affected
B. Relative sparing of glomeruli
C. Relative sparing of renal vessels
D. None of the above

Tubulointerstitial nephritis (TIN) is a group of disorders that primarily affect tubules & interstitium, with relative sparing of glomeruli & renal vessels. They can be acute and chronic.

1872. Tubulointerstitial diseases of the kidney can be due to?

Harrison's 20th Ed. Chapter 310 Page 2157 Table 310-1

A. Acute tubulointerstitial disorders
B. Chronic tubulointerstitial disorders
C. Cystic and hereditary disorders
D. All of the above

Tubulointerstitial diseases of the kidney can be due to acute tubulointerstitial disorders, chronic tubulointerstitial disorders, metabolic disturbances and cystic and hereditary disorders.

1873. Acute interstitial nephritis of the kidney can be due to?

Harrison's 20th Ed. Chapter 310 Page 2157 Table 310-1

A. Therapeutic agents
B. Infections
C. Autoimmune etiology
D. All of the above

Acute interstitial nephritis can be due to therapeutic agents, infections, autoimmune etiology, and acute obstructive causes.

1874. Which of the following about tubulointerstitial nephritis (TIN) is false?

Harrison's 20th Ed. Chapter 310 Page 2157

A. Acute TIN mostly presents as acute renal failure
B. Chronic TIN mostly presents as disorders of tubular function
C. Allergic reaction to a drug mostly cause acute interstitial nephritis (AIN)
D. None of the above

1875. Acute TIN caused by aggressive inflammatory infiltrates leads to?

Harrison's 20th Ed. Chapter 310 Page 2157

A. Tissue edema
B. Tubular cell injury
C. Compromised tubular flow
D. All of the above

1876. Frank obstruction of the tubules can be caused by?

Harrison's 20th Ed. Chapter 310 Page 2157

A. Casts
B. Cellular debris
C. Crystals
D. All of the above

Acute TIN that presents with acute renal failure is caused by aggressive inflammatory infiltrates that lead to tissue edema, tubular cell injury, and compromised tubular flow, or by Frank obstruction of the tubules with casts, cellular debris, or crystals.

1877. The clinical features of chronic TIN manifest with disorders of?

Harrison's 20th Ed. Chapter 310 Page 2157

A. Glomerular function
B. Tubular function
C. Interstitial function
D. All of the above

The clinical features of chronic TIN are more indolent and manifest with disorders of tubular function.

1878. Renal tubular dysfunction can manifest as?

Harrison's 20th Ed. Chapter 310 Page 2157

A. Polyuria
B. Non-anion-gap metabolic acidosis
C. Hyperkalemia
D. All of the above

1879. Which of the following is a feature of Fanconi's syndrome?

Harrison's 20th Ed. Chapter 310 Page 2157

A. Glycosuria
B. Phosphaturia
C. Aminoaciduria
D. All of the above

Disorders of tubular function can lead to polyuria from impaired concentrating ability (nephrogenic diabetes insipidus), defective proximal tubular reabsorption leading to features of Fanconi's syndrome (glycosuria, phosphaturia, aminoaciduria, hypokalemia and type II renal tubular acidosis [RTA] from bicarbonaturia) or non-anion-gap metabolic acidosis and hyperkalemia (type IV RTA) due to impaired ammonia genesis, as well as progressive azotemia (rising creatinine & blood urea nitrogen).

1880. On renal ultrasonography, which of the following is found in "medical renal disease"?

Harrison's 20th Ed. Chapter 310 Page 2157

A. Increased echogenicity of renal parenchyma
B. Loss of corticomedullary differentiation
C. Prominence of renal pyramids
D. All of the above

In Chronic TIN, renal ultrasonography may reveal "medical renal disease" which includes increased echogenicity of the renal parenchyma with loss of corticomedullary differentiation, prominence of the renal pyramids and cortical scarring.

1881. The predominant pathology in chronic TIN is?

Harrison's 20th Ed. Chapter 310 Page 2157

A. Interstitial fibrosis with patchy mononuclear cell infiltration
B. Widespread tubular atrophy & luminal dilation
C. Thickening of tubular basement membranes
D. All of the above

The predominant pathology in chronic TIN is interstitial fibrosis with patchy mononuclear cell infiltration & widespread tubular atrophy, luminal dilation, and thickening of tubular basement membranes.

1882. Which of the following is common in NSAID induced allergic interstitial nephritis?

Harrison's 20th Ed. Chapter 310 Page 2158

A. Fever
B. Rash
C. Eosinophilia
D. Proteinuria

In nonsteroidal anti-inflammatory drug (NSAID)-induced acute interstitial nephritis (AIN) fever, rash and eosinophilia are rare but acute renal failure with heavy proteinuria is common.

1883. Severe & rapid-onset allergic interstitial nephritis may occur on reintroduction after a drug-free period of which of the following drug?

Harrison's 20th Ed. Chapter 310 Page 2158

A. Proton pump inhibitors
B. Rifampin
C. Sulfasalazine
D. Indinavir

A particularly severe & rapid-onset AIN may occur upon reintroduction, after a drug-free period, of rifampin.

1884. Which of the following provide supporting evidence to the diagnosis of allergic interstitial nephritis?

Harrison's 20th Ed. Chapter 310 Page 2158

A. Peripheral blood eosinophilia
B. Pyuria with white blood cell casts
C. Hematuria
D. All of the above

1885. Which of the following may accelerate renal recovery in allergic interstitial nephritis?

Harrison's 20th Ed. Chapter 310 Page 2158

A. Diuretics
B. Glucocorticoids
C. N-acetyl cysteine
D. All of the above

Glucocorticoid therapy may accelerate renal recovery, but does not appear to impact long-term renal survival. It is best reserved for cases with severe renal failure in which dialysis is imminent or if renal function continues to deteriorate despite stopping the offending drug.

1886. Which of the following acute obstructive disorders cause acute interstitial nephritis?

Harrison's 20th Ed. Chapter 310 Page 2157 Table 310-1

A. Light chain cast nephropathy (myeloma kidney)
B. Acute phosphate nephropathy
C. Acute urate nephropathy
D. All of the above

1887. Which of the following autoimmune diseases can cause acute interstitial nephritis?

Harrison's 20th Ed. Chapter 310 Page 2157 Table 310-1

A. Sjogren's syndrome
B. Systemic lupus erythematosus
C. IgG4-related systemic disease
D. All of the above

1888. Which of the following drugs can cause chronic interstitial nephritis?

Harrison's 20th Ed. Chapter 310 Page 2157 Table 310-1

A. Rifampin
B. Acyclovir
C. Lithium
D. Valproate

1889. Which of the following can cause chronic interstitial nephritis?

Harrison's 20th Ed. Chapter 310 Page 2157 Table 310-1

A. Cyclosporine
B. Lead
C. Cadmium
D. All of the above

1890. Which of the following can cause chronic interstitial nephritis?

Harrison's 20th Ed. Chapter 310 Page 2157 Table 310-1

A. Radiation nephritis
B. Sickle cell disease
C. Nephronophthisis
D. All of the above

1891. Corticosteroids & immunosuppressives are absolutely indicated which of the following causes of interstitial nephritis?

Harrison's 20th Ed. Chapter 310 Page 2158 Table 310-2

A. Sjögren's syndrome
B. Sarcoidosis
C. SLE interstitial nephritis
D. All of the above

1892. Sjogren's syndrome is best related to?

Harrison's 20th Ed. Chapter 310 Page 2158

A. Dumping syndrome
B. Sinusoidal obstruction syndrome
C. Sicca syndrome
D. Tumor lysis syndrome

1893. Which of the following is false about Sjogren's syndrome?

Harrison's 20th Ed. Chapter 310 Page 2158

A. Autoimmune disorder that targets exocrine glands
B. Positive for anti-Ro (SS-A) & anti-La (SS- B) antibodies
C. Polyclonal hypergammaglobulinemia
D. None of the above

1894. Sjogren' s syndrome can be associated with?

Harrison's 20th Ed. Chapter 310 Page 2158

A. Aristolochic acid
B. Hyperuricemia
C. Nephrogenic diabetes insipidus
D. Nephrocalcinosis

1895. Sjogren' s syndrome can be associated with?

Harrison's 20th Ed. Chapter 310 Page 2158

A. Distal RTA
B. Nephrogenic diabetes insipidus
C. Renal failure
D. All of the above

Tubulointerstitial nephritis with a predominant lymphocytic infiltrate is the most common renal manifestation of Sjogren's syndrome and can be associated with distal RTA, nephrogenic diabetes insipidus and moderate renal failure.

1896. Which of the following drug is useful in Sjogren' s syndrome?
Harrison's 20th Ed. Chapter 310 Page 2158

A. Glucocorticoids
B. Azathioprine
C. Mycophenolate mofetil
D. All of the above

Treatment of Sjogren' s syndrome is initiated with glucocorticoids. Patients may require maintenance therapy with azathioprine or mycophenolate mofetil to prevent relapse.

1897. Which of the following about tubulointerstitial nephritis with uveitis (TINU) is false?
Harrison's 20th Ed. Chapter 310 Page 2158

A. Systemic autoimmune disease of unknown etiology
B. Affects females three times more often than males
C. Median age of onset is 15 years
D. None of the above

1898. Which of the following about tubulointerstitial nephritis with uveitis (TINU) is false?
Harrison's 20th Ed. Chapter 310 Page 2158

A. Posterior uveitis
B. Elevated creatinine, sterile pyuria, mild proteinuria
C. Features of Fanconi's syndrome
D. Clinical symptoms are self-limited in children

In addition to lymphocyte-predominant interstitial nephritis in TINU, the hallmark feature is a painful anterior uveitis, often bilateral and accompanied by blurred vision & photophobia. Ocular symptoms precede or accompany the renal disease.

1899. Cause of uveitis and renal disease is?
Harrison's 20th Ed. Chapter 310 Page 2158

A. Sjogren's syndrome
B. Sarcoidosis
C. Systemic lupus erythematosus
D. All of the above

Causes of uveitis and renal disease are tubulointerstitial nephritis with uveitis (TINU), Sjogren's syndrome, Behcet's disease, sarcoidosis and systemic lupus erythematosus.

1900. Chronic sclerosing sialadenitis is a feature of?
Harrison's 20th Ed. Chapter 310 Page 2158

A. Tubulointerstitial nephritis with uveitis (TINU)
B. Sarcoidosis
C. IgG4-related systemic disease
D. Systemic lupus erythematosus

1901. Urinalysis showing "sheaf of wheat" crystals best relates to?
Harrison's 20th Ed. Chapter 310 Page 2159

A. Intravenous acyclovir
B. Indinavir
C. Sulfonamide
D. Allopurinol

1902. Red-green birefringement needle-shaped crystals on urinalysis are of?
Harrison's 20th Ed. Chapter 310 Page 2159

A. Acyclovir
B. Indinavir
C. Sulfonamide
D. Allopurinol

1903. Oral phospho-soda best relates to?
Harrison's 20th Ed. Chapter 310 Page 2159

A. Diuretic
B. Antacid
C. Laxative
D. Sunscreen

Acute phosphate nephropathy is a serious complication of oral Phospho-soda used as a laxative or for bowel preparation for colonoscopy.

1904. Myeloma kidney best relates to?
Harrison's 20th Ed. Chapter 310 Page 2160

A. POEMS syndrome
B. Multiple myeloma
C. Waldenstrom's macroglobulinemia
D. All of the above

Myeloma kidney is also called light chain cast nephropathy (LCCN).

1905. Clinical clues to the diagnosis of myeloma cast nephropathy include?
Harrison's 20th Ed. Chapter 310 Page 2160

A. Hypercalcemia
B. Abnormally narrow anion gap
C. Hypoalbuminemia and hypergammaglobulinemia
D. All of the above

Clinical clues to the diagnosis of myeloma cast nephropathy include anemia, bone pain, hypercalcemia, and an abnormally narrow anion gap due to hypoalbuminemia and hypergammaglobulinemia.

1906. Chronic interstitial nephritis (CIN) occurs mostly due to?
Harrison's 20th Ed. Chapter 310 Page 2160

A. Secondary to a primary glomerular disease
B. Developmental anomalies
C. Inherited diseases
D. All of the above

Chronic interstitial nephritis (CIN) occurs mostly due to renal ischemia or secondary to a primary glomerular disease. Other important forms of CIN are the result of developmental anomalies or inherited diseases such as reflux nephropathy or sickle cell nephropathy.

1907. Tubulointerstitial disease affecting predominantly medullary & papillary structures is?
Harrison's 20th Ed. Chapter 310 Page 2160

A. Analgesic nephropathy
B. Lead nephropathy
C. Plasma cell dyscrasias
D. All of the above

Tubulointerstitial diseases that predominantly affect medullary & papillary structures are analgesic nephropathy & sickle cell disease.

1908. Renal papillary necrosis invariably produces?
Harrison's 20th Ed. Chapter 94 Page 693

A. Painless hematuria
B. Obstructive uropathy
C. Isosthenuria
D. Renal hematoma

Renal papillary necrosis invariably produces isosthenuria which refers to nonconcentrated urine that is isosmotic with plasma.

1909. Which of the following is a cause of papillary necrosis?
Harrison's 20th Ed. Chapter 310 Page 2162 Table 310-3

A. Analgesic nephropathy
B. Sickle cell nephropathy
C. Diabetes with urinary tract infection
D. All of the above

1910. "Ring sign" on the pyelogram is pathognomonic of?
J Clin Diagn Res. 2016;10(1):TD10-TD12

A. Polycystic kidney disease
B. Papillary necrosis
C. Transitional cell carcinoma
D. Medullary sponge kidney

"Ring sign" (radiolucent sloughed papilla surrounded by radiodense contrast material in calyx) on pyelogram is pathognomonic of papillary necrosis due to analgesic nephropathy. CT reveals papillary calcifications surrounding the central sinus complex in a "garland" pattern. Contrast-containing rice grain sized cavities in the papilla are the pathognomonic feature of the medullary form of renal papillary necrosis.

1911. Which of the following is false about aristolochic acid?
Harrison's 20th Ed. Chapter 310 Page 2162

A. Carcinogen, causes DNA damage
B. Cause of Balkan endemic nephropathy
C. Renal interstitial fibrosis with paucity of cellular infiltrates
D. None of the above

1912. Which of the following is false about aristolochic acid?
Harrison's 20th Ed. Chapter 310 Page 2162

A. Cause of Chinese herbal nephropathy
B. Causes severe anemia
C. Aristolactam-DNA adducts in kidney or urinary tract tissue
D. None of the above

1913. Which of the following gene is involved in karyomegalic tubulointerstitial nephritis?
Harrison's 20th Ed. Chapter 310 Page 2162

A. AGR2
B. cagA
C. FAN1
D. dupA

Karyomegalic tubulointerstitial nephritis is a recessive disorder caused by inheritance of two mutant copies of FAN1 gene. FAN1 encodes a component of a DNA repair machinery complex.

1914. Which of the following is the most common renal sequelae of lithium associated nephropathy?
Harrison's 20th Ed. Chapter 310 Page 2162

A. Secondary FSGS
B. Nephrogenic diabetes insipidus
C. Chronic tubulointerstitial nephritis
D. None of the above

Use of lithium salts has renal sequelae, the most common of which is nephrogenic diabetes insipidus.

1915. Lithium best relates to which of the following?
Harrison's 20th Ed. Chapter 310 Page 2162

A. Electroneutral thiazide-sensitive Na^+/Cl^- cotransporter
B. Epithelial sodium channel (ENaC)
C. Apical Ca^{++}-selective channels (TRPV5)
D. K^+/Cl^- cotransporter

Lithium accumulates in principal cells of collecting duct by entering through epithelial sodium channel (ENaC), where it inhibits glycogen synthase kinase 3β & downregulates vasopressin-regulated aquaporin water channels.

1916. Which of the following is highly characteristic of lithium associated nephropathy on renal biopsy?
Harrison's 20th Ed. Chapter 310 Page 2162

A. Glomerulosclerosis
B. Interstitial fibrosis
C. Tubular atrophy
C. Cysts or dilation of the distal tubule & collecting duct

1917. Which of the following is effective to prevent & treat lithium-induced nephrogenic diabetes insipidus?
Harrison's 20th Ed. Chapter 310 Page 2162

A. Amiloride
B. Thiazide diuretic
C. Dexamethasone
D. All of the above

The entry of lithium through amiloride-sensitive Na^+ channel ENaC is required for the effect of the drug on principal cells, such that combined therapy within lithium & amiloride can mitigate lithium-associated NDI.

1918. Which of the following cause blockade of epithelial sodium channel (ENaC)?
Harrison's 20th Ed. Chapter 49 Page 309 Table 49-5

A. Triamterene
B. Trimethoprim
C. Nafamostat
D. All of the above

Amiloride, triamterene, trimethoprim, pentamidine, & nafamostat cause blockade of epithelial sodium channel (ENaC).

1919. Acute renal injury with the use of calcineurin inhibitor (CNI) is due to?
Harrison's 20th Ed. Chapter 310 Page 2163

A. Vasoconstriction
B. Thrombotic microangiopathy
C. Toxic tubulopathy
D. All of the above

1920. Hyperkalemia as a complication of the use of calcineurin inhibitor (CNI) is caused by tubular resistance to?
Harrison's 20th Ed. Chapter 310 Page 2163

A. Renin
B. Aldosterone
C. Angiotensin II
D. All of the above

Hyperkalemia with use of calcineurin inhibitor (CNI) is caused by tubular resistance to aldosterone.

1921. Histologic change in renal tissue with the use of calcineurin inhibitor (CNI) is?
Harrison's 20th Ed. Chapter 310 Page 2163

A. Patchy interstitial fibrosis
B. Tubular atrophy in a "striped" pattern
C. Intrarenal vasculature hyalinosis
D. All of the above

The histologic changes in renal tissue include patchy interstitial fibrosis and tubular atrophy, in a "striped" pattern. In addition, the intrarenal vasculature demonstrates hyalinosis, and focal glomerulosclerosis.

1922. Lead exposure best relates to?
Harrison's 20th Ed. Chapter 310 Page 2163, Arch Intern Med. 1993;153(12):1501-4

A. Nip joint
B. Moonshine whiskey
C. Congener
D. Rum-running

Moonshine derives its name from production of illegal whiskey under cover of darkness with only the moon as a guide. It contained lead levels exceeding Environmental Protection Agency water guidelines of 15 parts per billion. Moonshine whiskey are distilled in lead-tainted containers & cause lead toxicity.

1923. Early signs of chronic lead intoxication are attributable to?
Harrison's 20th Ed. Chapter 310 Page 2163

A. Proximal tubule dysfunction
B. Loop of Henle dysfunction
C. Distal convoluted tubule dysfunction
D. Collecting duct dysfunction

Early signs of chronic lead intoxication are attributable to proximal tubule dysfunction.

1924. Which of the following is a characteristic finding in patients with chronic lead nephropathy?
Harrison's 20th Ed. Chapter 310 Page 2163

A. Hypokalemia
B. Hypercalcemia
C. Hyperuricemia
D. Hyponatremia

Patients with chronic lead nephropathy are characteristically hyperuricemic due to increased reabsorption of filtered urate leading to acute gouty arthritis called saturnine gout. Saturnine gout refers to development of hyperuricaemia & gout due to inhibiting effect of lead on the tubular urate transport.

1925. Which of the following is not a feature of lead intoxication?
Harrison's 20th Ed. Chapter 310 Page 2163

A. Chronic interstitial nephritis (CIN)
B. Gout
C. Hyperglycemia
D. Hypertension

1926. Lead exposure is likely if the diagnostic triad is present that consists of all except?
Harrison's 20th Ed. Chapter 310 Page 2163

A. Gout
B. Anemia
C. Hypertension
D. Renal insufficiency

1927. Chronic hypercalcemia occurs in?
Harrison's 20th Ed. Chapter 310 Page 2163

A. Sarcoidosis
B. Multiple myeloma
C. Metastatic bone disease
D. All of the above

Chronic hypercalcemia occurs in primary hyperparathyroidism, sarcoidosis, multiple myeloma, vitamin D intoxication, or metastatic bone disease. It causes tubulointerstitial disease & progressive renal failure.

1928. The earliest lesion in hypercalcemic nephropathy is?
Harrison's 20th Ed. Chapter 310 Page 2163

A. Calcium deposition in glomeruli
B. Calcium deposition in tubular cell
C. Calcium deposition in walls of renal arterioles
D. Focal degenerative change in renal epithelia

1929. In hypercalcemic nephropathy, initial focal degenerative change involves renal epithelia of?
Harrison's 20th Ed. Chapter 310 Page 2163

A. Collecting ducts
B. Distal tubules
C. Loops of Henle
D. All of the above

The earliest lesion in hypercalcemic nephropathy is a focal degenerative change in renal epithelia, primarily in collecting ducts, distal tubules & loops of Henle.

1930. Nephrocalcinosis refers to?
Harrison's 20th Ed. Chapter 310 Page 2163

A. Glomerular calcium deposition
B. Tubular calcium deposition
C. Interstitial calcium deposition
D. All of the above

Tubular epithelial cell necrosis leads to nephron obstruction and stasis of intrarenal urine, favoring precipitation of Ca^{++} salts and infection. Dilation & atrophy of tubules, interstitial fibrosis, mononuclear leukocyte infiltration, and interstitial calcium deposition eventually occur. Interstitial calcium deposition is called nephrocalcinosis.

1931. Which of the following occurs in hypercalcemic nephropathy?
Harrison's 20th Ed. Chapter 310 Page 2163

A. Reduced responsiveness to arginine vasopressin in CD
B. Defective transport of sodium & chloride in loop of Henle
C. Tubulointerstitial damage
D. All of the above

1932. Which of the following can cause prolonged and severe hypokalemia?
Harrison's 20th Ed. Chapter 310 Page 2163

A. Primary aldosteronism
B. Chronic laxative or diuretic abuse
C. Surreptitious vomiting
D. All of the above

Patients with prolonged and severe hypokalemia develop a reversible tubular lesion characterized by vacuolar degeneration of proximal and distal tubular cells.

Vascular Injury to the Kidney

1933. Thrombotic microangiopathy (TMA) is characterized by all except?

Harrison's 20th Ed. Chapter 311 Page 2164

A. Endothelial cell injury
B. Mainly of arterioles & capillaries
C. Occlusive platelet and hyaline thrombi
D. Thrombocytosis

TMA is usually accompanied by microangiopathic hemolytic anemia (MAHA) with its typical features of thrombocytopenia and schistocytes.

1934. Which of the following pattern is seen in the glomerulus in TMA?

Harrison's 20th Ed. Chapter 311 Page 2164

A. Minimal change
B. Membranous
C. Membranoproliferative
D. All of the above

1935. Which of the following is seen in the glomerulus in TMA?

Harrison's 20th Ed. Chapter 311 Page 2164

A. Endotheliosis
B. Fibrin thrombi & platelet plugs
C. Arterial intimal fibrosis
D. All of the above

In kidney, TMA is characterized by swollen endocapillary cells (endotheliosis), fibrin thrombi, platelet plugs, arterial intimal fibrosis and a membranoproliferative pattern in glomerulus. Fibrin thrombi may extend into arteriolar vascular pole, producing glomerular collapse and cortical necrosis. In kidneys that recover from acute TMA, secondary focal segmental glomerulosclerosis may develop.

1936. Diseases associated with TMA include?

Harrison's 20th Ed. Chapter 311 Page 2164

A. Antiphospholipid syndrome
B. HIV infection
C. Radiation nephropathy
D. All of the above

Diseases associated with TMA include thrombotic thrombocytopenic purpura (TTP), hemolytic-uremic syndrome (HUS), malignant hypertension, scleroderma renal crisis, antiphospholipid syndrome, preeclampsia/HELLP syndrome, HIV infection and radiation nephropathy.

1937. Thrombotic microangiopathy (TMA) can be seen in?

Harrison's 20th Ed. Chapter 311 Page 2164

A. Myeloproliferative neoplasm-related glomerulopathy
B. POEMS syndrome
C. Malignant hypertension
D. All of the above

TMA can be seen in myeloproliferative neoplasm (MPN)-related glomerulopathy and POEMS syndrome which are not associated with MAHA.

1938. Which of the following statements is false?

Harrison's 20th Ed. Chapter 311 Page 2164

A. HUS & TTP are the prototypes for MAHA
B. TTP develops more commonly in adults
C. HUS occurs more commonly in children
D. None of the above

TTP develops more commonly in adults and has more neurologic complications. HUS occurs more frequently in children, particularly when associated with hemorrhagic diarrhea.

1939. Shiga toxin is best related to which bacteria?

Harrison's 20th Ed. Chapter 311 Page 2164

A. Streptococcus viridans
B. Staphylococcus aureus
C. Escherichia coli
D. Enterococcus sp

Shiga toxins (Stx1 & Stx2) are also referred to as verotoxins. These toxins are produced by certain strains of E. coli and Shigella dysenteriae.

1940. Which is the most common variant of hemolytic-uremic syndrome (HUS)?

Harrison's 20th Ed. Chapter 311 Page 2164

A. Shiga toxin-producing Escherichia coli (STEC) HUS
B. D^+ HUS
C. Enterohemorrhagic E. coli (EHEC) HUS
D. All of the above

All of the above are the same entity.

1941. Hemolytic-uremic syndrome is associated with which pathotype of E. coli?

Harrison's 20th Ed. Chapter 311 Page 2164

A. STEC/EHEC/STEAEC
B. ETEC
C. EPEC
D. All of the above

ETEC (enterotoxigenic E. coli), STEAEC (Shiga toxin-producing enteroaggregative) E. coli, STEC (Shiga toxi n-producing E. coli), EPEC (enteropathogenic E. coli).

1942. Which of the following usually precedes MAHA?

Harrison's 20th Ed. Chapter 311 Page 2164

A. Diarrhea
B. Abdominal pain
C. Cramping
D. Vomiting

1943. Which of the following is typically absent in MAHA?

Harrison's 20th Ed. Chapter 311 Page 2164

A. Fever
B. Abdominal pain
C. Cramping
D. Vomiting

Diarrhea, often bloody, precedes MAHA within 1 week in >80% of cases. Abdominal pain, cramping, and vomiting are frequent whereas fever is typically absent.

1944. Verotoxin best relates to?

Harrison's 20th Ed. Chapter 311 Page 2164

A. Botulinum toxin
B. Hepatotoxin
C. Neurotoxin
D. Shiga toxin

1945. Which of the following is an action of Shiga toxin?

Harrison's 20th Ed. Chapter 311 Page 2164, Chapter 308 Page 2148

A. Binding to glycolipid surface receptor globotriaosylceramide (Gb3)
B. Inhibition of endothelial production of ADAMTS13
C. Inducing inflammatory cytokines & chemokine receptors
D. All of the above

1946. Which of the following is an inflammatory cytokine?

Harrison's 20th Ed. Chapter 311 Page 2164

A. Interleukin 8 (IL-8)
B. Monocyte chemotactic protein 1 (MCP-1)
C. Stromal cell–derived factor 1 (SDF-1)
D. All of the above

1947. Which of the following can also cause HUS?

Harrison's 20th Ed. Chapter 311 Page 2164

A. E. coli
B. Shigella dysenteriae
C. Streptococcus pneumoniae
D. All of the above

Streptococcus pneumoniae can also cause HUS.

1948. Which of the following about Thomsen-Friedenreich antigen is false?

Harrison's 20th Ed. Chapter 311 Page 2164

A. Present on platelets and endothelial cells
B. Normally covered by N-acetylneuraminic acid moieties
B. Exposure to preformed IgM results in severe MAHA
D. None of the above

1949. Thomsen–Friedenreich antigen best relates to?

Harrison's 20th Ed. Chapter 311 Page 2164, N Engl J Med. 2014; 371:1846-1848

A. S. pneumoniae-associated hemolytic-uremic syndrome
B. S. aureus-associated hemolytic-uremic syndrome
C. Enterococcus-associated hemolytic-uremic syndrome
D. Escherichia coli-associated hemolytic-uremic syndrome

1950. Thomsen-Friedenreich antigen (T-antigen) best relates to?

Harrison's 20th Ed. Chapter 311 Page 2164, Pediatr Infect Dis J 2011;30:1-4

A. Glucosaminidase
B. Neuraminidase
C. Hexosaminidase
D. Mannosidase

Streptococcus pneumoniae-associated hemolytic-uremic syndrome (SP-HUS) is a rare but severe complication that implicates binding of Thomsen–Friedenreich antigen (T-antigen) to preformed circulating IgM antibodies, owing to neuraminidase-mediated cleavage of sialic acid residues from the membrane of glomerular capillary endothelial cells, red cells, and platelets, leading to pneumococcal sepsis-mediated thrombotic microangiopathy and HUS. Neuraminidase-associated thrombotic microangiopathy is generally observed in pediatric patients with pneumonia and meningitis.

1951. Which STEC strain is mostly causes HUS?

Harrison's 20th Ed. Chapter 311 Page 2164

A. O157:H7
B. O145:H28
C. O157/H-
D. O111:H-

1952. Glomerular endotheliosis is a feature of?

Harrison's 20th Ed. Chapter 311 Page 2164

A. Preeclampsia
B. HELLP syndrome
C. HUS
D. All of the above

Glomerular endotheliosis is seen in HUS, preeclampsia/HELLP (hemolysis, elevated liver enzymes, and low platelet count syndrome), malignant hypertension and the antiphospholipid syndrome.

1953. Which of the following is related to "atypical HUS"?

Harrison's 20th Ed. Chapter 311 Page 2164

A. Complement dysregulation
B. Low C3 and normal C4 levels
C. Factor H deficiency
D. All of the above

The complement dysregulation can be congenital or acquired. Low C3 and a normal C4 levels are characteristic of alternative pathway activation.

1954. Which of the following about Factor H is false?

Harrison's 20th Ed. Chapter 311 Page 2164

A. Competes with factor B to prevent formation of C3bBb
B. Acts as a cofactor for factor I which degrades C3b
C. Deficiency linked to families with aHUS
D. None of the above

1955. DEAP HUS best relates to?

Harrison's 20th Ed. Chapter 311 Page 2165

A. Factor B
B. Factor H
C. Factor I
D. All of the above

DEAP refers to deficiency of CFHR plasma proteins and CFH autoantibody positive. HUS occurs when an autoantibody to factor H is formed, and blocks binding of factor H to C3b & surface-bound C3 convertase.

1956. Which of the following is not typical of TTP?

Harrison's 20th Ed. Chapter 311 Page 2165

A. Thrombocytopenia
B. Hemorrhagic tendency
C. Neurologic symptoms
D. Renal failure

Traditionally, TTP is characterized by the pentad: MAHA, thrombocytopenia, neurologic symptoms, fever and renal failure.

1957. Which of the following best relates to the pathophysiology of TTP?

Harrison's 20th Ed. Chapter 311 Page 2165

A. von Willebrand factor
B. Factor B
C. Factor H
D. All of the above

1958. Which of the following best relates to the pathophysiology of TTP?

Harrison's 20th Ed. Chapter 311 Page 2165

A. ADAMTS13
B. ADAMTS14
C. ADAMTS15
D. ADAMTS16

The pathophysiology of TTP involves accumulation of ultra-large multimers of von Willebrand factor due to the absence or markedly decreased activity of plasma protease ADAMTS13, a disintegrin and metalloproteinase with a thrombospondin type 1 motif, member 13. These ultra-large multimers form clots and damage erythrocytes, resulting in MAHA.

1959. TTP is defined as MAHA associated with ADAMTS13 activity of?

Harrison's 20th Ed. Chapter 311 Page 2165

A. < 5–10%
B. < 15–20%
C. < 35–40%
D. < 50–60%

TTP is defined as MAHA associated with ADAMTS13 activity of < 5–10%.

1960. Apart from low levels of ADAMTS13, which of the following is required to initiate clinical TTP?

Harrison's 20th Ed. Chapter 311 Page 2165

A. Infection
B. Surgery
C. Pregnancy
D. All of the above

Apart from low levels of ADAMTS13, an additional inflammatory trigger (infection, surgery, pancreatitis, or pregnancy) is required to initiate clinical TTP. This may be mediated by human neutrophil peptides that inhibit cleavage of von Willebrand factor by ADAMTS13.

1961. The median age of onset of TTP is?

Harrison's 20th Ed. Chapter 311 Page 2165

A. 20 years
B. 30 years
C. 40 years
D. 50 years

The median age of onset of TTP is 40 years.

1962. Which of the following about TTP is false?

Harrison's 20th Ed. Chapter 311 Page 2165

A. Incidence is higher among blacks than among non-blacks
B. Incidence is higher among women than among men
C. If untreated, TTP has a mortality rate exceeding 90%
D. None of the above

1963. Which of the following is a hereditary condition characterized by congenital deficiency of ADAMTS13?

Harrison's 20th Ed. Chapter 311 Page 2165

A. Boerhaave's syndrome
B. Upshaw-Schülman syndrome
C. Münchausen's syndrome
D. Chédiak-Higashi syndrome

Upshaw-Schülman syndrome is a hereditary condition characterized by congenital deficiency of ADAMTS13.

1964. TTP/HUS is seen in?

Harrison's 20th Ed. Chapter 311 Page 2165

A. Pregnancy
B. Use of oral contraceptives
C. HIV infection
D. All of the above

1965. TTP/HUS is seen with the use of?

Harrison's 20th Ed. Chapter 311 Page 2165

A. Quinine
B. Cyclosporine/tacrolimus
C. Ticlopidine/clopidogrel
D. All of the above

1966. Toxic or endothelial damage is the main cause of TMA produced by all of the following drugs except?

Harrison's 20th Ed. Chapter 311 Page 2165

A. Gemcitabine
B. Quinine
C. Interferon
D. Cyclosporine

1967. Quinine induces autoantibodies to all except?

Harrison's 20th Ed. Chapter 311 Page 2165

A. Granulocytes, lymphocytes
B. Endothelial cells
C. Platelet glycoprotein Ib/IX or IIb/IIIa complexes
D. ADAMTS13

Quinine induces autoantibodies to granulocytes, lymphocytes, endothelial cells, and platelet glycoprotein Ib/IX or IIb/IIIa complexes, but not to ADAMTS13.

1968. Autoantibody-mediated TTP and DEAP HUS respond to which of the following?

Harrison's 20th Ed. Chapter 311 Page 2165

A. Plasma exchange
B. Prednisone
C. Rituximab
D. All of the above

1969. Drug-induced TMA secondary to endothelial damage respond to?

Harrison's 20th Ed. Chapter 311 Page 2165

A. Plasma exchange
B. Prednisone
C. Rituximab
D. None of the above

Drug-induced TMA secondary to endothelial damage typically does not respond to plasma exchange and is treated primarily by discontinuing use of the offending agent and providing supportive care.

1970. STEC HUS respond to?

Harrison's 20th Ed. Chapter 311 Page 2165

A. Plasma exchange
B. Prednisone
C. Rituximab
D. None of the above

STEC HUS should be treated with supportive measures as plasma exchange is not effective.

1971. Which of the following is approved for use in aHUS?
Harrison's 20th Ed. Chapter 311 Page 2165

A. Golimumab
B. Bevacizumab
C. Eculizumab
D. Certolizumab pegol

Eculizumab is a monoclonal antibody to C5 that is approved for use in aHUS.

1972. Neuraminidase-associated HUS respond to?
Harrison's 20th Ed. Chapter 311 Page 2165

A. Antibiotics
B. Washed red cells
C. Plasmapheresis
D. All of the above

Antibiotics, washed red cells & plasmapheresis may be helpful in neuraminidase-associated HUS.

1973. Hematopoietic stem cell transplantation associated thrombotic microangiopathy (HSCT-TMA) usually occurs within how many days of HSCT?
Harrison's 20th Ed. Chapter 311 Page 2165

A. First 10 days
B. First 100 days
C. First 300 days
D. First 500 days

HSCT-TMA usually occurs within the first 100 days of HSCT.

1974. The incidence of HSCT-TMA developing after HSCT is?
Harrison's 20th Ed. Chapter 311 Page 2165

A. ~ 2%
B. ~ 4%
C. ~ 6%
D. ~ 8%

HSCT-TMA develops after HSCT, with an incidence of ~8%.

1975. Which of the following variables is not included in criteria for establishing microangiopathic kidney injury associated with HSCT by International Working Group?
Harrison's 20th Ed. Chapter 311 Page 2165 Table 311-1

A. Schistocytes in the blood
B. LDH concentration
C. Haptoglobin concentration
D. Coombs test

1976. Scleroderma renal crisis (SRC) includes?
Harrison's 20th Ed. Chapter 311 Page 2166

A. Accelerated hypertension
B. Rapid deterioration in renal function
C. Nephrotic proteinuria
D. All of the above

SRC is a rapid deterioration in renal function, usually accompanied by accelerated hypertension, oliguria, nephrotic range proteinuria, hematuria, fluid retention, microangiopathic hemolytic anemia, retinopathy and encephalopathy.

1977. Which of the following is rare in scleroderma renal crisis?
Harrison's 20th Ed. Chapter 311 Page 2166

A. Pericarditis
B. Retinopathy
C. Coagulopathy
D. Pulmonary edema

MAHA is present in > 50% patients of SRC, coagulopathy is rare.

1978. Renal lesion in scleroderma renal crisis is characterized by?
Harrison's 20th Ed. Chapter 311 Page 2166

A. Arcuate artery intimal proliferation
B. Arcuate artery medial proliferation
C. Luminal narrowing
D. All of the above

Renal lesion in scleroderma renal crisis is characterized by arcuate artery intimal and medial proliferation with luminal narrowing, described as "onion-skinning" and can be accompanied by glomerular collapse due to reduced blood flow.

1979. Onion-skin pattern best relates to?
Harrison's 20th Ed. Chapter 311 Page 2166

A. Intimal proliferation
B. Medial proliferation
C. Luminal narrowing
D. Hyalinosis

Patients with scleroderma renal crisis show acute fibrinoid necrosis of afferent arterioles, followed by intimal proliferation (onion-skin pattern), and ischemic collapse of glomeruli.

1980. Histologically, scleroderma renal crisis is indistinguishable from?
Harrison's 20th Ed. Chapter 311 Page 2166

A. Radiation nephropathy
B. HSCT-TMA
C. Malignant hypertension
D. HIV-related TMA

Histologically, scleroderma renal crisis is indistinguishable from malignant hypertension.

1981. Which of the following antibodies are strongly associated with scleroderma renal disease?
Harrison's 20th Ed. Chapter 311 Page 2166

A. P-ANCA
B. Smooth-muscle antibody (SMA)
C. anti-Jo-1 antibody
D. Anti-U3-RNP

Anti-U3-RNP antibodies are strongly associated with scleroderma renal disease. Anticentromere antibody is a negative predictor of this disorder.

1982. Which of the following is used for blood pressure management & improvement of renal perfusion in scleroderma renal crisis?
Harrison's 20th Ed. Chapter 311 Page 2166

A. Epoprostenol
B. Iloprost
C. Treprostinil
D. All of the above

Iloprost, epoprostenol & treprostinil are prostacyclin analogues.

1983. Which of the following is an antiphospholipid antibody?
Harrison's 20th Ed. Chapter 311 Page 2166

A. Anticardiolipin antibodies (IgG, IgM, IgA)
B. Lupus anticoagulant
C. Anti-β-2 glycoprotein I antibodies (antiβ2GPI)
D. All of the above

Patients with both anticardiolipin antibodies and antiβ2GPI have the highest risk of thrombosis.

1984. Anticardiolipin antibodies may belong to which of the following class of immunoglobulins?
Harrison's 20th Ed. Chapter 311 Page 2166

A. IgG
B. IgM
C. IgA
D. All of the above

1985. Which of the following is unusual in antiphospholipid syndrome?
Harrison's 20th Ed. Chapter 311 Page 2166

A. Systemic thrombosis (arterial and venous)
B. Fetal morbidity
C. Arteriosclerosis
D. Microangiopathic hemolytic anemia (MAHA)

In antiphospholipid syndrome, signs of MAHA and platelet consumption are usually absent.

1986. Which of the following is false about treatment in antiphospholipid syndrome?
Harrison's 20th Ed. Chapter 311 Page 2166

A. Lifelong anticoagulation
B. Glucocorticoids may be beneficial in accelerated hypertension
C. Immunosuppression and plasma exchange may be helpful
D. None of the above

1987. Which of the following about HELLP syndrome is false?
Harrison's 20th Ed. Chapter 311 Page 2166

A. Occurs in 0.2–0.9% of all pregnancies
B. Occurs in 10–20% of women with severe preeclampsia
C. Carries a mortality rate of 7.4–34%
D. None of the above

1988. Which of the following about HELLP syndrome is false?
Harrison's 20th Ed. Chapter 311 Page 2166

A. Most commonly develops in the third trimester
B. 10% of cases occur before week 27 of gestation
C. 30% cases occur post-partum
D. None of the above

1989. Risk factor HELLP syndrome is?
Harrison's 20th Ed. Chapter 311 Page 2166

A. Elevated levels of fetal mRNA for FLT1
B. Elevated levels of endoglin
C. Abnormal placentation
D. All of the above

1990. Patients with HELLP syndrome have higher levels of?
Harrison's 20th Ed. Chapter 311 Page 2166

A. C-reactive protein
B. IL-1 Ra
C. IL-6
D. All of the above

HELLP syndrome risk factors include abnormal placentation, family history, and elevated levels of fetal mRNA for FLT1 (vascular endothelial growth factor receptor 1) and endoglin. Patients with HELLP syndrome have higher levels of inflammatory markers (C-reactive protein, IL-1Ra, and IL-6) and soluble HLADR than do those with preeclampsia alone.

1991. Organ that defines HELLP syndrome is?
Harrison's 20th Ed. Chapter 311 Page 2166

A. Kidney
B. Lung
C. Liver
D. Brain

Although renal failure is common, the organ that defines HELLP syndrome is the liver.

1992. Potentially life-threatening complication of HELLP syndrome is?
Harrison's 20th Ed. Chapter 311 Page 2167

A. Spontaneous rupture of the liver
B. Cerebral infarction
C. Cerebral and brainstem hemorrhage
D. All of the above

In HELLP syndrome, subcapsular hepatic hematomas may produce spontaneous rupture of liver and can be life threatening.

1993. Which of the following is a complication of HELLP syndrome?
Harrison's 20th Ed. Chapter 311 Page 2167

A. Placental abruption
B. Permanent vision loss
C. Bleeding
D. All of the above

HELLP syndrome, nonfatal complications include placental abruption, permanent vision loss due to Purtscher-like retinopathy (hemorrhagic & vaso-occlusive vasculopathy), pulmonary edema, bleeding, and fetal demise.

1994. Which of the following can be triggered by pregnancy?
Harrison's 20th Ed. Chapter 311 Page 2167

A. HELLP syndrome
B. aHUS
C. TTP
D. All of the above

1995. Which of the following is false in HELLP syndrome?
Harrison's 20th Ed. Chapter 311 Page 2167

A. Serum levels of ADAMTS13 activity are reduced
B. Levels of antithrombin III are reduced
C. Levels of D-dimer are elevated
D. None of the above

Antithrombin III levels are decreased in HELLP syndrome (but not in TTP) and D-dimer levels are elevated in HELLP syndrome but not in TTP.

1996. Which of the following is a myeloproliferative neoplasm (MPN)?
Harrison's 20th Ed. Chapter 311 Page 2167

A. Chronic myelogenous leukemia (CML)
B. Polycythemia vera (PV)
C. Essential thrombocythemia (ET)
D. All of the above

1997. Which of the following is a myeloproliferative neoplasm (MPN)?
Harrison's 20th Ed. Chapter 311 Page 2167

A. Primary myelofibrosis (PMF)
B. Systemic mastocytosis
C. Chronic eosinophilic leukemia
D. All of the above

MPN represents a group of clonal disorders that includes chronic myelogenous leukemia (CML), polycythemia vera (PV), essential thrombocythemia (ET), primary myelofibrosis (PMF), systemic mastocytosis, chronic eosinophilic leukemia not otherwise specified, chronic neutrophilic leukemia, and unclassifiable MPN.

1998. Median time from diagnosis of MPN to MPN-related glomerulopathy is?
Harrison's 20th Ed. Chapter 311 Page 2167

A. ~ 1 year
B. ~ 3 years
C. ~ 5 years
D. ~ 7 years

MPN-related glomerulopathy usually occurs late in the course of the hematologic condition and median time from diagnosis of MPN to glomerulopathy is ~7.2 years.

1999. In POEMS syndrome, "O" stands for?
Harrison's 20th Ed. Chapter 311 Page 2167

A. Obesity
B. Organomegaly
C. Obstructive jaundice
D. Oliguria

POEMS syndrome is a systemic disease characterized by polyneuropathy, organomegaly, endocrinopathy, monoclonal gammopathy, and skin changes.

2000. Which of the following is the hallmark of POEMS syndrome?
Harrison's 20th Ed. Chapter 311 Page 2167

A. Peripheral neuropathy
B. Skin changes
C. Endocrinopathy
D. Monoclonal gammopathy

Peripheral neuropathy with severe motorsensory deficit is the hallmark of POEMS syndrome.

2001. In POEMS syndrome, majority of monoclonal light chain is of which isotype?
Harrison's 20th Ed. Chapter 311 Page 2167

A. Kappa
B. Lambda
C. Gamma
D. Theta

In POEMS syndrome, >95% of mono clonal light chain is of the lambda isotype. IgA also makes up about 50% of the monoclonal protein.

2002. Which of the following about POEMS syndrome is false?
Harrison's 20th Ed. Chapter 311 Page 2167

A. IgA constitutes ~50% of monoclonal protein
B. Lymphadenopathy is common
C. Unilateral hypertrophy of kidney frequent
D. None of the above

2003. Which of the following about POEMS syndrome is false?
Harrison's 20th Ed. Chapter 311 Page 2167

A. Glomerulomegaly
B. Low grade proteinuria
C. Progression to end stage renal disease is rare
D. None of the above

2004. Renal complications in sickle cell disease is due to occlusion of?
Harrison's 20th Ed. Chapter 311 Page 2167

A. Afferent arteriole
B. Efferent arteriole
C. Glomeruli
D. Vasa recta

Renal complications in sickle cell disease result from occlusion of the vasa recta in the renal medulla.

2005. Which of the following occur in sickle cell disease?
Harrison's 20th Ed. Chapter 311 Page 2167

A. Hyposthenuria
B. Hematuria
C. Papillary necrosis
D. All of the above

2006. Which of the following is true about sickle cell disease?
Harrison's 20th Ed. Chapter 311 Page 2167

A. Hypertension is uncommon
B. Glomeruli are typically enlarged
C. More prone to acute renal failure
D. All of the above

2007. Renal vein thrombosis can occur in?
Harrison's 20th Ed. Chapter 311 Page 2167

A. Antiphospholipid syndrome
B. Nephrotic syndrome
C. Proteins C, S and antithrombin deficiency
D. All of the above

2008. Renal vein thrombosis can occur in?
Harrison's 20th Ed. Chapter 311 Page 2167

A. Factor V Leiden
B. Disseminated malignancy
C. Oral contraceptives
D. All of the above

2009. Nephrotic syndrome due to which of the following predisposes to renal vein thrombosis?
Harrison's 20th Ed. Chapter 311 Page 2167

A. Minimal change disease
B. Membranous nephropathy
C. Membranoproliferative glomerulonephritis
D. Lupus nephropathy

Nephrotic syndrome due to membranous nephropathy predisposes to renal vein thrombosis.

2010. Which of the following threaten blood supply of the kidney?

N Engl J Med. 2009;361:1972-8

A. Fibromuscular diseases
B. Inflammatory disorders
C. Primary hematologic disorders
D. All of the above

Disorders that threaten blood supply of kidney include large vessel atherosclerosis, fibromuscular diseases, embolic, inflammatory, and primary hematologic disorders.

2011. Large-vessel renal artery occlusive disease result most commonly from?

N Engl J Med. 2009;361:1972-8

A. Extrinsic compression of the vessel
B. Fibromuscular dysplasias
C. Atherosclerotic disease
D. None of the above

Large vessel renal artery occlusive disease results most commonly from atherosclerotic disease and also from extrinsic compression of the vessel and fibromuscular dysplasias.

2012. What percentage of cases of hypertension are caused by renal artery stenosis (RAS)?

N Engl J Med. 2009;361:1972-8

A. ~ 1%
B. ~ 5%
C. ~ 7%
D. ~ 10%

~5% of cases of hypertension are caused by renal artery stenosis (RAS).

2013. Which of the following is not a characteristic of renal artery stenosis due to fibromuscular dysplasia?

N Engl J Med. 2009;361:1972-8

A. Usually young (<40 yr)
B. Usually male
C. Middle or distal lesion location
D. Good BP response to revascularization

Patients of RAS due to fibromuscular dysplasia are usually female (15–50 yrs).

2014. The clinical clues for the diagnosis of renal-artery stenosis include all except?

N Engl J Med. 2009;361:1972-8

A. Onset of stage 2 hypertension >30 years of age
B. Absence of family history of hypertension
C. Hypertension associated with renal insufficiency
D. Renal function worsens after ACE inhibitors

Classic clinical clues that suggest the diagnosis of RAS are onset of stage 2 hypertension (BP>160/100 mm Hg) after 50 years of age, absence of family history of HTN, HTN with renal insufficiency, renal function worsens after administration of renin–angiotensin–aldosterone system blocker, HTN with repeated hospital admissions for heart failure, and drug-resistant hypertension.

2015. Which of the following diagnostic imaging tests for renal-artery stenosis provide best image quality & anatomical information?

N Engl J Med. 2009;361:1972-8

A. Duplex ultrasonography
B. Magnetic resonance angiography
C. Computed tomographic angiography
D. Digital-subtraction angiography

2016. Which of the following is termed as renal enzyme?

N Engl J Med. 2009;361:1972-8

A. Serum aspartate aminotransferase (AST)
B. Serum lactate dehydrogenase (LDH)
C. Serum alkaline phosphatase
D. All of the above

Renal enzymes elevated in renal infarction are aspartate aminotransferase (AST), lactate dehydrogenase (LDH), and alkaline phosphatase.

2017. Most common cause of cholesterol crystal embolization in atheroembolic renal disease is?

N Engl J Med. 2009;361:1972-8

A. Vascular surgery
B. Arteriography
C. Anticoagulation with heparin
D. Thrombolytic therapy

Arteriographic procedures are the most common cause of cholesterol crystal embolization in atheroembolic renal disease.

2018. Which of the following is rare in cholesterol crystal embolization in atheroembolic renal disease?

N Engl J Med. 2009;361:1972-8

A. Livedo reticularis
B. "Purple" toes
C. Toe gangrene
D. Renal infarction

Renal infarction secondary to cholesterol embolization is rare.

2019. Lab. findings in cholesterol crystal embolization in atheroembolic renal disease include all except?

N Engl J Med. 2009;361:1972-8

A. Rising blood urea nitrogen & creatinine
B. Eosinopenia
C. Anemia
D. Hypocomplementemia

Lab. findings in cholesterol crystal embolization in atheroembolic renal disease include rising BUN & creatinine, eosinophilia, eosinophiluria, leukocytosis, elevated ESR, anemia & hypocomplementemia.

2020. Which of the following approaches in atheroembolic renal disease is not beneficial?

N Engl J Med. 2009;361:1972-8

A. Anticoagulation
B. Cholesterol-lowering agents
C. Steroid therapy
D. All of the above

Withdrawal of anticoagulation may be beneficial.

2021. In 'Benign arteriolar nephrosclerosis' the characteristic pathology 'Hyaline arteriolosclerosis' is in?

N Engl J Med. 2009;361:1972-8

A. Afferent arterioles
B. Capillaries
C. Efferent arterioles
D. All of the above

Characteristic pathology of arteriolar nephrosclerosis is in afferent arterioles that have thickened walls & narrowing of vascular lumen due to deposition of homogeneous eosinophilic material (hyaline arteriolosclerosis) resulting in ischemic injury to glomeruli & tubules.

2022. 'Flea-bitten appearance' of kidneys is seen in?

N Engl J Med. 2009;361:1972-8

A. Malignant arteriolar nephrosclerosis
B. Hemolytic uremic syndrome (HUS)
C. Thrombotic thrombocytopenic purpura (TTP)
D. All of the above

Flea-bitten appearance of kidneys is due to hemorrhages in surface capillaries.

2023. Which of the following is false regarding "onion-skin lesion"?

N Engl J Med. 2009;361:1972-8

A. Seen in malignant arteriolar nephrosclerosis
B. Involves interlobular arteries
C. Hyperplastic arteriolitis
D. None of the above

2024. In the natural course of malignant hypertension, death is almost always due to?

N Engl J Med. 2009;361:1972-8

A. CHF
B. Ischemic heart disease
C. Cerebrovascular accident
D. Uremia

Malignant hypertension is a medical emergency. Its natural course includes a death rate of 80–90% within 1 year of onset, almost always due to uremia.

2025. Acute bilateral cortical necrosis is associated with?

N Engl J Med. 2009;361:1972-8

A. Septic abortion
B. Abruptio placentae
C. Preeclampsia
D. All of the above

Acute bilateral cortical necrosis is associated with septic abortions, abruptio placentae & preeclampsia.

Nephrolithiasis

2026. Which of the following kidney stones are most common?

Harrison's 20th Ed. Chapter 312 Page 2168

A. Calcium oxalate
B. Calcium phosphate
C. Uric acid
D. Struvite

2027. Which of the following kidney stones is least common?

Harrison's 20th Ed. Chapter 312 Page 2168

A. Calcium oxalate
B. Calcium phosphate
C. Uric acid
D. Struvite

Calcium oxalate kidney stones are most common (~75%) followed by calcium phosphate (~15%), uric acid (~8%), struvite (~1%) and cystine (<1%).

2028. Kidney stones may be composed of which of the following medications?

Harrison's 20th Ed. Chapter 312 Page 2168

A. Acyclovir
B. Atazanavir
C. Triamterene
D. All of the above

Stones may be composed of medications like acyclovir, atazanavir and triamterene.

2029. Struvite best relates to?

Harrison's 20th Ed. Chapter 312 Page 2168

A. Calcium phosphate
B. Magnesium ammonium phosphate
C. Calcium oxalate dihydrate
D. Calcium oxalate monohydrate

2030. Apatite best relates to?

Harrison's 20th Ed. Chapter 312 Page 2168

A. Calcium phosphate
B. Magnesium ammonium phosphate
C. Calcium oxalate dihydrate
D. Calcium oxalate monohydrate

The main constituent of calcium stones is brushite (calcium hydrogen phosphate) or hydroxyapatite. Calcium oxalate crystals are of two types — the dihydrate (or Wedellite) and the monohydrate (or Whewellite).

2031. Which of the following duct is related to nephron?

Harrison's 20th Ed. Chapter 81 Page 616

A. Duct of Wirsung
B. Duct of Luschka
C. Duct of Rivinus
D. Duct of Bellini

2032. Which of the following about supersaturation (SS) is false?

Harrison's 20th Ed. Chapter 312 Page 2168

A. Driving force for crystallization in urine
B. Ratio of the concentration of dissolved salt to its solubility
C. Used to monitor response to medical & dietary interventions for stone prevention
D. None of the above

Supersaturation (SS) is the driving force for crystallization in urine and is defined as ratio of the concentration of dissolved salt to its solubility. The consequences of increased urinary SS are formation of crystalline particles that is the forerunner to stone formation. SSs are also used to monitor response to medical and dietary interventions for stone prevention.

2033. "Recurrent stone former" is defined as an increase in stone size during past?

Harrison's 20th Ed. Chapter 312 Page 2168

A. 1 year
B. 5 years
C. 10 years
D. 15 years

"Recurrent stone former" was defined as either a recurrent stone event or an increase in the stone size during the past five years confirmed by imaging modalities.

2034. Which of the following about nephrolithiasis is false?

Harrison's 20th Ed. Chapter 312 Page 2168

A. 19% men & 9% women will develop at least one stone in life
B. Prevalence is lower among black individuals than whites
C. Among white men, peak annual incidence at age 40
D. None of the above

2035. Which of the following about nephrolithiasis is false?

Harrison's 20th Ed. Chapter 312 Page 2168

A. Global disease
B. Systemic disorder
C. Incidence varies by age, sex, and race
D. None of the above

2036. Which of the following conditions predispose to stone formation?

Harrison's 20th Ed. Chapter 312 Page 2168

A. Crohn's disease
B. Gastric bypass surgery
C. Type 2 diabetes mellitus
D. All of the above

2037. Which of the following conditions predispose to stone formation?

Harrison's 20th Ed. Chapter 312 Page 2168

A. Gout
B. Cholelithiasis
C. Reduced bone mineral density
D. All of the above

Conditions that predispose to stone formation are Crohn's disease, gastric bypass surgery, primary hyperparathyroidism, obesity, type 2 diabetes mellitus and distal renal tubular acidosis. Medical conditions that are more likely to be present in individuals with a history of nephrolithiasis are hypertension, gout, cholelithiasis, reduced bone mineral density and chronic kidney disease.

2038. Term "pus under pressure" best relates to?
Harrison's 20th Ed. Chapter 312 Page 2168

A. Infected subcapsular renal infarct
B. Urinary tract infection in the setting of an obstructing stone
C. Urinary stone and renal papillary necrosis
D. All of the above

Nephrolithiasis does not directly cause upper urinary tract infections (UTIs). UTI in the setting of an obstructing stone is a urologic emergency and is referred to as "pus under pressure".

2039. Clinically, most important inhibitor of crystallization of calcium-containing stones is?
Harrison's 20th Ed. Chapter 312 Page 2168

A. Urine ammonia
B. Urine bicarbonate
C. Urine citrate
D. Urine phosphate

Clinically, most important inhibitor of calcium-containing stones is urine citrate.

2040. Renal biopsies of stone formers show which of the following?
Harrison's 20th Ed. Chapter 312 Page 2168

A. Calcium phosphate in the renal interstitium
B. Calcium phosphate in the renal glomerular mesangium
C. Calcium phosphate in the renal vessels
D. All of the above

Renal biopsies of stone formers reveal calcium phosphate in the renal interstitium.

2041. As an initial event, calcium phosphate deposits at?
Harrison's 20th Ed. Chapter 312 Page 2168

A. Thin limb of the loop of Henle
B. Thick limb of the loop of Henle
C. Distal convoluted tubuls
D. Collecting duct

It is hypothesized that as an initial event calcium phosphate deposits at the thin limb of loop of Henle, and then extends down to papilla and erodes through papillary epithelium, where it provides a site for deposition of calcium oxalate & calcium phosphate crystals.

2042. Randall's plaque best relates to?
Harrison's 20th Ed. Chapter 312 Page 2168

A. Renal interstitium
B. Renal papilla
C. Renal glomerulus
D. Renal vessels

Majority of calcium oxalate stones grow on calcium phosphate at the tip of renal papilla (Randall's plaque).

2043. Dietary factors that are associated with an increased risk of nephrolithiasis include all except?
Harrison's 20th Ed. Chapter 312 Page 2168

A. Dietary oxalate
B. Dietary sodium
C. Dietary calcium
D. Dietary sucrose

2044. Dietary factor associated with a lower risk of nephrolithiasis is?
Harrison's 20th Ed. Chapter 312 Page 2168

A. Calcium
B. Potassium
C. Phytate
D. All of the above

Dietary factors that are associated with an increased risk of nephrolithiasis include animal protein, oxalate, sodium, sucrose and fructose. Dietary factors associated with a lower risk include calcium, potassium and phytate. Higher dietary calcium intake is related to a lower risk of stone formation. Reduction in risk associated with higher calcium intake may be due to a reduction in intestinal absorption of dietary oxalate that results in lower urine oxalate.

2045. Which of the following increases the risk of stone formation?
Harrison's 20th Ed. Chapter 312 Page 2169

A. Vitamin C supplements
B. Sugar-sweetened carbonated beverage consumption
C. Higher intake of animal protein
D. All of the above

2046. Higher intake of animal protein leads to?
Harrison's 20th Ed. Chapter 312 Page 2169

A. Increased excretion of calcium
B. Increased excretion of uric acid
C. Decreased urinary excretion of citrate
D. All of the above

2047. Which of the following reduces risk of renal stones in type 1 primary hyperoxaluria?
Harrison's 20th Ed. Chapter 312 Page 2169

A. Supplemental vitamin B1
B. Supplemental vitamin B3
C. Supplemental vitamin B6
D. Supplemental vitamin B12

High doses of supplemental vitamin B6 may be beneficial in selected patients with type 1 primary hyperoxaluria, the risk is not reduced in other patients.

2048. Which of the following is false about renal stones?
Harrison's 20th Ed. Chapter 312 Page 2169

A. Risk increases as urine volume decreases
B. Higher dietary Ca^{++} intake lowers risk of stone formation
C. Urinary oxalate is a risk factor for Ca^{++} oxalate stone formation
D. Lower urine citrate excretion decreases the risk

When the urine output is <1 L/day, the risk of stone formation more than doubles. Lower urine volume results in higher concentrations of lithogenic factors and is a common & readily modifiable risk factor. Lower urine citrate excretion increases the risk.

2049. Which of the following is false about renal stones?
Harrison's 20th Ed. Chapter 312 Page 2169

A. Higher potassium intake decreases calcium excretion
B. Higher sodium & sucrose intake increases calcium excretion
C. Magnesium & phytate lower renal stone risk include
D. Higher urine uric acid increases risk of Ca^{++} oxalate stones

Higher urine levels of uric acid is a risk factor for uric acid stone formation but is not associated with the risk of calcium oxalate stone formation.

2050. Which of the following reduces risk of renal stones?
Harrison's 20th Ed. Chapter 312 Page 2169

A. Tea
B. Beer
C. Orange juice
D. All of the above

Coffee, tea, beer, wine, and orange juice are associated with a reduced risk of renal stone formation.

2051. Which of the following about urine pH and kidney stones is false?

Harrison's 20th Ed. Chapter 312 Page 2169

A. Uric acid stones form when urine pH is consistently ≤ 5.5
B. Ca^{++} phosphate stones form when urine pH is ≥ 6.5
C. Ca^{++} oxalate stones are not influenced by urine pH
D. None of the above

2052. Which of the following disorders cause nephrolithiasis?

Harrison's 20th Ed. Chapter 312 Page 2169

A. Hartnup disorder
B. Homocystinuria
C. Cystinuria
D. Dent disease

Two most common monogenic disorders that lead to kidney stone formation are primary hyperoxaluria and cystinuria.

2053. Which of the following about primary hyperoxaluria is false?

Harrison's 20th Ed. Chapter 312 Page 2169

A. Autosomal recessive disorder
B. Excessive endogenous oxalate generation by liver
C. Ca^{++} oxalate stone formation & crystal deposition in organs
D. None of the above

Primary hyperoxaluria is an autosomal recessive disorder that causes excessive endogenous oxalate generation by liver, with consequent calcium oxalate stone formation and crystal deposition in organs.

2054. Which of the following about cystinuria is false?

Harrison's 20th Ed. Chapter 312 Page 2169

A. Autosomal recessive disorder
B. Abnormal reabsorption of filtered basic amino acids
C. Excessive urinary excretion of cysteine
D. Cysteine stones are visible on plain radiographs and often manifest as staghorn calculi or multiple bilateral stones

Cystinuria is an autosomal recessive disorder that causes abnormal reabsorption of filtered basic amino acids. The excessive urinary excretion of cystine, which is poorly soluble, leads to cystine stone formation. Cystine stones are visible on plain radiographs and often manifest as staghorn calculi or multiple bilateral stones.

2055. Which of the following is a common presentation for individuals with an acute stone event?

Harrison's 20th Ed. Chapter 312 Page 2169

A. Syncope
B. Painless gross hematuria
C. Urinary urgency
D. Urinary burning

2056. Which of the following is false about renal colic?

Harrison's 20th Ed. Chapter 312 Page 2169

A. Sudden onset of unilateral flank pain
B. No alleviating factors
C. Accompanied by nausea and vomiting
D. None of the above

2057. Differential diagnosis of renal colic include?

Harrison's 20th Ed. Chapter 312 Page 2170

A. Acute cholecystitis
B. Acute appendicitis
C. Acute diverticulitis
D. All of the above

2058. Urinary urgency and frequency appear when the renal stone lodges at?

Harrison's 20th Ed. Chapter 312 Page 2170

A. Ureteral pelvic junction
B. Pelvic brim
C. Ureterovesical junction
D. All of the above

If the stone lodges in ureter at ureterovesical junction, patient experiences urinary urgency & frequency.

2059. Renal colic may be confused as acute diverticulitis when the stone lodges at?

Harrison's 20th Ed. Chapter 312 Page 2170

A. Ureteral pelvic junction
B. Pelvic brim
C. Ureterovesical junction
D. All of the above

2060. Renal colic may be confused as acute appendicitis when the stone lodges at?

Harrison's 20th Ed. Chapter 312 Page 2170

A. Ureteral pelvic junction
B. Pelvic brim
C. Ureterovesical junction
D. All of the above

2061. Which of the following stone is radiolucent?

Harrison's 20th Ed. Chapter 312 Page 2170

A. Calcium
B. Cystine
C. Struvite
D. Uric acid

Calcium, cystine & struvite stones are radiopaque on standard X-rays. Uric acid stones are radiolucent.

2062. The "gold standard" diagnostic test in nephrolithiasis is?

Harrison's 20th Ed. Chapter 312 Page 2170

A. Helical CT without contrast
B. Helical CT with contrast
C. Renal ultrasound
D. MRI

The "gold standard" diagnostic test in nephrolithiasis is helical CT without contrast. Helical CT detects stones as small as 1 mm.

2063. In helical CT, which of the following is the evidence of recent passage of a ureteral stone?

Harrison's 20th Ed. Chapter 312 Page 2170

A. Irregular ureteral lumen
B. Irregular urinary bladder neck
C. Perinephric stranding
D. All of the above

2064. In helical CT, which of the following is the evidence of recent passage of a ureteral stone?

Harrison's 20th Ed. Chapter 312 Page 2170

A. Irregular ureteral peristalsis
B. Hydronephrosis
C. Vesicoureteral reflux
D. All of the above

Helical CT reveals ureteral stone or evidence of recent passage (perinephric stranding or hydronephrosis).

2065. Use of which of the following may increase the rate of spontaneous renal stone passage?

Harrison's 20th Ed. Chapter 312 Page 2170

A. Alpha blocker
B. Beta blocker
C. NSAID
D. PDE-5 inhibitor

Use of alpha blockers (tamsulosin) may increase the rate of spontaneous renal stone passage.

2066. Renal stones of what size have a low probability of spontaneous passage?

Harrison's 20th Ed. Chapter 312 Page 2170

A. ≥ 3 mm
B. ≥ 6 mm
C. ≥ 8 mm
D. ≥ 10 mm

Renal stones measuring ≥ 6 mm have a low probability of spontaneous passage.

2067. Which of the following states suggest a low probability of spontaneous passage of renal stones?

Harrison's 20th Ed. Chapter 312 Page 2170

A. Renal stone measuring ≥ 6 mm
B. An urological anatomic abnormality
C. Intractable pain
D. All of the above

2068. More than half of first-time stone formers will have a recurrence within?

Harrison's 20th Ed. Chapter 312 Page 2171

A. 3 years
B. 5 years
C. 7 years
D. 10 years

More than half of first-time stone formers will have a recurrence within 10 years.

2069. Which of the following is a high-oxalate food?

Harrison's 20th Ed. Chapter 312 Page 2171

A. Spinach
B. Rhubarb
C. Potatoes
D. All of the above

High-oxalate foods are spinach, rhubarb, almonds, and potatoes.

2070. Levels of which of the following must be measured in concert with PTH?

Harrison's 20th Ed. Chapter 312 Page 2171

A. Calcium
B. Phosphorus
C. 25-hydroxy vitamin D
D. Uric acid

Elevated serum levels of parathyroid hormone (PTH) and a normal 25-hydroxy vitamin D level is rare. 25-hydroxy vitamin D is measured in concert with PTH to investigate the possible role of secondarily elevated PTH levels in the setting of vitamin D insufficiency. Similarly, primary renal Ca^{++} loss with lower serum Ca^{++} concentrations is rare.

2071. Which of the following renal stones can be identified by low Hounsfield units on CT?

Harrison's 20th Ed. Chapter 312 Page 2171

A. Calcium oxalate
B. Calcium phosphate
C. Uric acid
D. Struvite

Pure uric acid stones can be identified by low Hounsfield units on CT.

2072. Which of the following statements is false?

Harrison's 20th Ed. Chapter 312 Page 2171

A. ↑ed urine Ca^{++} excretion causes ↑ed absorption of ingested Ca^{++}
B. Crystalluria is a strong risk factor for new stone formation
C. Consistently diluted urine reduces likelihood of crystal formation
D. None of the above

Calcium oxalate dihydrate crystals are bipyramidally shaped, and cystine crystals are hexagonal

2073. For prevention of stone formation, urine volume should be?

Harrison's 20th Ed. Chapter 312 Page 2171

A. 1 liter per day
B. 2 liters per day
C. 3 liters per day
D. 4 liters per day

Urine volume goal is of 2 L/day for prevention of stone formation.

2074. Risk factor for calcium oxalate stones is?

Harrison's 20th Ed. Chapter 312 Page 2171

A. Higher urine calcium
B. Higher urine oxalate
C. Lower urine citrate
D. All of the above

Risk factors for calcium oxalate stones include higher urine calcium, higher urine oxalate, and lower urine citrate. This stone type is insensitive to pH in physiologic range.

2075. What quantity of calcium is recommended for a patient with or history of calcium oxalate stone?

Harrison's 20th Ed. Chapter 312 Page 2172

A. 400 mg/day
B. 800 mg/day
C. 1200 mg/day
D. 1600 mg/day

In men with high urine calcium & recurrent calcium oxalate stones, a diet of 1200 mg/day of calcium with low intake of sodium & animal protein significantly reduced subsequent stone formation from that with a low-calcium diet (400 mg/day). Excessive calcium intake (>1200 mg/day) should be avoided.

2076. Which of the following can substantially lower urine calcium excretion?

Harrison's 20th Ed. Chapter 312 Page 2172

A. Furosemide
B. Thiazide
C. Triamterene
D. Spironolactone

Thiazide diuretic (chlorthalidone), in doses higher than those used to treat hypertension (with sodium restriction), can substantially lower urine calcium excretion and consequently can reduce calcium oxalate stone recurrence.

2077. Which of the following is the only known strategy that reduces endogenous oxalate production?

Harrison's 20th Ed. Chapter 312 Page 2172

A. Overhydration
B. Avoiding nondairy animal protein
C. Avoiding high-dose vitamin C supplements
D. All of the above

Avoiding high-dose vitamin C supplements is the only known strategy that reduces endogenous oxalate production.

2078. Which of the following about calcium phosphate renal stones is false?

Harrison's 20th Ed. Chapter 312 Page 2172

A. ↑ed occurrence with higher urine pH (≥ 6.5)
B. More common in patients with distal renal tubular acidosis
C. More common in patients with primary hyperparathyroidism
D. None of the above

2079. Nephrocalcinosis best relates to?

Harrison's 20th Ed. Chapter 312 Page 2172

A. Primary hyperparathyroidism
B. Type 1 RTA
C. Primary oxalosis
D. All of the above

Multiple papillary calcifications are called nephrocalcinosis.

2080. Main risk factors for uric acid stones is?

Harrison's 20th Ed. Chapter 312 Page 2172

A. Persistently low urine pH
B. Persistently high urine pH
C. Persistently normal urine pH
D. All of the above

Two main risk factors for uric acid renal stones are persistently low urine pH & higher uric acid excretion.

2081. Mainstay of prevention of uric acid stone formation is?

Harrison's 20th Ed. Chapter 312 Page 2172

A. Avoiding nondairy animal protein
B. Increasing urine pH
C. Allopurinol therapy
D. All of the above

Mainstay of prevention of uric acid stone formation entails increasing urine pH. Recommended urine pH goal is of 6.5 throughout day and night.

2082. Which of the following drug increases cystine solubility and prevents cystine stone formation?

Harrison's 20th Ed. Chapter 312 Page 2172

A. Vitamin B6
B. Tiopronin
C. Terbinafine
D. Zinc

Tiopronin & penicillamine covalently bind to cystine.

2083. Which of the following are the most common cause of renal stones in children?

Harrison's 20th Ed. Chapter 414 Page 3022

A. Calcium oxalate
B. Calcium phosphate
C. Cystine
D. Struvite

Cystine stones account for 1–2% of all urinary tract calculi but are the most common cause of renal stones in children.

2084. Which of the following about struvite stones is false?

Harrison's 20th Ed. Chapter 312 Page 2172

A. Also known as infection stones or triple-phosphate stones
B. Grow quickly & fill the renal pelvis (staghorn calculi)
C. Form only when the upper urinary tract is infected with urease-producing bacteria
D. None of the above

2085. Which of the following renal stones form only when upper urinary tract is infected with urease-producing bacteria?

Harrison's 20th Ed. Chapter 312 Page 2172

A. Calcium oxalate
B. Calcium phosphate
C. Cystine
D. Struvite

Struvite stones, also known as infection stones or triple-phosphate stones, form only when the upper urinary tract is infected with urease-producing bacteria such as Proteus mirabilis, Klebsiella pneumoniae, or Providencia species. Urease produced by these bacteria hydrolyzes urea and may elevate the urine pH to a supraphysiologic level (>8.0).

2086. Infection due to bacteria that possess enzyme urease can cause stones composed of?

Harrison's 20th Ed. Chapter 312 Page 2172

A. Calcium
B. Cystine
C. Struvite
D. Uric acid

Infection due to bacteria that possess the enzyme urease can cause stones composed of struvite.

2087. Which of the following is false about 'Struvite stones'?

Harrison's 20th Ed. Chapter 312 Page 2172

A. Occur mainly in men
B. Occur in patients with chronic bladder catheterization
C. Due to UTI with urease-producing bacteria
D. May grow to produce a "staghorn" appearance

Struvite stones occur mainly in women.

2088. Which of the following is an urease inhibitor?
Harrison's 20th Ed. Chapter 312 Page 2172

A. Acetohydroxamic acid
B. Tranexamic acid
C. ε-aminocaproic acid
D. Pyroglutamic acid

2089. The element in 'Struvite' is?
Harrison's 20th Ed. Chapter 313 Page 2174

A. Calcium
B. Aluminium
C. Magnesium
D. Zinc

The chemical formula of struvite is Magnesium Ammonium Phosphate ($MgNH_4PO_4$).

2090. Causes of 'Hypercalciuria' include all except?
Harrison's 20th Ed. Chapter 403 Page 2932

A. Hypothyroidism
B. Cushing syndrome
C. Sarcoidosis
D. Immobilization

2091. Causes of 'Hypercalciuria' include?
Harrison's 20th Ed. Chapter 403 Page 2932

A. Vitamin D intoxication
B. Rapidly progressive bone disease
C. Paget's disease
D. All of the above

Hyperthyroidism, Cushing syndrome, sarcoidosis, malignant tumors, immobilization, vitamin D intoxication, rapidly progressive bone disease, and Paget's disease cause hypercalciuria.

2092. Basic constituents of most kidney stones include all except?
Nephrol Dial Transplant 1996;11:379-387

A. Alumina
B. Uric acid
C. Cystine
D. Struvite

2093. Urine crystals that are rectangular prisms and resemble 'coffin lids' are of?
Nephrol Dial Transplant 1996;11:379-387

A. Calcium
B. Uric acid
C. Cystine
D. Struvite

The typical shape of triple phosphate crystals is that of prisms ('coffin lid'), which are always strongly birefringent. Triple phosphate crystals are typical of infected urine, especially that caused by urea-splitting bacteria. For this reason they are frequently found also in patients with infected calculi.

2094. Urine crystals that are flat, rhomboidal shaped are of?
Nephrol Dial Transplant 1996;11:379-387

A. Calcium
B. Uric acid
C. Cystine
D. Struvite

Uric acid crystals are very pleiomorphic, but the amber coloured, constant polychromatic birefringence rhomboidal shape is the most frequent.

2095. Urine crystals that are rectangular prism shaped are of?
Nephrol Dial Transplant 1996;11:379-387

A. Calcium
B. Uric acid
C. Cystine
D. Struvite

2096. Urine crystals that are Hexagonal plate shaped are of?
Nephrol Dial Transplant 1996;11:379-387

A. Calcium
B. Uric acid
C. Cystine
D. Struvite

Cystine crystals precipitate as symmetrical hexagons, mostly aggregated, and are constantly birefringent.

2097. Urine crystals that are of dumbbell shape are of?
Nephrol Dial Transplant 1996;11:379-387

A. Calcium oxalate monohydrate
B. Calcium oxalate dihydrate
C. Cystine
D. Struvite

2098. Urine crystals that are of bipyramidal shape are of?
Nephrol Dial Transplant 1996;11:379-387

A. Calcium oxalate monohydrate
B. Calcium oxalate dihydrate
C. Calcium phosphate
D. Mixed calcium oxalate/uric acid

2099. Urine crystals that are of elongated, narrow shape are of?
Nephrol Dial Transplant 1996;11:379-387

A. Calcium oxalate monohydrate
B. Calcium oxalate dihydrate
C. Calcium phosphate
D. Mixed calcium oxalate/uric acid

Calcium phosphate crystals are pleiomorphic, appearing as birefringent stars or needles, in isolation or in clumps. Calcium phosphate crystals were the most frequent crystals in both normals and stone formers.

2100. 'Maltese crosses' urine crystals best relate to?
Nephrol Dial Transplant 1996;11:379-387

A. Acyclovir
B. Sulphadiazine
C. Triamterene
D. Primidone

Triamterene crystals are spherical & predominantly brown in colour, under polarized light they appear as 'Maltese crosses'. These crystals are associated with brown casts, which are also due to triamterene.

2101. Calcium oxalate monohydrate crystals in the urinary sediment are typical of?
N Engl J Med. 2006;354:1065-72

A. Antacid overdose
B. Ethylene glycol ingestion
C. Blunt abdominal trauma
D. Fat embolism

ANSWERS

1. C
2. D
3. B
4. D
5. B
6. D
7. C
8. B
9. C
10. D
11. D
12. B
13. C
14. A
15. D
16. C
17. B
18. B
19. A
20. A
21. A
22. A
23. D
24. D
25. D
26. D
27. B
28. A
29. D
30. C
31. D
32. B
33. B
34. D
35. D
36. D
37. A
38. B
39. B
40. D
41. D
42. D
43. D
44. D
45. A
46. D
47. B
48. D
49. C
50. B
51. D
52. D
53. D
54. D
55. C
56. D
57. D
58. D
59. B
60. D
61. B
62. D
63. D
64. D
65. C
66. C
67. C
68. D
69. D
70. C
71. A
72. A
73. A
74. D
75. D
76. B
77. C
78. D
79. D
80. C
81. D
82. D
83. D
84. A
85. A
86. D
87. C
88. D
89. D
90. D
91. A
92. C
93. B
94. D
95. B
96. D
97. B
98. D
99. D
100. D
101. D
102. D
103. C
104. D
105. D
106. B
107. A
108. B
109. C
110. B
111. C
112. C
113. B
114. A
115. A
116. D
117. D
118. A
119. C
120. D
121. D
122. B
123. C
124. D
125. B
126. C
127. D
128. B
129. A
130. C
131. D
132. D
133. D
134. B
135. D
136. D
137. A
138. D
139. B
140. C
141. D
142. C
143. A
144. A
145. B
146. B
147. C
148. D
149. D
150. C
151. D
152. D
153. A
154. D
155. B
156. B
157. B
158. A
159. D
160. A
161. B
162. C
163. D
164. D
165. B
166. A
167. D
168. C
169. D
170. D
171. A
172. B
173. D
174. C
175. A
176. D
177. A
178. C
179. D
180. D
181. B
182. D
183. C
184. A
185. D
186. C
187. A
188. D
189. D
190. D
191. D
192. B
193. C
194. B
195. D
196. C
197. D
198. B
199. D
200. D
201. A
202. B
203. D
204. C
205. A
206. D
207. B
208. D
209. A
210. B
211. C
212. B
213. B
214. D
215. D
216. D
217. D
218. C
219. D
220. D
221. D
222. D
223. D
224. D
225. A
226. B
227. B
228. D
229. D
230. A
231. D
232. D
233. D
234. D
235. C
236. A
237. D
238. A
239. D
240. D
241. D
242. D
243. D
244. D
245. D
246. D
247. A
248. A
249. B
250. C
251. D
252. A
253. D
254. B
255. A
256. D
257. D
258. B
259. A
260. D
261. A
262. D
263. A
264. D

ANSWERS

265. B
266. D
267. A
268. D
269. C
270. B
271. C
272. A
273. D
274. D
275. C
276. A
277. D
278. D
279. C
280. D
281. D
282. C
283. B
284. B
285. D
286. D
287. D
288. D
289. A
290. B
291. C
292. C
293. C
294. D
295. C
296. D
297. C
298. B
299. A
300. B
301. D
302. A
303. C
304. D
305. A
306. D
307. D
308. D
309. D
310. C
311. B
312. D
313. C
314. B
315. B
316. D
317. D
318. D
319. D
320. D
321. D
322. D
323. D
324. D
325. C
326. B
327. C
328. C
329. D
330. C
331. C
332. D
333. D
334. A
335. D
336. C
337. A
338. B
339. C
340. C
341. C
342. C
343. B
344. D
345. A
346. D
347. B
348. D
349. B
350. D
351. B
352. A
353. A
354. A
355. A
356. B
357. D
358. B
359. D
360. D
361. B
362. A
363. D
364. C
365. B
366. D
367. D
368. D
369. C
370. D
371. A
372. D
373. A
374. A
375. D
376. D
377. D
378. B
379. B
380. D
381. D
382. D
383. D
384. D
385. D
386. D
387. D
388. D
389. B
390. C
391. D
392. D
393. C
394. C
395. D
396. D
397. D
398. D
399. D
400. D
401. D
402. C
403. D
404. A
405. A
406. D
407. D
408. D
409. D
410. D
411. D
412. D
413. D
414. A
415. B
416. A
417. A
418. D
419. D
420. D
421. D
422. D
423. D
424. A
425. C
426. D
427. A
428. D
429. D
430. D
431. A
432. A
433. B
434. D
435. D
436. A
437. B
438. A
439. C
440. C
441. D
442. D
443. A
444. A
445. D
446. D
447. C
448. B
449. D
450. D
451. D
452. D
453. D
454. C
455. D
456. C
457. B
458. C
459. D
460. C
461. D
462. D
463. B
464. D
465. D
466. C
467. D
468. D
469. A
470. C
471. D
472. A
473. D
474. C
475. D
476. B
477. A
478. D
479. C
480. C
481. B
482. D
483. D
484. D
485. D
486. D
487. D
488. C
489. D
490. C
491. D
492. B
493. B
494. D
495. D
496. C
497. C
498. D
499. D
500. D
501. A
502. D
503. B
504. B
505. D
506. B
507. B
508. B
509. B
510. B
511. B
512. D
513. D
514. D
515. D
516. D
517. B
518. C
519. D
520. D
521. D
522. C
523. D
524. D
525. A
526. D
527. B
528. D

ANSWERS

529. D
530. D
531. D
532. D
533. B
534. C
535. D
536. C
537. D
538. D
539. D
540. D
541. D
542. A
543. D
544. C
545. C
546. D
547. B
548. C
549. D
550. D
551. A
552. D
553. D
554. A
555. D
556. D
557. B
558. B
559. B
560. B
561. C
562. D
563. B
564. D
565. B
566. B
567. C
568. A
569. D
570. D
571. B
572. B
573. D
574. D
575. A
576. D
577. D
578. D
579. D
580. D
581. A
582. B
583. C
584. C
585. D
586. C
587. B
588. C
589. C
590. A
591. D
592. C
593. C
594. A
595. C
596. B
597. D
598. A
599. D
600. A
601. D
602. B
603. A
604. C
605. D
606. B
607. C
608. A
609. B
610. C
611. D
612. C
613. D
614. C
615. B
616. D
617. D
618. A
619. D
620. C
621. D
622. A
623. A
624. D
625. D
626. D
627. A
628. C
629. D
630. D
631. D
632. D
633. C
634. B
635. A
636. A
637. D
638. D
639. D
640. A
641. C
642. C
643. D
644. D
645. D
646. D
647. C
648. A
649. A
650. D
651. A
652. C
653. C
654. A
655. D
656. B
657. D
658. C
659. C
660. A
661. D
662. A
663. C
664. D
665. B
666. A
667. A
668. D
669. D
670. C
671. D
672. D
673. C
674. B
675. C
676. B
677. B
678. D
679. B
680. A
681. D
682. D
683. C
684. C
685. D
686. D
687. D
688. A
689. C
690. D
691. D
692. D
693. B
694. C
695. D
696. D
697. D
698. C
699. B
700. A
701. A
702. B
703. C
704. D
705. C
706. A
707. D
708. D
709. D
710. D
711. B
712. D
713. D
714. A
715. D
716. D
717. D
718. C
719. D
720. D
721. D
722. D
723. C
724. D
725. D
726. D
727. A
728. C
729. A
730. D
731. B
732. B
733. D
734. B
735. D
736. D
737. C
738. D
739. D
740. A
741. A
742. A
743. C
744. A
745. A
746. A
747. C
748. B
749. C
750. B
751. D
752. B
753. B
754. A
755. B
756. C
757. D
758. D
759. B
760. A
761. D
762. A
763. C
764. C
765. A
766. A
767. D
768. D
769. D
770. D
771. D
772. C
773. D
774. D
775. C
776. C
777. D
778. D
779. D
780. D
781. D
782. D
783. D
784. D
785. D
786. D
787. C
788. A
789. B
790. D
791. D
792. C

ANSWERS

793. D
794. D
795. C
796. D
797. D
798. B
799. B
800. D
801. B
802. A
803. A
804. D
805. B
806. A
807. A
808. D
809. A
810. C
811. A
812. D
813. D
814. A
815. C
816. C
817. B
818. B
819. B
820. A
821. B
822. C
823. B
824. A
825. B
826. B
827. D
828. C
829. D
830. B
831. D
832. B
833. B
834. A
835. D
836. D
837. C
838. D
839. B
840. D
841. B
842. A
843. A
844. D
845. A
846. A
847. B
848. B
849. C
850. A
851. A
852. A
853. B
854. D
855. D
856. B
857. D
858. D
859. D
860. B
861. A
862. C
863. D
864. B
865. A
866. D
867. D
868. D
869. D
870. C
871. C
872. C
873. D
874. C
875. D
876. D
877. D
878. B
879. B
880. D
881. D
882. D
883. D
884. C
885. D
886. B
887. C
888. D
889. D
890. D
891. A
892. B
893. C
894. D
895. D
896. D
897. D
898. C
899. C
900. A
901. B
902. D
903. D
904. D
905. A
906. D
907. B
908. D
909. D
910. D
911. D
912. B
913. B
914. D
915. B
916. A
917. D
918. B
919. D
920. D
921. D
922. D
923. D
924. D
925. B
926. B
927. B
928. D
929. C
930. B
931. C
932. D
933. D
934. D
935. A
936. C
937. D
938. D
939. A
940. B
941. A
942. A
943. C
944. B
945. D
946. C
947. B
948. B
949. D
950. A
951. A
952. A
953. A
954. D
955. D
956. C
957. D
958. D
959. C
960. D
961. D
962. A
963. B
964. B
965. D
966. D
967. C
968. C
969. D
970. B
971. D
972. C
973. A
974. D
975. B
976. D
977. D
978. D
979. D
980. D
981. C
982. A
983. B
984. D
985. A
986. A
987. D
988. A
989. B
990. D
991. D
992. D
993. C
994. D
995. D
996. C
997. D
998. D
999. B
1000. D
1001. D
1002. A
1003. D
1004. A
1005. D
1006. D
1007. B
1008. D
1009. D
1010. D
1011. C
1012. C
1013. A
1014. D
1015. D
1016. D
1017. B
1018. D
1019. D
1020. D
1021. D
1022. C
1023. C
1024. D
1025. D
1026. C
1027. A
1028. D
1029. D
1030. D
1031. D
1032. D
1033. D
1034. B
1035. D
1036. C
1037. D
1038. D
1039. D
1040. D
1041. D
1042. A
1043. D
1044. D
1045. B
1046. D
1047. B
1048. B
1049. A
1050. D
1051. D
1052. B
1053. D
1054. A
1055. C
1056. B

ANSWERS

1057. A
1058. A
1059. A
1060. D
1061. D
1062. D
1063. D
1064. B
1065. D
1066. A
1067. B
1068. C
1069. C
1070. D
1071. D
1072. D
1073. D
1074. D
1075. D
1076. D
1077. D
1078. D
1079. D
1080. D
1081. D
1082. D
1083. D
1084. D
1085. D
1086. A
1087. C
1088. D
1089. D
1090. D
1091. D
1092. D
1093. D
1094. D
1095. A
1096. D
1097. C
1098. D
1099. D
1100. C
1101. D
1102. D
1103. D
1104. D
1105. D
1106. D
1107. D
1108. D
1109. D
1110. D
1111. D
1112. D
1113. B
1114. D
1115. D
1116. D
1117. C
1118. C
1119. B
1120. B
1121. C
1122. D
1123. A
1124. D
1125. D
1126. D
1127. C
1128. D
1129. D
1130. A
1131. A
1132. A
1133. A
1134. D
1135. C
1136. D
1137. C
1138. C
1139. D
1140. D
1141. D
1142. D
1143. B
1144. D
1145. D
1146. C
1147. A
1148. D
1149. D
1150. D
1151. D
1152. D
1153. D
1154. D
1155. D
1156. D
1157. A
1158. D
1159. D
1160. C
1161. D
1162. B
1163. D
1164. D
1165. D
1166. D
1167. D
1168. A
1169. A
1170. D
1171. D
1172. D
1173. C
1174. C
1175. D
1176. A
1177. A
1178. D
1179. C
1180. C
1181. B
1182. D
1183. D
1184. D
1185. D
1186. A
1187. D
1188. B
1189. D
1190. D
1191. D
1192. B
1193. D
1194. B
1195. D
1196. D
1197. D
1198. C
1199. C
1200. C
1201. B
1202. D
1203. D
1204. D
1205. B
1206. D
1207. D
1208. B
1209. C
1210. C
1211. D
1212. B
1213. C
1214. D
1215. D
1216. D
1217. B
1218. D
1219. D
1220. D
1221. A
1222. C
1223. D
1224. D
1225. D
1226. B
1227. D
1228. D
1229. B
1230. D
1231. A
1232. D
1233. D
1234. D
1235. B
1236. D
1237. D
1238. D
1239. D
1240. D
1241. A
1242. B
1243. D
1244. C
1245. B
1246. D
1247. C
1248. C
1249. D
1250. B
1251. D
1252. C
1253. B
1254. D
1255. D
1256. D
1257. D
1258. B
1259. D
1260. D
1261. A
1262. B
1263. D
1264. D
1265. D
1266. D
1267. D
1268. D
1269. B
1270. A
1271. D
1272. D
1273. A
1274. B
1275. B
1276. A
1277. D
1278. D
1279. D
1280. B
1281. D
1282. D
1283. D
1284. B
1285. B
1286. D
1287. D
1288. B
1289. C
1290. A
1291. A
1292. B
1293. A
1294. C
1295. D
1296. D
1297. C
1298. B
1299. B
1300. B
1301. A
1302. D
1303. D
1304. D
1305. B
1306. D
1307. D
1308. A
1309. B
1310. D
1311. C
1312. D
1313. D
1314. D
1315. D
1316. D
1317. D
1318. A
1319. D
1320. D

ANSWERS

1321. A
1322. B
1323. D
1324. D
1325. D
1326. D
1327. D
1328. D
1329. D
1330. D
1331. D
1332. B
1333. D
1334. D
1335. D
1336. D
1337. B
1338. D
1339. D
1340. D
1341. C
1342. D
1343. A
1344. B
1345. D
1346. D
1347. B
1348. A
1349. C
1350. D
1351. D
1352. D
1353. D
1354. D
1355. B
1356. C
1357. C
1358. D
1359. B
1360. C
1361. B
1362. A
1363. D
1364. C
1365. D
1366. D
1367. B
1368. A
1369. D
1370. B
1371. D
1372. C
1373. D
1374. B
1375. C
1376. A
1377. D
1378. D
1379. C
1380. D
1381. B
1382. D
1383. B
1384. B
1385. D
1386. C
1387. B
1388. C
1389. B
1390. D
1391. A
1392. B
1393. A
1394. B
1395. A
1396. D
1397. B
1398. D
1399. D
1400. A
1401. D
1402. B
1403. B
1404. D
1405. A
1406. D
1407. D
1408. D
1409. A
1410. D
1411. D
1412. B
1413. D
1414. D
1415. C
1416. B
1417. D
1418. A
1419. B
1420. B
1421. C
1422. C
1423. D
1424. D
1425. D
1426. C
1427. B
1428. D
1429. D
1430. D
1431. D
1432. D
1433. D
1434. D
1435. C
1436. B
1437. A
1438. D
1439. D
1440. B
1441. C
1442. C
1443. D
1444. B
1445. D
1446. A
1447. B
1448. D
1449. A
1450. D
1451. A
1452. A
1453. B
1454. C
1455. D
1456. D
1457. A
1458. C
1459. A
1460. B
1461. D
1462. B
1463. C
1464. B
1465. D
1466. B
1467. D
1468. D
1469. C
1470. B
1471. A
1472. D
1473. B
1474. D
1475. D
1476. D
1477. D
1478. D
1479. C
1480. B
1481. D
1482. A
1483. C
1484. D
1485. D
1486. D
1487. B
1488. D
1489. D
1490. D
1491. B
1492. C
1493. A
1494. C
1495. B
1496. C
1497. C
1498. D
1499. C
1500. D
1501. D
1502. C
1503. A
1504. C
1505. D
1506. D
1507. D
1508. B
1509. D
1510. D
1511. D
1512. A
1513. B
1514. A
1515. C
1516. D
1517. D
1518. D
1519. D
1520. D
1521. B
1522. D
1523. B
1524. D
1525. D
1526. B
1527. D
1528. B
1529. D
1530. D
1531. D
1532. D
1533. A
1534. A
1535. D
1536. B
1537. D
1538. B
1539. C
1540. D
1541. D
1542. D
1543. D
1544. B
1545. D
1546. A
1547. D
1548. D
1549. B
1550. B
1551. B
1552. C
1553. B
1554. C
1555. D
1556. B
1557. D
1558. B
1559. D
1560. C
1561. D
1562. D
1563. C
1564. B
1565. C
1566. D
1567. D
1568. D
1569. A
1570. B
1571. B
1572. D
1573. D
1574. D
1575. D
1576. C
1577. D
1578. B
1579. A
1580. D
1581. D
1582. A
1583. D
1584. D

ANSWERS

1585. D
1586. D
1587. D
1588. B
1589. D
1590. A
1591. D
1592. B
1593. D
1594. B
1595. D
1596. D
1597. D
1598. D
1599. D
1600. D
1601. D
1602. C
1603. B
1604. D
1605. D
1606. D
1607. D
1608. D
1609. A
1610. C
1611. B
1612. C
1613. A
1614. D
1615. D
1616. B
1617. B
1618. B
1619. B
1620. D
1621. D
1622. C
1623. D
1624. A
1625. D
1626. D
1627. D
1628. D
1629. A
1630. B
1631. D
1632. D
1633. D
1634. A
1635. A
1636. C
1637. B
1638. D
1639. D
1640. A
1641. D
1642. D
1643. D
1644. D
1645. D
1646. D
1647. C
1648. D
1649. D
1650. D
1651. D
1652. B
1653. D
1654. A
1655. C
1656. C
1657. D
1658. D
1659. D
1660. D
1661. D
1662. D
1663. C
1664. C
1665. A
1666. B
1667. D
1668. D
1669. B
1670. A
1671. C
1672. D
1673. D
1674. D
1675. C
1676. D
1677. C
1678. A
1679. D
1680. C
1681. D
1682. D
1683. B
1684. A
1685. D
1686. D
1687. D
1688. B
1689. B
1690. C
1691. D
1692. B
1693. C
1694. B
1695. D
1696. C
1697. D
1698. D
1699. D
1700. D
1701. D
1702. C
1703. A
1704. D
1705. B
1706. C
1707. A
1708. D
1709. D
1710. D
1711. B
1712. C
1713. D
1714. B
1715. A
1716. B
1717. D
1718. A
1719. A
1720. D
1721. D
1722. D
1723. D
1724. D
1725. D
1726. D
1727. D
1728. D
1729. D
1730. D
1731. D
1732. D
1733. D
1734. D
1735. D
1736. B
1737. D
1738. A
1739. A
1740. A
1741. C
1742. D
1743. D
1744. D
1745. D
1746. D
1747. D
1748. D
1749. D
1750. D
1751. D
1752. B
1753. B
1754. B
1755. C
1756. C
1757. C
1758. B
1759. B
1760. D
1761. D
1762. D
1763. D
1764. A
1765. A
1766. D
1767. D
1768. C
1769. D
1770. D
1771. B
1772. C
1773. A
1774. D
1775. C
1776. C
1777. B
1778. C
1779. D
1780. B
1781. B
1782. D
1783. B
1784. D
1785. D
1786. D
1787. D
1788. D
1789. B
1790. D
1791. C
1792. A
1793. D
1794. A
1795. B
1796. C
1797. B
1798. D
1799. D
1800. D
1801. D
1802. B
1803. D
1804. D
1805. D
1806. D
1807. D
1808. D
1809. D
1810. D
1811. D
1812. D
1813. D
1814. B
1815. D
1816. A
1817. D
1818. C
1819. C
1820. B
1821. D
1822. D
1823. D
1824. D
1825. A
1826. D
1827. B
1828. D
1829. A
1830. D
1831. C
1832. C
1833. D
1834. D
1835. C
1836. A
1837. B
1838. A
1839. D
1840. A
1841. A
1842. D

ANSWERS

1843. A
1844. A
1845. D
1846. D
1847. A
1848. B
1849. D
1850. D
1851. D
1852. D
1853. A
1854. D
1855. C
1856. D
1857. D
1858. B
1859. B
1860. D
1861. D
1862. D
1863. B
1864. B
1865. B
1866. B
1867. B
1868. C
1869. B
1870. D
1871. D
1872. D
1873. D
1874. D
1875. D
1876. D
1877. B
1878. D
1879. D
1880. D
1881. D
1882. D
1883. B
1884. D
1885. B
1886. D
1887. D
1888. C
1889. D
1890. B
1891. D
1892. C
1893. D
1894. C
1895. D
1896. D
1897. D
1898. A
1899. D
1900. C
1901. C
1902. A
1903. C
1904. B
1905. D
1906. A
1907. A
1908. C
1909. D
1910. B
1911. D
1912. D
1913. C
1914. B
1915. B
1916. C
1917. A
1918. D
1919. D
1920. B
1921. D
1922. B
1923. A
1924. C
1925. C
1926. B
1927. D
1928. D
1929. D
1930. C
1931. D
1932. D
1933. D
1934. C
1935. D
1936. D
1937. D
1938. D
1939. C
1940. D
1941. A
1942. A
1943. A
1944. D
1945. D
1946. D
1947. D
1948. D
1949. A
1950. B
1951. A
1952. D
1953. D
1954. D
1955. B
1956. B
1957. A
1958. A
1959. A
1960. D
1961. C
1962. D
1963. B
1964. D
1965. D
1966. B
1967. D
1968. D
1969. D
1970. D
1971. C
1972. D
1973. B
1974. D
1975. D
1976. D
1977. C
1978. D
1979. A
1980. C
1981. D
1982. B
1983. D
1984. D
1985. D
1986. D
1987. D
1988. D
1989. D
1990. D
1991. C
1992. D
1993. D
1994. D
1995. D
1996. D
1997. D
1998. D
1999. B
2000. A
2001. B
2002. D
2003. D
2004. D
2005. D
2006. D
2007. D
2008. D
2009. B
2010. D
2011. C
2012. B
2013. B
2014. A
2015. D
2016. D
2017. B
2018. D
2019. B
2020. A
2021. A
2022. D
2023. D
2024. D
2025. D
2026. A
2027. D
2028. D
2029. B
2030. A
2031. D
2032. D
2033. B
2034. D
2035. D
2036. D
2037. D
2038. B
2039. C
2040. A
2041. A
2042. B
2043. C
2044. D
2045. D
2046. D
2047. C
2048. D
2049. D
2050. D
2051. D
2052. C
2053. D
2054. A
2055. B
2056. D
2057. D
2058. C
2059. B
2060. B
2061. D
2062. A
2063. C
2064. B
2065. A
2066. B
2067. D
2068. D
2069. D
2070. C
2071. C
2072. D
2073. B
2074. D
2075. C
2076. B
2077. C
2078. D
2079. D
2080. A
2081. B
2082. B
2083. C
2084. D
2085. D
2086. C
2087. A
2088. A
2089. C
2090. A
2091. D
2092. A
2093. D
2094. B
2095. D
2096. C
2097. A
2098. B
2099. C
2100. C
2101. B